Benefits of the Mediterranean Diet–Wine Association: Role of Components

Benefits of the Mediterranean Diet–Wine Association: Role of Components

Editors

Paula Silva
Norbert Latruffe

MDPI • Basel • Beijing • Wuhan • Barcelona • Belgrade • Manchester • Tokyo • Cluj • Tianjin

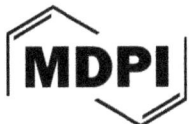

Editors
Paula Silva
University of Porto
Portugal

Norbert Latruffe
University Bourgogne Franche Comte
France

Editorial Office
MDPI
St. Alban-Anlage 66
4052 Basel, Switzerland

This is a reprint of articles from the Special Issue published online in the open access journal *Molecules* (ISSN 1420-3049) (available at: https://www.mdpi.com/journal/molecules/special_issues/wine_diet_benefit).

For citation purposes, cite each article independently as indicated on the article page online and as indicated below:

LastName, A.A.; LastName, B.B.; LastName, C.C. Article Title. *Journal Name* **Year**, *Volume Number*, Page Range.

ISBN 978-3-0365-3561-6 (Hbk)
ISBN 978-3-0365-3562-3 (PDF)

© 2022 by the authors. Articles in this book are Open Access and distributed under the Creative Commons Attribution (CC BY) license, which allows users to download, copy and build upon published articles, as long as the author and publisher are properly credited, which ensures maximum dissemination and a wider impact of our publications.

The book as a whole is distributed by MDPI under the terms and conditions of the Creative Commons license CC BY-NC-ND.

Contents

About the Editors vii

Paula Silva and Norbert Latruffe
Benefits of the Mediterranean Diet–Wine Association: The Role of Ingredients
Reprinted from: *Molecules* **2022**, *27*, 1273, doi:10.3390/molecules27041273 1

Benazir Abbasi, Yan Dong and Rong Rui
Resveratrol Hinders Postovulatory Aging by Modulating Oxidative Stress in Porcine Oocytes
Reprinted from: *Molecules* **2021**, *26*, 6346, doi:10.3390/molecules26216346 3

Clarisse Cornebise, Flavie Courtaut, Marie Taillandier-Coindard, Josep Valls-Fonayet, Tristan Richard, David Monchaud, Virginie Aires and Dominique Delmas
Red Wine Extract Inhibits VEGF Secretion and Its Signaling Pathway in Retinal ARPE-19 Cells to Potentially Disrupt AMD
Reprinted from: *Molecules* **2020**, *25*, 5564, doi:10.3390/molecules25235564 17

You-Lin Tain, Li-Cheng Jheng, Sam K. C. Chang, Yu-Wei Chen, Li-Tung Huang, Jin-Xian Liao and Chih-Yao Hou
Synthesis and Characterization of Novel Resveratrol Butyrate Esters That Have the Ability to Prevent Fat Accumulation in a Liver Cell Culture Model
Reprinted from: *Molecules* **2020**, *25*, 4199, doi:10.3390/molecules25184199 31

Laura Lossi, Adalberto Merighi, Vittorino Novello and Alessandra Ferrandino
Protective Effects of Some Grapevine Polyphenols against Naturally Occurring Neuronal Death
Reprinted from: *Molecules* **2020**, *25*, 2925, doi:10.3390/molecules25122925 45

Aline Yammine, Thomas Nury, Anne Vejux, Norbert Latruffe, Dominique Vervandier-Fasseur, Mohammad Samadi, Hélène Greige-Gerges, Lizette Auezova and Gérard Lizard
Prevention of 7-Ketocholesterol-Induced Overproduction of Reactive Oxygen Species, Mitochondrial Dysfunction and Cell Death with Major Nutrients (Polyphenols, $\omega 3$ and $\omega 9$ Unsaturated Fatty Acids) of the Mediterranean Diet on N2a Neuronal Cells
Reprinted from: *Molecules* **2020**, *25*, 2296, doi:10.3390/molecules25102296 63

Sajad Fakhri, Mohammad Mehdi Gravandi, Sadaf Abdian, Esra Küpeli Akkol, Mohammad Hosein Farzaei and Eduardo Sobarzo-Sánchez
The Neuroprotective Role of Polydatin: Neuropharmacological Mechanisms, Molecular Targets, Therapeutic Potentials, and Clinical Perspective
Reprinted from: *Molecules* **2021**, *26*, 5985, doi:10.3390/molecules26195985 83

Josip Vrdoljak, Marko Kumric, Tina Ticinovic Kurir, Ivan Males, Dinko Martinovic, Marino Vilovic and Josko Bozic
Effects of Wine Components in Inflammatory Bowel Diseases
Reprinted from: *Molecules* **2021**, *26*, 5891, doi:10.3390/molecules26195891 103

Celestino Santos-Buelga, Susana González-Manzano and Ana M. González-Paramás
Wine, Polyphenols, and Mediterranean Diets. What Else Is There to Say?
Reprinted from: *Molecules* **2021**, *26*, 5537, doi:10.3390/molecules26185537 117

Simona Minzer, Ramon Estruch and Rosa Casas
Wine Intake in the Framework of a Mediterranean Diet and Chronic Non-Communicable Diseases: A Short Literature Review of the Last 5 Years
Reprinted from: *Molecules* **2020**, *25*, 5045, doi:10.3390/molecules25215045 139

Francesco Visioli, Stefan-Alexandru Panaite and Joao Tomé-Carneiro
Wine's Phenolic Compounds and Health: A Pythagorean View
Reprinted from: *Molecules* **2020**, *25*, 4105, doi:10.3390/molecules25184105 161

Paula Silva, Norbert Latruffe and Giovanni de Gaetano
Wine Consumption and Oral Cavity Cancer: Friend or Foe, Two Faces of Janus
Reprinted from: *Molecules* **2020**, *25*, 2569, doi:10.3390/molecules25112569 179

About the Editors

Paula Silva, Ph.D., is an assistant professor at the Laboratory of Histology and Embryology, Department of Microscopy, in the Institute of Biomedical Sciences Abel Salazar (ICBAS) of the University of Porto (UPorto) and a researcher at iNOVA Media Lab, ICNOVA of NOVA University Lisbon. Her teaching experience covers: Histology and Embryology (Human and Comparative), Animal Models of Human Disease, and Science Communication. She is the director of the continuing training course "Science communication—Life and health sciences" (6ECTS) and the continuing training unit "Animal Models of Human Disease" (6ECTS). She obtained her PhD in Biomedical Sciences from UPorto. In her CV, Paula Silva presents 28 original articles published in journals indexed in the Science Citation Index (SCI), 1 book chapter, participation in some I&DT projects, and numerous works in many national and international congress. At present, her main research topic is the influence of the moderate consumption of wine on chronic diseases, particularly neurodegenerative diseases, and health science communication. She is the editor of the Science & Wine blog (http://science-and-wine.com/).

Norbert Latruffe defended his PhD in 1977 and, having been appointed in 1989, is currently a Research Professor in Biochemistry at the University of Burgundy, where he installed and headed the Laboratory of Molecular and Cellular Biology until 2006. Then, he was in charge of a team working on Biochemistry of Metabolism and Nutrition in the INSERM research center, UMR 866 of Dijon until 2011. Since 2013, he has been an emeritus Professor at the University of Bourgogne. He graduated with his undergraduate degree from the University of Besançon, and then graduated from the University of Lyon I. Then, he became interested in the following research topics: energetic metabolism of lipids (UA CNRS 531, Besançon); phospholipid-dependent membrane enzymes (Post-doc at Vanderbilt University, Nashville TN, USA 1978–1979); collaboration as a visitor at different foreign universities (Stockholm, Bern, Himeji...); and on the toxicology of peroxisome proliferators when he arrived in Dijon in 1989. Starting in 1998, he launched a new challenge regarding the preventative role of resveratrol, a well-known phytophenol from grape and wine, against age-related pathologies: cancer, inflammation, and cardiovascular diseases. With his collaborators, he was one of the first to explore resveratrol metabolism (2004 BBRC) and its pro-apoptotic properties (2004 J Biol Chem) and discovered a new resveratrol signaling pathway through micro RNA's modulation (2010 Carcinogenesis). N. Latruffe is currently (or a past) an expert member of several national evaluation councils (CNRS, AFSSA, AERES, CNU, Cancer League...) and at international level (UE). He has been awarded several distinctions (Prize at the 16th Oncology and Molecular Medicine at Rhodes, laureate of the APICIL foundation, Palmes academic award and s.o.). Scientific production: H-index of 32. Citations: 4393. He is the author of 450 international contributions, including 190 peer review papers, 8 books, 36 book chapters, 180 congresses communications, 2 scientific films, and 150 lectures or seminars at invitation He has helped more than 25 PhD students in developing great scientific careers. In 2015, he founded the Mediterranean diet and health association, providing academic bursaries for PhD students.

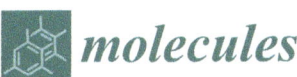

Editorial

Benefits of the Mediterranean Diet–Wine Association: The Role of Ingredients

Paula Silva [1,2,*] and Norbert Latruffe [3,*]

1. Laboratory of Histology and Embryology, Institute of Biomedical Sciences Abel Salazar (ICBAS), Rua de Jorge Viterbo Ferreira n°228, 4050-313 Porto, Portugal
2. iNOVA Media Lab, ICNOVA-NOVA Institute of Communication, NOVA School of Social Sciences and Humanities, Universidade NOVA de Lisboa, 1069-061 Lisbon, Portugal
3. BioPeroxIL, INSERM, Biochemistry of Peroxisome and Inflammation & Lipid Metabolism, EA7270, University Bourgogne-Franche Comte, F-21000 Dijon, France
* Correspondence: psilva@icbas.up.pt (P.S.); norbert.latruffe@u-bourgogne.fr (N.L.)

Citation: Silva, P.; Latruffe, N. Benefits of the Mediterranean Diet–Wine Association: The Role of Ingredients. *Molecules* **2022**, *27*, 1273. https://doi.org/10.3390/molecules27041273

Received: 20 January 2022
Accepted: 8 February 2022
Published: 14 February 2022

Publisher's Note: MDPI stays neutral with regard to jurisdictional claims in published maps and institutional affiliations.

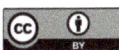

Copyright: © 2022 by the authors. Licensee MDPI, Basel, Switzerland. This article is an open access article distributed under the terms and conditions of the Creative Commons Attribution (CC BY) license (https://creativecommons.org/licenses/by/4.0/).

The cultural and nutritional aspects of the multi-secular Mediterranean civilization include diet as a central element of health and well-being, including wine if it is used in moderation. Indeed, Mediterranean meals provide food microcomponents including polyphenols, vitamins, fibers, polyunsaturated fatty acids, and oligoelements present in fruits, vegetables, olive oil, fish, infusions, etc. In addition, wine, especially the red variety, provide additional unique polyphenols with antioxidant properties, such as resveratrol, procyanidins, and monophenols, including hydroxytyrosol and tyrosol [1].

The Mediterranean diet is a model of eating based on the traditional foods and drinks of the countries surrounding the Mediterranean Sea. In recent decades, it has been promoted worldwide (UNESCO 2010) as one of the healthiest dietary patterns and has been reported to have benefits regarding chronic diseases, i.e., cardiovascular illness [2,3], breast [4] and colon cancer [5], cognition [6] and longevity [7]. Many consumers do not know what to believe when it comes to the health effects of drinking wine. Some researchers have associated moderate drinking with various health benefits, especially since wine is rich in antioxidants. Others, on the other hand, claim that even an occasional drink is harmful to health.

The publication of a Special Issue in the journal *Molecules* that focuses on the role of wine ingredients in the health benefits associated with the Mediterranean diet was a good opportunity to clarify this issue. Researchers were invited to submit manuscripts related to polyphenols, resveratrol, ageing, antioxidant, wine, health, the Mediterranean diet, nutrition, diseases, welfare, behavior, etc. at the level of mechanisms, analysis, and experimental and epidemiological studies.

The objective of this Special Issue is to highlight wine as part of the Mediterranean diet, especially through the perspectives of policymakers, the medical world, and the vectors of image.

The valuable accepted and published papers contributing to this Special Issue are as follows:

Original papers include 'Resveratrol Hinders Postovulatory Aging by Modulating Oxidative Stress in Porcine Oocytes' by Benazir Abbasi et al.; 'Red Wine Extract Inhibits VEGF Secretion and Its Signaling Pathway in Retinal ARPE-19 Cells to Potentially Disrupt AMD' by Clarisse Cornebise et al.; 'Synthesis and Characterization of Novel Resveratrol Butyrate Esters That Have the Ability to Prevent Fat Accumulation in a Liver Cell Culture Model' by You Lin Tain; 'Protective Effects of Some Grapevine Polyphenols against Naturally Occurring Neuronal Death' by Laura Lossi et al.; 'Prevention of 7-Ketocholesterol-Induced Overproduction of Reactive Oxygen Species, Mitochondrial Dysfunction and Cell Death with Major Nutrients (Polyphenols, ω3 and ω9 Unsaturated Fatty Acids) of the Mediterranean Diet on N2a Neuronal Cells' by Aline Yammine et al.

Additionally, several review papers are included—namely, 'The Neuroprotective Role of Polydatin: Neuropharmacological Mechanisms, Molecular Targets, Therapeutic Potentials, and Clinical Perspective' by Sajad Fakhri et al.; 'Effects of Wine Components in Inflammatory Bowel Diseases' by Josip Vrdoljak et al.; 'Wine, Polyphenols, and Mediterranean Diets. What Else Is There to Say?' by Celestino Santos-Buelga et al.; 'Wine Intake in the Framework of a Mediterranean Diet and Chronic Non-Communicable Diseases: A Short Literature Review of the Last 5 Years' by Simona Minzer et al.; 'Wine's Phenolic Compounds and Health: A Pythagorean View' by Francesco Visioli et al.; 'Wine Consumption and Oral Cavity Cancer: Friend or Foe, Two Faces of Janus' by Paula Silva et al.

Many readers would be interested in the content amassed in this Special Issue, including scientists in nutrition, medical doctors, wine biochemists, wine tasting associations, winemakers, researchers in Vin viticulture and in enology, etc.

Notably, the topic of this Special Issue induced Science & Wine to promote the Second World Congress "Wine and Olive Oil Production: The Fluid Aspect of Mediterranean Diet" held on 2 to 3 June 2021, https://www.science-and-wine-conferences.com.

Author Contributions: Conceptualization, P.S. and N.L.; writing—original draft preparation, N.L.; writing—review and editing, P.S. All authors have read and agreed to the published version of the manuscript.

Funding: The management of this Special Issue did not need any special funding.

Acknowledgments: The authors acknowledge the NMS association (Mediterranean Diet and Health), the UNESCO Chair, culture and wine tradition (France), and The Science & Wine Conference (Portugal) for their continuous interest.

Conflicts of Interest: The authors declare no conflict of interest, financial or otherwise.

References

1. Latruffe, N. *Wine, Mediterranean Nutrition and Health, a Virtuous Association*; EUD Editions (Universitaires de Dijon): Dijon, France, 2017; 204p, ISBN 978-2-36441-199-9. (In French)
2. Sofi, F.; Macchi, C.; Abbate, R.; Gensini, G.F.; Casini, A. Mediterranean diet and health status: An updated meta-analysis and a proposal for a literature-based adherence score. *Public Health Nutr.* **2014**, *17*, 2769–2782. [CrossRef] [PubMed]
3. Estruch, R.; Ros, E.; Salas-Salvadó, J.; Covas, M.I.; Corella, D.; Arós, F.; Gómez-Gracia, E.; Ruiz-Gutiérrez, V.; Fiol, M.; Lapetra, J.; et al. PREDIMED Study Investigators. Primary Prevention of Cardiovascular Disease with a Mediterranean Diet Supplemented with Extra-Virgin Olive Oil or Nuts. *N. Engl. J. Med.* **2018**, *378*, e34. [CrossRef] [PubMed]
4. Villarini, M.; Lanari, C.; Nucci, D.; Gianfredi, V.; Marzulli, T.; Berrino, F.; Borgo, A.; Bruno, E.; Gargano, G.; Moretti, M.; et al. Community-based participatory research to improve life quality and clinical outcomes of patients with breast cancer (DianaWeb in Umbria pilot study). *BMJ Open* **2016**, *6*, e009707. [CrossRef] [PubMed]
5. Grosso, G.; Antonio Biondi, A.; Galvano, F.; Mistretta, A.; Marventano, S.; Buscemi, S.; Drago, F.; Basile, F. Factors associated with colorectal cancer in the context of the Mediterranean diet: A case-control study. *Nutr. Cancer* **2014**, *66*, 558–565. [CrossRef] [PubMed]
6. McEvoy, C.T.; Hoang, T.; Sidney, S.; Steffen, L.M.; Jacobs, D.R., Jr.; Shikany, J.M.; Wilkins, J.T.; Yaffe, K. Dietary patterns during adulthood and cognitive performance in midlife: The CARDIA study. *Neurology* **2019**, *92*, e1589–e1599. [CrossRef] [PubMed]
7. Boccardi, V.; Esposito, A.; Rizzo, M.R.; Marfella, R.; Barbieri, M.; Paolisso, G. Mediterranean diet, telomere maintenance and health status among elderly. *PLoS ONE* **2013**, *8*, e62781. [CrossRef] [PubMed]

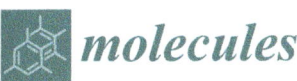

Article

Resveratrol Hinders Postovulatory Aging by Modulating Oxidative Stress in Porcine Oocytes

Benazir Abbasi, Yan Dong and Rong Rui *

College of Veterinary Medicine, Nanjing Agricultural University, Nanjing 210095, China; benazirabbassi@gmail.com (B.A.); 2016107099@njau.edu.cn (Y.D.)
* Correspondence: rrui@njau.edu.cn; Tel.: +86-25-843-955-95

Abstract: Postovulatory aging of the mammalian oocytes causes deterioration of oocytes through several factors including oxidative stress. Keeping that in mind, we aimed to investigate the potential of a well-known antioxidant, resveratrol (RV), to evaluate the adverse effects of postovulatory aging in porcine oocytes. After in vitro maturation (IVM), a group of (25–30) oocytes (in three replicates) were exposed to 0, 1, 2, and 4 µmol/L of RV, respectively. The results revealed that the first polar body (PB1) extrusion rate of the oocytes significantly increased when the RV concentration reached up to 2 µmol/L ($p < 0.05$). Considering optimum RV concentration of 2 µmol/L, the potential of RV was evaluated in oocytes aged for 24 and 48 h. We used fluorescence microscopy to detect the relative level of reactive oxygen species (ROS), while GHS contents were measured through the enzymatic method. Our results revealed that aged groups (24 h and 48 h) treated with RV (2 µmol/L) showed higher ($p < 0.05$) ROS fluorescence intensity than the control group, but lower ($p < 0.05$) than untreated aged groups. The GSH content in untreated aged groups (24 h and 48 h) was lower ($p < 0.05$) than RV-treated groups, but both groups showed higher levels than the control. Similarly, the relative expression of the genes involved in antioxidant activity (*CAT*, *GPXGSH-Px*, and *SOD1*) in RV-treated groups was lower ($p < 0.05$) as compared to the control group but higher than that of untreated aged groups. Moreover, the relative mRNA expression of caspase-3 and Bax in RV-treated groups was higher ($p < 0.05$) than the control group but lower than untreated groups. Furthermore, the expression of *Bcl-2* in the RV-treated group was significantly lower than control but higher than untreated aged groups. Taken together, our findings revealed that the RV can increase the expression of antioxidant genes by decreasing the level of ROS, and its potent antiapoptotic effects resisted against the decline in mitochondrial membrane potential in aged oocytes.

Keywords: resveratrol; postovulatory aging; oocyte quality; oxidative stress; reactive oxygen species

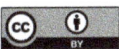

1. Introduction

The postovulation oocyte quality is the main factor that affects the efficiency of assisted reproductive technologies (ART) such as somatic cell nuclear transfer (SCNT), intracytoplasmic sperm injection (ICSI), and in vitro fertilization (IVF) [1,2]. The quality of an oocyte is mainly affected by structural and functional changes induced during aging including chromosome and spindle anomalies [3], cortical granule exocytosis [4], lower fertilization rates [5], zona pellucida (ZP) hardening [6], and abnormal or retarded development of embryos/fetuses [7,8]. The exact molecular mechanism underlying the reduced competence of an oocyte due to postovulatory aging is not fully understood. However, there are some major factors that mediate time dependent reduction in oocyte competence such as oxidative stress [9], chromosomal abnormalities [10], and modification of poly (A) tails (Deadenylation) of genes responsible for maternal effects [11] and epigenetic alteration [12,13]. Therefore, it is imperative to better understand the various mechanisms responsible for the postovulatory aging process to devise effective strategies to delay oocyte aging process and increase the time required for performing normal reproductive functions [9,14]. Oxidative stress is strongly associated with a deterioration in oocyte quality because it significantly reduces the glutathione (GSH) contents and assists in the accumulation of reactive oxygen species (ROS). The ROS such as superoxide anions (O^{-2}), hydroxyl radicals (OH^-), and hydrogen peroxide (H_2O_2) are released during normal metabolic (intermediate steps of oxygen reduction) processes [15,16]. The mitochondrion is the major cell organelle responsible for ROS production [17,18]. A dynamic balance is required between ROS production and antioxidant enzymes to ensure proper cellular homeostasis including cell proliferation, host defense, signal transduction, and gene expression [19]. The antioxidant defense system disrupted through the overproduction of ROS, which, in turn, causes oxidative stress. Excessive load of ROS results in proapoptotic signaling, subsequently leading to the activation of cell apoptosis [20]. Postovulatory aging is associated with excessive accumulation of ROS leading to oxidative stress, which predisposes aged oocytes to the apoptotic process [9,21]. The mitochondria as the major "energy generators" have a significant role in regulating proper function and survival of oocytes. However, being a prime source of ROS production, mitochondria are susceptible to ROS-induced damage [22], which results in the decreased ATP synthesis, altered mitochondrial membrane potential, oxidative stress, and early onset of apoptosis [23,24]. The excessive accumulation of ROS can affect the permeability of mitochondrial membranes to open MPTP (1-methyl-4-phenyl-1,2,3,6-tetrahydropyridine) and promote the flow of calcium ions [25], which subsequently induces the release of cytochrome C and caspase 3 activation leading to the apoptosis [26,27]. The apoptotic activation is mainly induced by the glutathione efflux [28], which leads to several morphological changes including cell shrinkage, progressive DNA, and cell membrane damage, ultimately leading to the cell death [29]. Therefore, one of the major challenges in reproductive embryology is to prevent oocytes' degeneration to maintain their developmental competences [30]. To avoid oxidative damage by maintaining a robust antioxidant defense system in the oocyte, supplementation of exogenous antioxidants can be used as the most effective strategy.

Resveratrol (3,5,4'-trihydroxyl-Trans-stilbene) (RV) is a stilbenoid, a type of natural polyphenolic compound with excellent antioxidant and free radical scavenging capacity. It is associated with reduced ROS accumulation, scavenges superoxide radicals, inhibits lipid peroxidation, and regulates the expression of antioxidant cofactors and enzymes [31]. Natural antioxidants that are effective may provide novel and safe interventional strategies to delay or prevent oocyte aging and related diseases. Porcine oocytes can be used as an ideal model in the field of reproductive biology, as they have much similar developmental and physiological properties as with human oocytes [32]. Therefore, this study was conducted to evaluate the effect of RV on pig oocytes during aging and to provide mechanistic insights regarding its potential of protecting oocytes against ROS attack. Reducing oxidative stress in the oocytes is an important way to slow down oocyte aging. Still, there is lack of data regarding the rescue of oocytes during aging. The underlying mechanisms of oxidative stress during oocyte aging as well as the protective mechanisms of the natural antioxidants in antiaging are thoroughly explored in the present study.

2. Results

2.1. RV Treatment Reverses Aging-Induced Impairment in Aged Porcine Oocytes

For determining the optimal concentration of RV, which can delay oocyte age dependent impairments, the cumulus cells incubated for 44 h were removed with 0.1% (w/v) hyaluronidase using 37 °C for 3 min. The oocytes with even granular cytoplasm and a first polar body were selected for the subsequent experiments. During in vitro maturation, a total of 25–30 oocytes (in three replicates) for each group were cultured with 0, 1, 2, and 4 µmol/L RV, respectively. After maturation, the proliferation rate of cumulus oocyte complexes (COCs) was observed under a stereomicroscope. As shown in Figure 1a, most of the COCs showed fully expanded peripheral layers of cumulus in 1 and 2 µmol/L RV-treated groups, whereas the cumulus proliferation of COCs was significantly decreased in the control and 4 µmol/L of RV-treated group. In addition, a large proportion of the RV-treated oocytes failed to extrude the PB1 in a dose-dependent manner. As shown in Figure 1b, percentage of the PB1 extrusion rate was significantly higher in the 2 µmol/L RV-treated group (78.99 ± 1.07) as compared to the control group (71.26 ± 1.02%). However, there was no significant difference observed for these parameters in 1 and 4 µmol/L RV-treated groups (73.95 ± 1.05% and 73.76 ± 1.02, respectively).

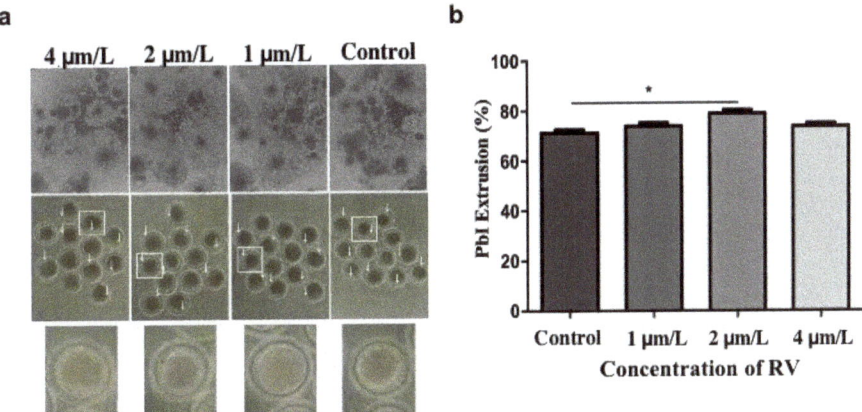

Figure 1. RV treatment reverses aging-induced impairment in aged porcine oocytes. (a) The representative images showing degrees of cumulus spread and first polar body extrusion rate, as indicated by white arrows. (b) The graph showing PB1 extrusion percentage rate at various concentrations (0, 1, 2, and 4 µmol/L RV). Significant difference (* $p < 0.05$).

2.2. RV Suppresses the Increasing Perivitaline Space (PVS) in Aged Porcine Oocytes

As shown in Figure 2a, arrows indicate the significantly increased perivitaline space in oocytes of 24 h and 48 h aged groups (15.98 ± 0.60 and 21.51 ± 1.16, respectively) as compared to the control group (10.94 ± 0.53). Moreover, the treatment with 2 µmol/L of RV prolonged oocyte culture (24 h and 48 h) can significantly suppress the perivitaline space when compared with untreated (24 h and 48 h) aged groups.

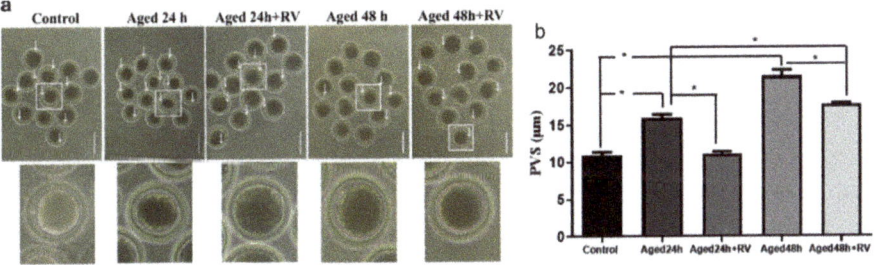

Figure 2. RV suppresses the increasing perivitaline space (PVS) in aged porcine oocytes (a) The representative images of perivitaline space in aged porcine oocytes with visible space indicated by white arrows under the microscope, scale bar = 180 µm. (b) The graph indicates the percent increase in perivitaline space after the oocytes treated with 2 µmol/L RV. Significant difference (* $p < 0.05$).

2.3. RV Reduces the Apoptosis Extent in Aged Porcine Oocytes

The apoptosis includes a series of cellular apoptotic events that occur during oocyte aging during in vitro maturation [33]. As shown in Figure 3 the mRNA expression of apoptosis related genes (Caspase-3, Bax, and Bcl-2) were analyzed through qRT-PCR to determine the cellular activities during the RV treatment. The results showed that the mRNA levels of Caspase-3 and Bax treated with 2 µmol/L RV were significantly higher than those in the control group but significantly lower than those in the 24 h and 48 h aged groups, while the expression of Bcl-2 was significantly lower. Moreover, the expression of Bcl-2 group oocytes treated with 2 µmol/L RV was significantly lower than that in control but significantly higher than that in the untreated aged groups.

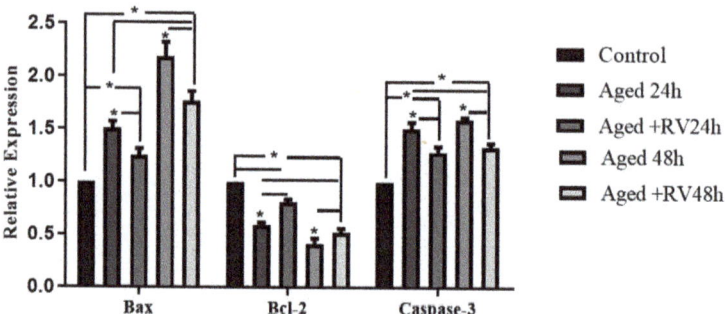

Figure 3. The relative mRNA expression of apoptosis related (Caspase-3, Bcl-2, and Bax) genes in aged porcine oocytes at different time periods. Significant difference (* $p < 0.05$).

2.4. RV Alleviates the Oxidative Stress in Aged Porcine Oocytes

RV is known to protect cells against oxidative stress and to determine whether RV can protect porcine oocyte against oxidative stress. We first measured the levels of intracellular ROS, as shown in Figure 4a,b; the levels of ROS were significantly higher in the 24 h and 48 h untreated aged groups when compared with the control group, while the oocytes treated with 2 µmol/L RV (24 and 48 h) showed significantly higher fluorescence intensity levels as compared to the control group but significantly lower intensity as compared to the untreated aged groups. The glutathione (GSH) is an important intracellular antioxidant because it exerts powerful functions for protecting the cells from the oxidative stress-induced damage, and so the GSH and GSSG kits were used to detect the ROS levels. Surprisingly, our analysis for ROS levels using GSH and GSSG kit shows that the intracellular levels of GSH in the 24 h and 48 h untreated aged groups were significantly lower when compared with the control group (Figure 4c). The GSH content in the 24 h and 48 h groups treated with 2 µmol/L of RV was significantly higher than that in the 24 h and 48 h untreated aged groups. In addition, we also determined the mRNA expression of antioxidant and oxidative stress related genes (CAT, GPX, and SOD1) by qRT-PCR analysis. Our results (Figure 4d) showed that the mRNA transcript levels of CAT and SOD1 groups' oocytes treated with 2 µmol/L RV were significantly higher than those in the untreated aged groups; however, the expression of CAT and SOD1 was lower as compared to the control group. Likewise, there was a significant increase in the treated groups of GPX, and no difference was found between the untreated aged GPX and control groups.

2.5. RV Rescues the Mitochondrial Membrane Potential in Aged Porcine Oocytes

It is well-known that oxidative stress is associated with mitochondrial membrane potential (MMP) changes and cell apoptosis. Therefore, we intended to determine the mitochondrial membrane potential state during porcine oocyte aging. To investigate the mitochondrial membrane potential, we analyzed the ratio of red/green fluorescence. As shown in Figure 5c,e,h,j,k, the oocytes treated with 2 µmol/L RV (24 and 48 h) aged groups showed lower ratios than those in the untreated aged groups. Moreover, oocytes in control (Figure 5a,f,k) showed the lowest values. Based on our findings, this is concluded that RV has remarkable efficacy on keeping mitochondrial membrane potential in porcine oocyte aging.

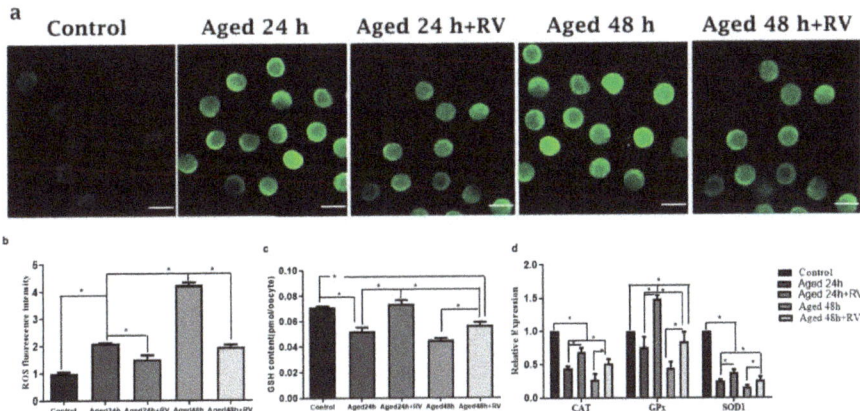

Figure 4. RV alleviates the oxidative stress in aged porcine oocytes. (**a**) The representative images of ROS in aged porcine oocytes. (**b,c**) The graphs showing quantified intracellular levels of ROS and GSH in aged porcine oocytes. (**d**) The graph showing relative mRNA expression of oxidative stress related *(CAT, GPX,* and *SOD1)* genes in aged porcine oocytes. ROS levels were quantified by relative fluorescence intensity in porcine oocytes, scale bar = 280 μm. Each experiment was independently repeated at least three times. Significant difference (* $p < 0.05$).

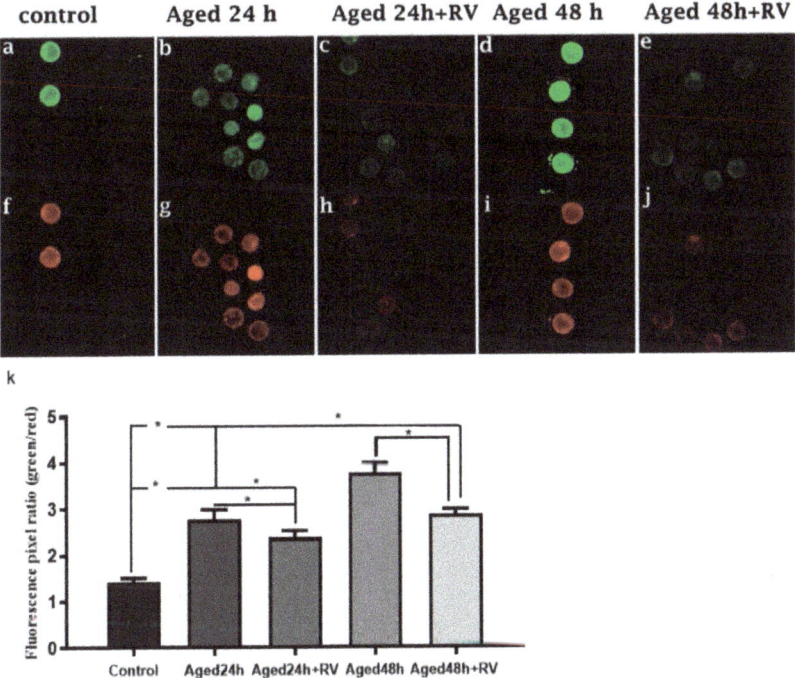

Figure 5. RV rescues the mitochondrial membrane potential in aged porcine oocytes. Representative Fluorescent images of JC-1-stained oocytes. Cultured in the absence or presence of 2 μmol/L RV. (**a,f**) Control; (**b,g**) aged 24 h; (**c,h**) aged 24 h + RV; (**d,i**) aged 48 h; (**e,j**) aged 48 h + RV. (**k**) Quantitative analysis of JC-1 red/green fluorescence intensity ratio in porcine oocytes. Membrane potential was calculated as the ratio of red fluorescence, which corresponds to activated mitochondria (J-aggregates), and to green fluorescence, which corresponds to less-activated mitochondria (J-monomers). Fluorescence emitted from each oocyte was analyzed using the ImageJ software. Significant difference (* $p < 0.05$).

3. Discussion

One of the main aspects of ovarian aging is the decline in fertility over time, which is characterized by the decline in the quality and quantity of oocytes [34]. However, some evidence suggests that an imbalance between ROS and antioxidants causes a decline in oocyte quality, which is a critical factor in the success of ART and is linked to the aging of the ovaries. Furthermore, the RV as an antioxidant has been proved to alleviate oxidative stress in various cell types including oocytes. Moreover, RV has shown to prevent mitochondrial damage in cardiomyocytes through the upregulation of the deacetylation of apoptotic proteins. Studies have revealed that treatment of porcine oocytes with 2 μmol/L RV significantly reduced the levels of intracellular ROS while increased GSH contents during in vitro maturation [35,36]. In our study, we revealed that, under in vitro conditions, 2 μmol/L RV was able to delay postovulatory oocyte aging, owing to possible mechanisms mediated by reducing oxidative stress. RV could significantly increase the GSH content in 24 h and 48 h aged groups treated with 2 μmol/L of RV as compared with the control group ($p < 0.05$). The certain survival factors and antiapoptosis factors lead to oocyte maturation disorder or apoptosis by a decrease in mature-promoting factor (MPF) stability [37]. Furthermore, induced oxidative stress can adversely affect a variety of reproductive processes including sperm capacitation, ovulation, and corpus luteum production and can also trigger oocyte apoptosis. The accumulation of ROS has serious manifestation regarding the quality and aging of oocytes [38]. The uncontrolled and excessive production of free radicals may harm DNA, proteins, and lipids, which can severely compromise cell health and contribute to the disease development [39–41]. Our results showed that RV can significantly reduce the ROS level in aged oocytes (24 and 48 h), which is consistent with previous findings [42]. Similarly, RV (at concentrations ≥ 100 μM) has been shown to scavenge O2 directly in a nonenzymatic, cell-free system [43]. Findings in the present study indicate the potential of RV to delay oocyte aging by reducing ROS levels owing to its reported antioxidant [44], antiapoptosis [45], and antiaging [42] activities. Moreover, RV has also shown to reduce lipid peroxidation by eliminating free radicals and thus achieve the effect of protecting cells [46]. The main antioxidant enzymes are *SOD*, catalase (*CAT*), and glutathione peroxidase (*GPX*). Moreover, O_2 is converted by *SOD* to H_2O_2, which is decomposed to water and oxygen by *CAT*, preventing the production of hydroxyl radicals. In addition, *GPX* transforms peroxides and hydroxyl radicals into nontoxic forms by oxidizing reduced glutathione (GSH) into glutathione disulfide and triggers reduction to GSH by glutathione reductase [47]. When Cu^{+2} or Fe^{+2} are available, H_2O_2 reacts with these ions to form unstable hydroxyl radicals. Previous studies have shown that RV can increase the expression of various antioxidant genes such as *CAT*, *SOD*, and *GPX* in cells [48,49]. When low-dose of RV was used to treat cardiomyocytes, the catalytic activity of *CAT* and *SOD* increased significantly with no effect on glutathione activity. Moreover, *SOD* can reduce intracellular superoxide levels and potentially resist against cell apoptosis, membrane permeability changes, and mitochondrial dysfunction [50]. Previous studies in our laboratory have demonstrated that RV can eliminate mitochondrial injury while delaying oocyte aging and improving the expression of sirtuin-1 (sirt1) and thus the quality of aged porcine oocytes [1]. Similarly, in the present study, RV treatment increased the expression of *GPX* gene in 24 h aged groups as compared to the control and untreated aged groups ($p < 0.01$). However, the expression of *CAT* and *SOD1* genes was lower than that of the control group ($p < 0.05$) but still higher than their untreated counterparts. Likewise, RV increases GSH content in primary keratinocytes and in epidermis of a reconstructed skin model as reported previously [51]. The antioxidant response of RV was further confirmed through enhanced activity of SOD with administration of 2-NP in a rat model conducted by Lodovici et al. [52]. Our findings revealed that RV can effectively mediate oxidative stress induced by the aging oocytes during in vitro culture through increasing the antioxidant gene expression. Progesterone causes elongation of the Mos poly (A) tail via cytoplasmic polyadenylation, and this polyadenylation increases the rate of Mos translation leading to the accumulation of Mos protein [53]. Mos protein is essentially required for the initiation of oocyte germinal vesicle breakdown [54]. In our study, we observed an increase in cumulus spread after treatment of oocytes with different concentrations of RV (0, 1, 2, and 4 µmol/L), which is consistent with previous findings, as mentioned earlier. Furthermore, PB1 extrusion rate with 2 µmol/L of RV group was also significantly higher than other groups, indicating the potential of RV to increase oocyte maturation rate in a dose-dependent manner. During this study, we found that oocytes treated with RV showed a significant decrease in perivitaline spaces during 24 h and 48 h of aging. However, differences were nonsignificant compared with the control group. A full expansion of cumulus cells is mandatory for the proper maturation of the oocyte. The beneficial effects of RV might depend upon its ability to improve oocyte quality. Therefore, it can be concluded that RV (2 µmol/L) can inhibit the increase of perivitaline space of oocytes aged for 24 h and 48 h, indicating its ability to alleviate the adverse effects of postovulatory oocyte aging by improving the quality, which is necessary for its development during fertilization. Apoptosis is well-known for exogenous (mediated by death receptors) and mitochondria-guided endogenous pathways. Both of these pathways participate in the activation of certain members of the Caspase family to trigger apoptosis. The proteins involved in the mitochondria-mediated endogenous pathway include the member of the Bcl-2 family, which comprises both antiapoptotic and proapoptotic proteins. The antiapoptotic proteins (Bcl-XL, Bcl-2, and Mcl-1) potentially inhibit the activation of the Caspase family and block the transduction of apoptotic signals, while proapoptotic proteins (Bcl XS, Bak, Bax, and Bad) promote and initiate an apoptotic response. Caspase 3 acts as a key effector in the process of apoptosis and directly hydrolyzes specific substrates. When there is apoptosis, Bax acts on the outer mitochondrial membrane of cell causing the release of mitochondrial cytochrome C (Cytc) that activates Caspase 3 and triggers Caspase cascade. The nucleated cytoskeleton recombines and degrades cytoskeletal structure [33]. However, Bcl 2 inhibits Cytc and Caspase, causing an antiapoptotic effect. The recruitment of Bax, which is knocked out, restricts the expression of Bax and leads to an increase in the number of ovarian oocytes [55]. Deacetylated Sirt1 and Sirt-3 inhibit the apoptotic pathway by affecting 1-methyl-4-phenyl-1, 2, 3, 6-tetrahydropyridine (MPTP) pores of the mitochondrial membrane [56]. Furthermore, downregulation of caspase 3 upregulates the expression of the antiapoptotic protein such as Bcl-2 that subsequently inhibits apoptosis. We observed lower expression of Bax and Caspase 3 in RV-treated aged oocytes in the present study. Moreover, relative mRNA expression of Bcl-2 was significantly lower in the RV-treated group than the control but was significantly higher as compared to untreated aged groups. Our findings suggested that RV can effectively inhibit mitochondrial apoptotic pathway through downregulation of the Bax and Caspase 3 while upregulating the expression of Bcl-2 in aged oocytes, eventually reducing the adverse effects of aging in porcine oocytes. Mitochondria are responsible for maintaining cellular metabolic functions, and their physiological efficiency can be assessed by examining the mitochondrial membrane potential state. In this regard, fluorescence probes such as JC-1 tend to accumulate in the mitochondrial matrix (by forming I-J-aggregates) and produce red excitation light when the mitochondrial membrane potential is maintained high. However, if mitochondrial membrane potential is maintained low, JC-1 cannot accumulate in the mitochondrial matrix and, hence, forms monomers and generates green excitation light. On the basis of these results is suggested a remarkable efficacy of RV on keeping mitochondrial membrane potential in porcine oocyte aging. During the present study, inclusion of RV in the oocyte culture medium maintained the mitochondrial membrane potential of aged oocytes in a state consistent with nonaged counterparts. Furthermore, RV significantly increased the expression of Bcl-2 in 24 and 48 h aged oocytes, which subsequently can modulate the mitochondrial apoptotic pathway by controlling the permeability of the outer mitochondrial membrane [57]. Consequently, the RV-regulated follicular development primarily through increased expression of mitochondrial-related Bcl-2 gene, which might have played its role in the maintenance of mitochondrial membrane potential in its normal position in 24 and 48 h aged oocytes. However, further in vivo studies are required to elucidate its potential mechanism of action.

4. Materials and Methods

4.1. Ethics Statement

The present study (short title: "Resveratrol hinders postovulatory aging by modulating oxidative stress in porcine oocytes") was carried out in strict accordance with the recommendation of the National Ethical commission of (Nanjing, Jiangsu, China). All the experiments and procedures compiled with the guideline and were approved by the local ethical committee of the Nanjing Agricultural University (Nanjing, Jiangsu, China) with respect to animal experimentation and care of animal under study.

4.2. Reagents

Resveratrol (R5010, Sigma, purity $\geq$ 99%), Dulbecco's PBS (DPBS), Hyaluronidase H-3506, DMSO D2650, paraformaldehyde 158127, poly vinyl alcohol (PVA) 046K0086, D-Mannitol M-9647, and Sodium pyruvate 100M12532V were purchased from Sigma–Aldrich (St. Louis, MO, USA), unless otherwise mentioned.

4.3. Oocytes Collection and IVM

The porcine ovaries were collected from prepubertal gilts at a local slaughterhouse of (Nanjing Yuan-run Group Co., Ltd., Nanjing, China) and transported to our laboratory at 37 °C in 0.9% NaCl (w/v) physiological saline within 2 h postcollection. Follicular fluid from superficial follicles of 3–6 mm in diameter was aspirated using a disposable syringe with an 18-guage needle, and the fluid was immediately transferred into conical tubes to allow COCs to settle down at the bottom for quick (pick up purpose) of COCs. After 10–12 min, the whole bottom sediment was placed down in petri dish. Follicular contents containing COCs that had more than 3 unexpanded cumulus cell layers with uniform cytoplasm were selected under a stereomicroscope (Olympus, Tokyo, Japan) and washed thrice in HEPES buffered Tyrode's medium containing 0.05% (w/v) PVA (TLH–PVA). A group of approximately 50–70 of COCs was placed in each well in a 4-well plate (Nunclon, Roskilde, Denmark) containing 500 µL pre-equilibrated TCM199 medium (Gibco NY, USA) supplemented with 3.05 Mm D-glucose, 0.91 Mm sodium pyruvate, 0.57 Mm cysteine, 10 ng/mL epidermal growth factor, 10 IU/mL PMSG and hCG (Ningbo Hormonal Reagents Co., Ltd., Ningbo, Zhejiang, China), 75 µg/mL penicillin, 50 µg/mL streptomycin, 0.1% (w/v) polyvinyl alcohol, and 10% (v/v) porcine follicular fluid (pFF) [58], covered with 150 µL of mineral oil at 38.5 °C in an atmosphere of 5% CO_2 in humidified air for 44 h.

4.4. RV Concentration and In Vitro Aging

RV was dissolved in 10 mmol/L of Dimethyl Sulfoxide (DMSO) as a stock solution and was stored at −20 °C before use. At the start of each culture, the stock solution was diluted with TCM-199 in vitro maturation medium to adjust a final concentration of 2 µmol/L for the RV treatments. For in vitro aging analysis, oocytes were cultured in IVM medium supplemented with or without 2 µmol/L RV (Control, Aged 24 h, Aged 24 h + RV, Aged 48 h, and Aged 48 h+ RV groups, respectively) for an additional 24 h and 48 h prolonged aging period at 38.5 °C supplemented with 5% CO_2 in the humidified air for 44 h. The fresh oocytes without any prolonged culture were used as control group.

4.5. RNA Isolation and Quantitative Real-Time Polymerase Chain Reaction (qRT-PCR)

According to the time-based group differentiation and after maturation (44 h) of oocytes, the denuded oocytes were collected and washed thrice in DPBS solution and stored at −80 °C until the RNA was extracted. A total of 100 oocytes were used for total RNA extraction (in three replicates) from each group using the Trizol™ Reagent (Thermo Fisher scientific, Waltham, MA, USA). The extracted RNA was quantified using Nano-Drop and stored at −80 °C until further use. The first strand of cDNA was synthesized from 2 ug of total RNA with Primer Script™ RT Master Mix (Takara, Dalian, China) following the manufacturer's described reaction protocol: 37 °C for 15 min, 85 °C for 5 s, and hold at 4 °C. The synthesized cDNA was subjected to real-time PCR using TB Green® Premix Ex

Taq™ (TaKaRa, Dalian, China). The forward and reverse primer sequences for real-time PCR are listed in Table 1. The reaction conditions were 30 s at 95 °C, followed by 40 cycles of 95 °C for 5 s and 60 °C for 30 s. Ultimately, they were quantified at 95 °C for 15 s, 60 °C for 1 min, and 95 °C for 15 s. At least three replications were performed for each reaction and data were analyzed using the $2^{-\triangle\triangle CT}$ method [58].

Table 1. Primer sequences of the target genes used for RT-qPCR.

Target Gene	Forward and Reverse Sequence	Product Size (bp)	Accession Number
GAPDH	F: 5'-GTCGGTTGTGGATCTGACCT-3' R: 5'-TTGACGAAGTGGTCGTTGAG-3'	207	NM_001206359
Caspase-3	F: 5'-CGTGCTTCTAAGCCATGGTG-3' R: 5'-GTCCCACTGTCCGTCTCAAT-3'	186	NM_214131
Bcl-2	F:5'-AGGGCATTCAGTGACCTGAC-3' R: 5'-CGATCCGACTCACCAATACC-3'	193	NM_214285
Bax	F:5'-TGCCTCAGGATGCATCTACC-3' R: 5'-AAGTAGAAAAGCGCGACCAC-3'	199	XM_003127290
CAT	F-5'-AACTGTCCCTTCCGTGCTA-3' R-5'-CCTGGGTGACATTATCTTCG-3'	195	XM_021081498
GPX	F:GAGCCCTTCAACCTGTCCTC R:GTCGGACGTACTTCAGGCAA	210	NC_010455.5
SOD1	F-5'-ACCTGGGCAATGTGACTG-3' R-5'-TCCAGCATTTCCCGTCT-3	131	NM_001190422

4.6. Measurement of Reactive Oxygen Species (ROS) Intensity

To measure the level of intracellular ROS, DCFH-DA (2, 7-Dichlorodi-hydrofluorescein diacetate) and 10 µM working solution (with TCM199 medium), after diluting together, were equilibrated in the incubator at 37 °C for 30 min subsequently, and the oocytes were incubated in the DCFH-DA working solution at 37 °C for 1 h under total darkness. After incubation, oocytes were washed three times in PBS, and the fluorescence signals were detected and imaged using confocal microscope (Zeiss LSM 700META, Oberkochen, Germany) that was fluorescence intensity of ROS (Excitation wavelength: 450–490 nm and Emission wavelength: 515–565 nm). The relative fluorescence intensity was measured with ImageJ 1.5 software (Bethesda, Maryland, USA). Total numbers of 25–30 oocytes (in three replicates) were used for ROS measurement, respectively.

4.7. Determination of Intracellular GSH Contents

The contents of total glutathione (T-GSH) were examined through an enzymatic method by using a GSH/GSSG assay kit (Beyotime, Shanghai, China) according to the manufacturer's instructions. A total of 50 oocytes from each group were placed into a small conical tube containing 30 µL of protein scavenger M solution supplied with the kit. Afterward, tube contents were vortexed thoroughly for 5 min, then the mixture was frozen at liquid nitrogen for 2 min and thawed in a water bath at 37 °C repeatedly for 3 times. Subsequently, mixture was centrifuged at 10,000 rpm for 10 min at 4°C and placed on ice for 5 min using a 96-well plate. The samples or standard in the sequence were added and mixed accordingly. Immediately, absorbance was observed at 405 nm with a microplate reader, for 25 min, with a reading recorded for every 5 min. A standard curve was developed for the determination of the GSH content of each sample. The GSH concentration was calculated by dividing the total concentration of each sample by the total number of oocytes present in the sample (pmol/oocyte).

4.8. Mitochondrial Membrane Potential Assay

The mitochondrial membrane potential (MMP, $\Delta\varphi m$) of the aged and fresh oocytes was evaluated using mitochondrial membrane potential assay kit JC-1 (Beyotime, Shanghai, China). The oocytes were exposed to 10 µL JC-1 in 100 µL working solution at 38.5 °C in 5% CO_2 for 20 min under total darkness. To remove surface fluorescence, oocytes were washed three times in PBS and then mounted on glass slides using D-PBS for microscopy. Laser excitation was set at 488 nm for green and 525 nm for red fluorescence, respectively. The fluorescence microscope (Zeiss LSM 700 META, Oberkochen, Germany) with the same scan settings for each sample was used to measure the fluorescence intensity of each oocyte. ImageJ 1.5 software (Bethesda, Maryland, USA) was used to analyze the normal fluorescence pixel intensities of each oocyte. The ratio of green to red fluorescence pixels was used to analyze mitochondrial membrane potential.

4.9. Statistical Analysis

Each treatment group had a minimum of 3 replicates, and the images of oocytes stained in the same dye were captured with the same scan settings. The average value of fluorescence intensity in each group of oocytes was analyzed after deduction of the background fluorescence through ImageJ software (National Institutes of Health, Bethesda, MD, USA). The obtained data were analyzed by the Statistical Package for Social Sciences (SPSS) software (version18.0) by using one-way analysis of variance (ANOVA). The treatment means were compared by the least significant difference (LSD) test at 1% and 5% probability levels. The p-value of <0.05 was considered a significant difference, while $p < 0.01$ was considered as highly significant, and $p < 0.001$ was considered as extremely significant.

5. Conclusions

Findings of the present study revealed that RV can effectively alleviate the adverse effects of oocyte aging by increasing the expression of antioxidant enzymes while decreasing the ROS level. Additionally, the RV treatment resisted against the decline in mitochondrial membrane potential in aged oocytes. Moreover, RV showed potent antiapoptotic effects by potentially upregulating the expression of Bcl-2 while downregulating the Bax and Caspase 3 transcript levels. Collectively, our findings lead to the evidence that RV may be one of the important constituents in improving the oocyte quality by delaying the antiaging effects through its antioxidant properties on porcine oocytes.

Author Contributions: Conceptualization, B.A. and Y.D.; Methodology, B.A.; Software, B.A.; Validation, B.A., Y.D. and R.R.; Formal analysis, B.A.; Investigation, B.A.; Resources, Y.D.; Data curation, B.A.; Writing—original draft preparation, B.A.; Writing—review and editing, Y.D. and R.R.; Visualization, Y.D.; Supervision, R.R.; Project administration, R.R.; Funding acquisition, R.R. All authors have read and agreed to the published version of the manuscript.

Funding: This study was supported by the Doctoral Program of the Ministry of Education of China (20130097110020) and the Priority Academic Program Development of Jiangsu higher education institutions (PAPD).

Institutional Review Board Statement: All the experiments and procedures compiled with the guideline and were approved by the local ethical committee of the Nanjing Agricultural University (Jiangsu Province, China) with respect to animal experimentation and care of animal under study.

Informed Consent Statement: Informed consent was not required for this experiment.

Data Availability Statement: The data that support the findings of this study are available on a reasonable request from the corresponding author.

Conflicts of Interest: The authors declare no conflict of interest.

Sample Availability: Samples of the compounds are not available from the authors.

References

1. Ma, W.; Zhang, D.; Hou, Y.; Li, Y.-H.; Sun, Q.-Y.; Sun, X.-F.; Wang, W.-H. Reduced Expression of MAD2, BCL2, and MAP Kinase Activity in Pig Oocytes after In Vitro Aging Are Associated with Defects in Sister Chromatid Segregation During Meiosis II and Embryo Fragmentation After Activation. *Biol. Reprod.* **2005**, *72*, 373–383. [CrossRef]
2. Mukherjee, A.; Malik, H.; Saha, A.P.; Dubey, A.; Singhal, D.K.; Boateng, S.; Saugandhika, S.; Kumar, S.; De, S.; Guha, S.K.; et al. Resveratrol treatment during goat oocytes maturation enhances developmental competence of parthenogenetic and hand-made

cloned blastocysts by modulating intracellular glutathione level and embryonic gene expression. *J. Assist. Reprod. Genet.* **2014**, *31*, 229–239. [CrossRef] [PubMed]
3. Saito, H.; Koike, K.; Saito, T.; Nohara, M.; Kawagoe, S.; Hiroi, M. Aging Changes in the Alignment of Chromosomes after Human Chorionic Gonadotropin Stimulation May Be a Possible Cause of Decreased Fertility in Mice. *Horm. Res.* **1993**, *39*, 28–31. [CrossRef] [PubMed]
4. Díaz, H.; Esponda, P. Ageing-induced changes in the cortical granules of mouse eggs. *Zygote* **2004**, *12*, 95–103. [CrossRef]
5. Goud, P.; Goud, A.; Laverge, H.; De Sutter, P.; Dhont, M. Effect of post-ovulatory age and calcium in the injection medium on the male pronucleus formation and metaphase entry following injection of human spermatozoa into golden hamster oocytes. *Mol. Hum. Reprod.* **1999**, *5*, 227–233. [CrossRef]
6. Díaz, H.; Esponda, P. Postovulatory ageing induces structural changes in the mouse zona pellucida. *J. Submicrosc. Cytol. Pathol.* **2004**, *36*, 211.
7. Kovacic, P.; Somanathan, R. Multifaceted Approach to Resveratrol Bioactivity: Focus on Antioxidant Action, Cell Signaling and Safety. *Oxid. Med. Cell. Longev.* **2010**, *3*, 86–100. [CrossRef] [PubMed]
8. Tarín, J.J.; Pérez-Albalá, S.; Aguilar, A.; Miñarro, J.; Hermenegildo, C.; Cano, A. Long-term effects of postovulatory aging of mouse oocytes on offspring: A two-generational study. *Biol. Reprod.* **1999**, *61*, 1347–1355. [CrossRef]
9. Lord, T.; Aitken, R.J. Oxidative stress and ageing of the post-ovulatory oocyte. *Reproduction* **2013**, *146*, R217–R227. [CrossRef]
10. Mailhes, J.B.; Young, D.; London, S.N. Postovulatory Ageing of Mouse Oocytes in Vivo and Premature Centromere Separation and Aneuploidy. *Biol. Reprod.* **1998**, *58*, 1206–1210. [CrossRef]
11. Dankert, D.; Demond, H.; Trapphoff, T.; Heiligentag, M.; Rademacher, K.; Eichenlaub-Ritter, U.; Horsthemke, B.; Grümmer, R. Pre- and Postovulatory Aging of Murine Oocytes Affect the Transcript Level and Poly(A) Tail Length of Maternal Effect Genes. *PLoS ONE* **2014**, *9*, e108907. [CrossRef]
12. Huang, J.-C.; Yan, L.-Y.; Lei, Z.-L.; Miao, Y.-L.; Shi, L.-H.; Yang, J.-W.; Wang, Q.; Ouyang, Y.-C.; Sun, Q.-Y.; Chen, D.-Y. Changes in Histone Acetylation During Postovulatory Aging of Mouse Oocyte. *Biol. Reprod.* **2007**, *77*, 666–670. [CrossRef]
13. Trapphoff, T.; Heiligentag, M.; Dankert, D.; Demond, H.; Deutsch, D.; Fröhlich, T.; Arnold, G.; Grümmer, R.; Horsthemke, B.; Eichenlaub-Ritter, U. Postovulatory aging affects dynamics of mRNA, expression and localization of maternal effect proteins, spindle integrity and pericentromeric proteins in mouse oocytes. *Hum. Reprod.* **2016**, *31*, 133–149. [CrossRef]
14. Wang, T.; Gao, Y.-Y.; Chen, L.; Nie, Z.-W.; Cheng, W.; Liu, X.; Schatten, H.; Zhang, X.; Miao, Y.-L. Melatonin prevents postovulatory oocyte aging and promotes subsequent embryonic development in the pig. *Aging* **2017**, *9*, 1552–1564. [CrossRef] [PubMed]
15. Arain, M.; Mei, Z.; Hassan, F.; Saeed, M.; Alagawany, M.; Shar, A.; Rajput, I. Lycopene: A natural antioxidant for prevention of heat-induced oxidative stress in poultry. *World's Poult. Sci. J.* **2018**, *74*, 89–100. [CrossRef]
16. Kim, W.-J.; Lee, S.-E.; Park, Y.-G.; Jeong, S.-G.; Kim, E.-Y.; Park, S.-P. Antioxidant hesperetin improves the quality of porcine oocytes during aging in vitro. *Mol. Reprod. Dev.* **2019**, *86*, 32–41. [CrossRef] [PubMed]
17. Inoue, M.; Sato, E.F.; Nishikawa, M.; Park, A.-M.; Kira, Y.; Imada, I.; Utsumi, K. Mitochondrial Generation of Reactive Oxygen Species and its Role in Aerobic Life. *Curr. Med. Chem.* **2003**, *10*, 2495–2505. [CrossRef] [PubMed]
18. Liu, Y.; Fiskum, G.; Schubert, D. Generation of reactive oxygen species by the mitochondrial electron transport chain. *J. Neurochem.* **2002**, *80*, 780–787. [CrossRef]
19. Dröge, W. Free Radicals in the Physiological Control of Cell Function. *Physiol. Rev.* **2002**, *82*, 47–95. [CrossRef]
20. Redza-Dutordoir, M.; Averill-Bates, D.A. Activation of apoptosis signalling pathways by reactive oxygen species. *Biochim. Biophys. Acta BBA Bioenerg.* **2016**, *1863*, 2977–2992. [CrossRef]
21. Liang, S.; Guo, J.; Choi, J.-W.; Shin, K.-T.; Wang, H.-Y.; Jo, Y.-J.; Kim, N.-H.; Cui, X.-S. Protein phosphatase 2A regulatory subunit B55α functions in mouse oocyte maturation and early embryonic development. *Oncotarget* **2017**, *8*, 26979–26991. [CrossRef] [PubMed]
22. Ramalho-Santos, J.; Varum, S.; Amaral, S.; Mota, P.C.; Sousa, A.P.; Amaral, A. Mitochondrial functionality in reproduction: From gonads and gametes to embryos and embryonic stem cells. *Hum. Reprod. Updat.* **2009**, *15*, 553–572. [CrossRef] [PubMed]
23. Babayev, E.; Wang, T.; Szigeti-Buck, K.; Lowther, K.; Taylor, H.S.; Horvath, T.; Seli, E. Reproductive aging is associated with changes in oocyte mitochondrial dynamics, function, and mtDNA quantity. *Maturitas* **2016**, *93*, 121–130. [CrossRef] [PubMed]
24. Wang, T.; Han, J.; Duan, X.; Xiong, B.; Cui, X.-S.; Kim, N.-H.; Liu, H.-L.; Sun, S.-C. The toxic effects and possible mechanisms of Bisphenol A on oocyte maturation of porcine in vitro. *Oncotarget* **2016**, *7*, 32554–32565. [CrossRef]
25. Zhang, D.; Ma, W.; Li, Y.-H.; Hou, Y.; Li, S.-W.; Meng, X.-Q.; Sun, X.-F.; Sun, Q.-Y.; Wang, W.-H. Intra-oocyte Localization of MAD2 and Its Relationship with Kinetochores, Microtubules, and Chromosomes in Rat Oocytes During Meiosis. *Biol. Reprod.* **2004**, *71*, 740–748. [CrossRef]
26. Suzuki, Y.; Imai, Y.; Nakayama, H.; Takahashi, K.; Takio, K.; Takahashi, R. A Serine Protease, HtrA2, Is Released from the Mitochondria and Interacts with XIAP, Inducing Cell Death. *Mol. Cell* **2001**, *8*, 613–621. [CrossRef]
27. Verhagen, A.M.; Ekert, P.; Pakusch, M.; Silke, J.; Connolly, L.M.; Reid, G.; Moritz, R.L.; Simpson, R.; Vaux, D.L. Identification of DIABLO, a Mammalian Protein that Promotes Apoptosis by Binding to and Antagonizing IAP Proteins. *Cell* **2000**, *102*, 43–53. [CrossRef]

28. Fico, A.; Manganelli, G.; Cigliano, L.; Bergamo, P.; Abrescia, P.; Franceschi, C.; Martini, G.; Filosa, S. 2-deoxy-d-ribose induces apoptosis by inhibiting the synthesis and increasing the efflux of glutathione. *Free Radic. Biol. Med.* **2008**, *45*, 211–217. [CrossRef]
29. Papaliagkas, V.; Anogianaki, A.; Anogianakis, G.; Ilonidis, G. The proteins and the mechanisms of apoptosis: A mini-review of the fundamentals. *Hippokratia* **2007**, *11*, 108–113.
30. Hoffmann, P.R.; Decathelineau, A.M.; Ogden, C.A.; Leverrier, Y.; Bratton, D.L.; Daleke, D.L.; Ridley, A.; Fadok, V.A.; Henson, P.M. Phosphatidylserine (PS) induces PS receptor–mediated macropinocytosis and promotes clearance of apoptotic cells. *J. Cell Biol.* **2001**, *155*, 649–660. [CrossRef]
31. Pervaiz, S.; Holme, A.L. Resveratrol: Its Biologic Targets and Functional Activity. *Antioxid. Redox Signal.* **2009**, *11*, 2851–2897. [CrossRef] [PubMed]
32. Jia, B.-Y.; Xiang, D.-C.; Shao, Q.-Y.; Zhang, B.; Liu, S.-N.; Hong, Q.-H.; Quan, G.-B.; Wu, G.-Q. Inhibitory effects of astaxanthin on postovulatory porcine oocyte aging in vitro. *Sci. Rep.* **2020**, *10*, 20217. [CrossRef] [PubMed]
33. Nutt, L.K.; Gogvadze, V.; Uthaisang, W.; Mirnikjoo, B.; McConkey, D.J.; Orrenius, S. Research paper indirect effects of Bax and Bak initiate the mitochondrial alterations that lead to cytochrome c release during arsenic trioxide-induced apoptosis. *Cancer Biol. Ther.* **2005**, *4*, 459–467. [CrossRef]
34. May-Panloup, P.; Boucret, L.; De La Barca, J.-M.C.; Desquiret-Dumas, V.; Ferré-L'Hotellier, V.; Morinière, C.; Descamps, P.; Procaccio, V.; Reynier, P. Ovarian ageing: The role of mitochondria in oocytes and follicles. *Hum. Reprod. Updat.* **2016**, *22*, 725–743. [CrossRef]
35. Kim, E.N.; Lim, J.H.; Kim, M.Y.; Ban, T.H.; Jang, I.-A.; Yoon, H.E.; Park, C.W.; Chang, Y.S.; Choi, B.S. Resveratrol, an Nrf2 activator, ameliorates aging-related progressive renal injury. *Aging* **2018**, *10*, 83–99. [CrossRef] [PubMed]
36. Kwak, S.-S.; Cheong, S.-A.; Jeon, Y.; Lee, E.; Choi, K.-C.; Jeung, E.-B.; Hyun, S.-H. The effects of resveratrol on porcine oocyte in vitro maturation and subsequent embryonic development after parthenogenetic activation and in vitro fertilization. *Theriogenology* **2012**, *78*, 86–101. [CrossRef] [PubMed]
37. Zuo, L.; Prather, E.R.; Stetskiv, M.; Garrison, D.E.; Meade, J.R.; Peace, T.I.; Zhou, T. Inflammaging and Oxidative Stress in Human Diseases: From Molecular Mechanisms to Novel Treatments. *Int. J. Mol. Sci.* **2019**, *20*, 4472. [CrossRef]
38. Yang, L.; Chen, Y.; Liu, Y.; Xing, Y.; Miao, C.; Zhao, Y.; Chang, X.; Zhang, Q. The Role of Oxidative Stress and Natural Antioxidants in Ovarian Aging. *Front. Pharmacol.* **2021**, *11*, 617843. [CrossRef]
39. Birben, E.; Sahiner, U.M.; Sackesen, C.; Erzurum, S.; Kalayci, O. Oxidative stress and antioxidant defense. *World Allergy Organ. J.* **2012**, *5*, 9–19. [CrossRef]
40. McCord, J.M. The evolution of free radicals and oxidative stress. *Am. J. Med.* **2000**, *108*, 652–659. [CrossRef]
41. Therond, P. Oxidative stress and damages to biomolecules (lipids, proteins, DNA). *Ann. Pharm. Fr.* **2006**, *64*, 383–389. [CrossRef]
42. Liang, Q.-X.; Lin, Y.-H.; Zhang, C.-H.; Sun, H.-M.; Zhou, L.; Schatten, H.; Sun, Q.-Y.; Qian, W.-P. Resveratrol increases resistance of mouse oocytes to postovulatory aging in vivo. *Aging* **2018**, *10*, 1586–1596. [CrossRef]
43. Jia, Z.; Zhu, H.; Misra, B.R.; Mahaney, J.E.; Li, Y.; Misra, H.P. EPR studies on the superoxide-scavenging capacity of the nutraceutical resveratrol. *Mol. Cell. Biochem.* **2008**, *313*, 187–194. [CrossRef] [PubMed]
44. De La Lastra, C.A.; Villegas, I. Resveratrol as an antioxidant and pro-oxidant agent: Mechanisms and clinical implications. *Biochem. Soc. Trans.* **2007**, *35*, 1156–1160. [CrossRef] [PubMed]
45. Park, J.-W.; Choi, Y.-J.; Suh, S.-I.; Baek, W.-K.; Suh, M.-H.; Jin, I.-N.; Min, D.S.; Woo, J.-H.; Chang, J.-S.; Passaniti, A.; et al. Bcl-2 overexpression attenuates resveratrol-induced apoptosis in U937 cells by inhibition of caspase-3 activity. *Carcinogenesis* **2001**, *22*, 1633–1639. [CrossRef]
46. Wenzel, E.; Soldo, T.; Erbersdobler, H.; Somoza, V. Bioactivity and metabolism of trans-resveratrol orally administered to Wistar rats. *Mol. Nutr. Food Res.* **2005**, *49*, 482–494. [CrossRef]
47. Wu, J.Q.; Kosten, T.R.; Zhang, X.Y. Free radicals, antioxidant defense systems, and schizophrenia. *Prog. Neuro Psychopharmacol. Biol. Psychiatry* **2013**, *46*, 200–206. [CrossRef]
48. Meng, Q.; Guo, T.; Li, G.; Sun, S.; He, S.; Cheng, B.; Shi, B.; Shan, A. Dietary resveratrol improves antioxidant status of sows and piglets and regulates antioxidant gene expression in placenta by Keap1-Nrf2 pathway and Sirt1. *J. Anim. Sci. Biotechnol.* **2018**, *9*, 34. [CrossRef]
49. Wu, C.-C.; Huang, Y.-S.; Chen, J.-S.; Huang, C.-F.; Su, S.-L.; Lu, K.-C.; Lin, Y.-F.; Chu, P.; Lin, S.-H.; Sytwu, H.-K. Resveratrol Ameliorates Renal Damage, Increases Expression of Heme Oxygenase-1, and Has Anti-Complement, Anti-Oxidative, and Anti-Apoptotic Effects in a Murine Model of Membranous Nephropathy. *PLoS ONE* **2015**, *10*, e0125726. [CrossRef]
50. Movahed, A.; Yu, L.; Thandapilly, S.J.; Louis, X.; Netticadan, T. Resveratrol protects adult cardiomyocytes against oxidative stress mediated cell injury. *Arch. Biochem. Biophys.* **2012**, *527*, 74–80. [CrossRef] [PubMed]
51. Soeur, J.; Eilstein, J.; Léreaux, G.; Jones, C.; Marrot, L. Skin resistance to oxidative stress induced by resveratrol: From Nrf2 activation to GSH biosynthesis. *Free Radic. Biol. Med.* **2015**, *78*, 213–223. [CrossRef] [PubMed]
52. Lodovici, M.; Bigagli, E.; Luceri, C.; Manni, E.; Zaid, M. Protective Effect of Resveratrol against Oxidation Stress Induced by 2-Nitropropane in Rat Liver. *Pharmacol. Pharm.* **2011**, *2*, 127–135. [CrossRef]
53. Gebauer, F.; Xu, W.; Cooper, G.; Richter, J. Translational control by cytoplasmic polyadenylation of c-mos mRNA is necessary for oocyte maturation in the mouse. *EMBO J.* **1994**, *13*, 5712–5720. [CrossRef] [PubMed]

54. Yew, N.; Mellini, M.L.; Martinez, C.K.; Woude, G.F.V. Meiotic initiation by the mos protein in Xenopus. *Nature* **1992**, *355*, 649–652. [CrossRef]
55. Pascuali, N.; Scotti, L.; Abramovich, D.; Irusta, G.; Di Pietro, M.; Bas, D.; Tesone, M.; Parborell, F. Inhibition of platelet-derived growth factor (PDGF) receptor affects follicular development and ovarian proliferation, apoptosis and angiogenesis in prepubertal eCG-treated rats. *Mol. Cell. Endocrinol.* **2015**, *412*, 148–158. [CrossRef]
56. Tong, Z.; Xie, Y.; He, M.; Ma, W.; Zhou, Y.; Lai, S.; Meng, Y.; Liao, Z. VDAC1 deacetylation is involved in the protective effects of resveratrol against mitochondria-mediated apoptosis in cardiomyocytes subjected to anoxia/reoxygenation injury. *Biomed. Pharmacother.* **2017**, *95*, 77–83. [CrossRef] [PubMed]
57. Brunelle, J.K.; Letai, A. Control of mitochondrial apoptosis by the Bcl-2 family. *J. Cell Sci.* **2009**, *122*, 437–441. [CrossRef]
58. Shi, F.; Li, W.; Zhao, H.; He, Y.; Jiang, Y.; Ni, J.; Abbasi, B.; Rui, R.; Ju, S. Microcystin-LR exposure results in aberrant spindles and induces apoptosis in porcine oocytes. *Theriogenology* **2020**, *158*, 358–367. [CrossRef]

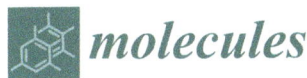

Article

Red Wine Extract Inhibits VEGF Secretion and Its Signaling Pathway in Retinal ARPE-19 Cells to Potentially Disrupt AMD

Clarisse Cornebise [1,2,†], Flavie Courtaut [1,2,†], Marie Taillandier-Coindard [1,2], Josep Valls-Fonayet [3], Tristan Richard [3], David Monchaud [1,4], Virginie Aires [1,2] and Dominique Delmas [1,2,5,*]

1. Université de Bourgogne Franche-Comté, F-21000 Dijon, France; clarisse.cornebise@gmail.com (C.C.); flavie.courtaut@gmail.com (F.C.); marie.taillandiercoindard@gmail.com (M.T.-C.); david.monchaud@u-bourgogne.fr (D.M.); virginie.aires02@u-bourgogne.fr (V.A.)
2. INSERM Research Center U1231—Cancer and Adaptive Immune Response Team, Bioactive Molecules and Health Research Group, F-21000 Dijon, France
3. Unité de Recherche Oenologie, EA 4577, USC 1366 INRA-ISVV, F-33882 Villenave d'Ornon, France; Josep.Valls-Fonayet@U-Bordeaux.Fr (J.V.-F.); tristan.richard@u-bordeaux.fr (T.R.)
4. Institut de Chimie Moléculaire (ICMUB), CNRS UMR6302, UBFC, F-21078 Dijon, France
5. Centre Anticancéreux Georges François Leclerc, F-21000 Dijon, France
* Correspondence: dominique.delmas@u-bourgogne.fr; Tel.: +33-380-39-32-26
† These authors contributed equally to this work.

Academic Editors: Paula Silva and Norbert Latruffe
Received: 5 November 2020; Accepted: 25 November 2020; Published: 27 November 2020

Abstract: Age-related macular degeneration (AMD) is a degenerative disease of the retina where the molecular mechanism involves the production of vascular endothelial growth factor (VEGF), a factor of poor prognosis of the progression of the disease. Previous studies have shown that resveratrol, a polyphenol of grapevines, can prevent VEGF secretion induced by stress from retinal cells. Considering the fundamental role played by VEGF in development and progression of AMD, we investigate the potential effect of red wine extract (RWE) on VEGF secretion and its signaling pathway in human retinal cells ARPE-19. To examine the effect of RWE in ARPE-19, a quantitative and qualitative analysis of the RWE was performed by HPLC MS/MS. We show for the first time that RWE decreased VEGF-A secretion from ARPE-19 cells and its protein expression in concentration-dependent manner. RWE-induced alteration in VEGF-A production is associated with a down of VEGF-receptor 2 (VEGF-R2) protein expression and its phosphorylated intracytoplasmic domain. Subsequently, the activation of kinase pathway is disturbing and RWE prevents the phosphorylation of MEK and ERK 1/2 in human retinal cells ARPE-19. Finally, this study sheds light on the interest that the use of polyphenolic cocktails could represent in a prevention strategy.

Keywords: polyphenols; red wine extract; AMD; retinal cells; ARPE-19; degenerative diseases; ocular diseases

---

1. Introduction

Since the last decade, several epidemiological studies have shown an inverse relation between the incidence of coronary diseases and wine consumption, compared to wine abstinence [1,2]. In France, despite of a fat-containing diet, the incidence of coronary heat diseases is lower than other western countries with a similar diet, which is partly attributed to the moderation consumption of red wine [3]. This apparent discrepancy is called the "French paradox". However, since the 1990s, some studies have shown that this "French paradox" is more likely resulting from a Mediterranean-type diet [4,5].

In this context, we have previously shown in a controlled environment in hospital that a moderate consumption of red wine (250 mL/day), even for a short period (2 weeks), associated with a "Western prudent" diet, improves various blood parameters in the lipid and antioxidative status in patients with previous coronary ischemic accidents in comparison to patients receiving water [6]. This "Western prudent" diet has also been proposed to prevent other pathologies such as degenerative diseases or diseases linked to oxidative stress or even cancer. Very recently, we were able to demonstrate that a red wine extract (RWE) made it possible to act on inflammation by reducing the level of certain proinflammatory cytokines produced by immune cells [7] but also by reducing the formation of an inflammatory complex in macrophages such as NLRP3 (NOD-like receptor family, pyrin domain containing 3) [8], or to reduce intestine polyp preneoplasia development in mice [9]. These effects have been confirmed in other studies, where RWE can reduce tumoral C26 growth in BALB/c mice and vascular endothelial growth factor (VEGF) [10]. The latter factor is not only important for the neoangiogenesis, which is necessary for tumor growth and the spread of metastatic cells, but it is also involved in other disease processes such as age-related macular degeneration (AMD).

Indeed, AMD is a degenerative disease of the retina characterized by progressive loss of central vision. This disease selectively affects the macula, which is the central region of the retina, which explains why only the central vision is affected, and not the peripheral vision. The formation of new blood vessels through the membrane destroys the cells lining the back of the retina. These cells serve as an anchor for the cones and rods, which allow vision, their destruction leads to a localized and permanent loss of this vision. Thus the overexpression of this vascular factor is a factor of poor prognosis of the progression of the disease and many strategies are put in place to counter the production of VEGF in particular the use of anti-VEGF antibodies. Alongside these pharmacological strategies for which resistance sometimes appears, numerous studies have been able to show the influence of nutrition on the occurrence of this type of pathology and its evolution [11,12]. Among natural compounds, polyphenols could present interest to counteract AMD. Indeed, some studies have performed in order to prove the effect of several preparations enriched with polyphenol grape extract or wine polyphenols on age-related degenerative diseases [13] and ocular diseases [14–16]. More specifically, we have shown that resveratrol, a polyphenol of grapevines, prevented VEGF secretion induced by oxysterols from human retinal cells [15]. However, what about a more polyphenolic complex mixture such as red wine, which contains a wide variety of polyphenols? Considering the fundamental role played by VEGF in development and progression of AMD, we investigated the potential effect of a red wine extract (RWE) on VEGF-A secretion in human retinal cells ARPE-19 having an AMD phenotype. The main goal is to determine whether RWE could decrease VEGF-A secretion and alter this signaling pathway and thus influence the progression of AMD. We show here for the first time that RWE inhibits VEGF-A secretion in a dose-dependent manner in human retinal cells. This reduction is associated with a decrease in VEGF-A protein expression. Very interestingly, RWE affects the signaling pathway leading VEGF production, particularly, RWE decreases activation of the receptor to VEGF-A, VEGF-R2 and the associated-protein kinases such as the mitogen-activated protein kinase (MEK) and extracellular regulated kinase 1/2 (ERK 1/2).

2. Results

2.1. Qualitative and Quantitative Analysis of RWE and Its Toxicity on ARPE-19 Retinal Cells

The wine vinification processes can affect, by many factors, the wine. Indeed, the climate, the vine, the country and the year can alter the quantity and the quality of polyphenols in wine, which also varies between white and red wines. Red wine present a higher quantity of polyphenols estimated to be around 900–2500 mg/L in contrary to white wine composition estimated to be around 190–290 mg/L. As we previously demonstrated in a previous study, the quantitative and qualitative wine composition of bioactive molecules such as polyphenolic compounds is essential in the biological effects that can be observed whether there are antagonistic or synergistic [9]. The Figure 1 summarizes the extraction of red wine (Santenay 1er cru Les Gravières 2012 (Côte d'Or, France), to obtain a power of red wine namely red wine extract (RWE), which was diluted in 70% ethanol at a rate of 100 mg/mL.

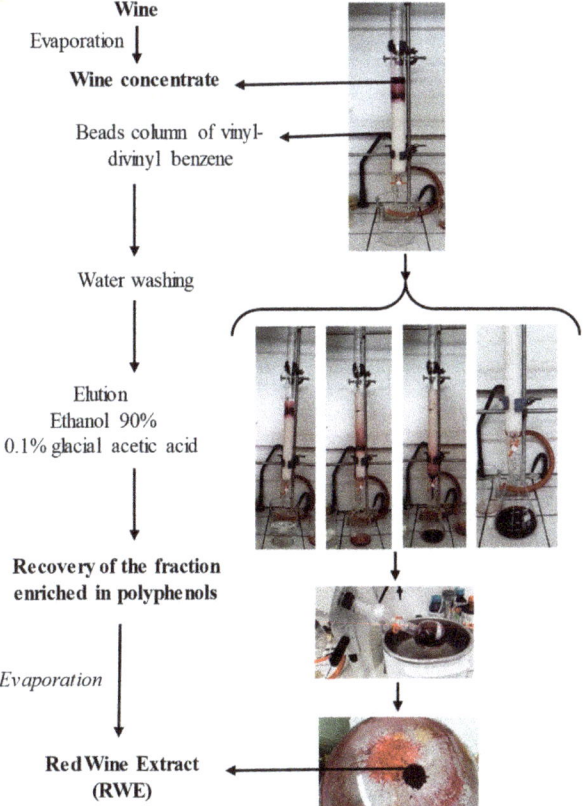

Figure 1. A preparative column was used to adsorb phenolic compounds present in red wine, and after alcohol evaporation, the concentrated residue was lyophilized to be finally sprayed in order to obtain the phenolic extract dry powder.

A qualitative and quantitative analysis performed by HPLC of the RWE was carried out in order to determine its polyphenolic content. As illustrated in Figure 2, we obtained different spectra allowing identifying with MRM transitions and by UV (λ = 520 nm) the main compounds contained in the extract by differentiating the main phenolic non-anthocyanin compounds (Figure 2a) and the main anthocyanins (Figure 2b).

The qualitative and quantitative determination of polyphenolic compounds in RWE is crucial to evaluate its biological activities since we have previously demonstrated that composition of bioactive compounds of the wine could impact its antiproliferative and anti-inflammatory activities [7,8]. In fact, we have shown that an association of resveratrol and quercetin can have a synergetic effect against the proliferation of colon cancer cells, which is not the case for other combinations such as resveratrol/catechin or resveratrol/catechin/quercetin [9]. The evaluation of the polyphenolic content revealed an important proportion of phenolic acids and flavan-3-ols. Indeed, we identified 49% of phenolic acids (gallic acid, caftaric acid and caffeic acid) and 36% of flavan 3-ols (catechin, epicatechin, procyanidins B1, B2, B3 and B4) of the total content (Figure 3). To this is added in a smaller but not insignificant quantity, 9% of anthocyanins (delphinidin 3-glucoside, cyanidin 3-glucoside, petunidin 3-glucoside, peonidin 3-glucoside and malvidin 3-glucoside); 2% of flavonols (quercetin, quercetin-3-glucoside and quercetin-3-rhamnoside) and 4% of stilbenes (*cis*- and *trans*-resveratrol, emphcis- and *trans*-piceid, *trans*-piceatannol, ε-viniferin, Ω-viniferin, pallidol and isohopeaphenol).

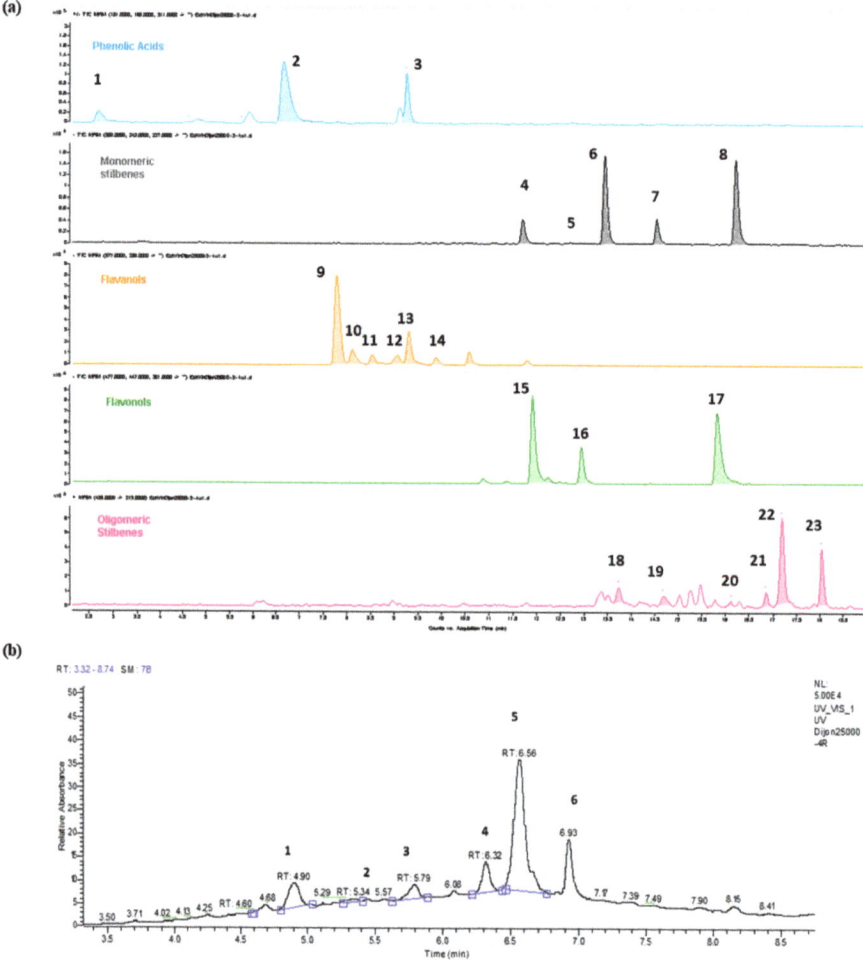

Figure 2. (a) Extracted ion chromatogram of the MRM transitions belonging to the main phenolic non-anthocyanin compounds detected in the wine extract. 1 = Gallic Acid; 2 = Caftaric Acid; 3 = Caffeic Acid; 4 = *t*-Piceid; 5 = *t*-Piceatannol; 6 = *c*-Piceid; 7 = *t*-Resveratrol; 8 = *c*-Resveratrol; 9 = Procyanidin B1; 10 = Procyanidin B3; 11 = Catechin; 12 = Procyanidin B4; 13 = Procyanidin B2; 14 = Epicatechin; 15 = Quercetin-3-glucuronide; 16 = Quercetin-3-rhamnoside; 17 = Quercetin; 18 = Pallidol; 19 = Parthenocisin A; 20 = Isohopeaphenol; 21 = *c*-E-viniferin; 22 = *t*-E-viniferin, 23 = *t*-w-viniferin. (b) UV520 Chromatogram of the main anthocyanins detected in the red wine extract. 1 = Delphinidin 3-glucoside; 2 = Cyanidin 3-glucoside; 3= Petunidin 3-glucoside; 4= Peonidin 3-glucoside; 5= Malvidin 3-glucoside; 6 = Malvidin acylated derivative.

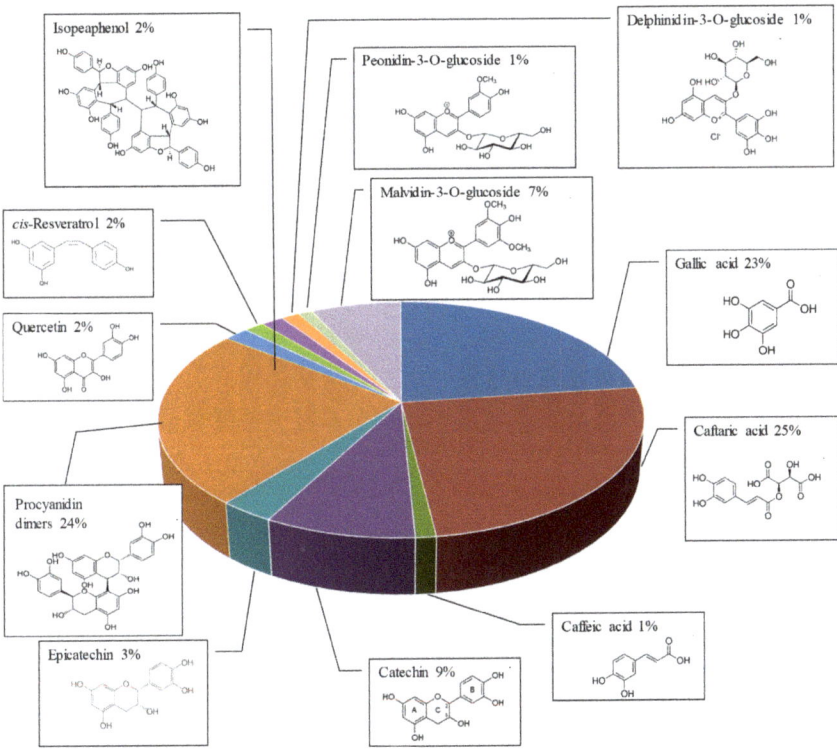

Figure 3. Quantitative analysis of red wine extract content and chemical structures of the main polyphenolic compounds.

To specify the potential role of RWE in AMD and more particularly against VEGF, we first evaluated its toxicity on undifferentiated ARPE-19 retinal cells mimicking cells affected by AMD [17]. As revealed by cytotoxic curves that whatever the time of treatment, 24 and 48 h, RWE had no significant impact on the cellular viability of human retinal cells ARPE-19 with a game of increasing concentrations of RWE to 0 up to 250 µg/mL (Figure 4a). In the same manner, resveratrol (RSV) used in our experiment as a reference compound, presented no significant toxicity at the time of treatment and concentrations used (Figure 4b). In the following experiments, RWE was therefore used at three concentrations namely 30, 50 and 100 µg/mL in ARPE-19 cell lines. These concentrations were chosen both because they are noncytotoxic on retinal cells and because we have previously shown with these same concentrations that RWE was able to present significative properties (i.e., inhibition of proinflammatory cytokines production from macrophages [8], prevention of naïve T lymphocytes differentiation into proinflammatory T helper 17 cells [7] and inhibition of polyps development [9]). Furthermore, the secretion of VEGF by retinal cells being a rapid process with an early response of the kinase cascade activation, we explored the effect of RWE after 24 h of treatment of APRE-19 cells. In this experiment, RSV was used as a comparison at a concentration of 30 µM, which is non cytotoxic on the cell line ARPE-19. Indeed, we have previously shown a protective effect of RSV against toxic effects of oxysterols in retinal cells after 24 h and 48 h of treatment [15].

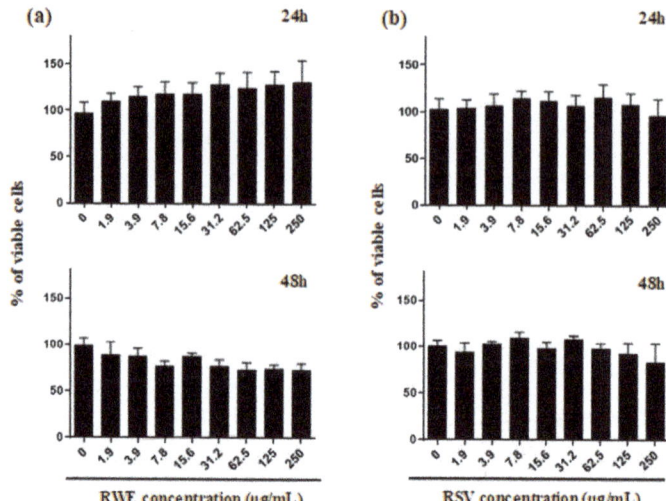

Figure 4. Safety assessment of red wine extract (RWE) and RSV on human retinal cell line ARPE-19. Crystal violet staining was performed in order to analyzed the cell viability of ARPE-19 after 24, 48 and 72 h of the (**a**) RWE treatment (starting concentration up to 250 µg/mL, 1:2 serial dilutions) and (**b**) RSV (starting concentration up to 250 µg/mL, 1:2 serial dilutions). Data are expressed as mean percentages ± s.d. of three independent experiments.

2.2. RWE Prevents VEGF Secretion from ARPE-19 Cells and Its Protein Expression

Since VEGF is the main factor involved in the neoangiogenesis and the progression of AMD, we firstly determined whether RWE was able to affect its expression. Immunoblotting analysis shown that after 24 h of treatment, RWE strongly decreased VEGF protein expression in ARPE-19 cells in a concentration-dependent manner as compared to the control (Figure 5a). Interestingly, RWE at 50 µg/mL presented the same inhibitory effect of VEGF expression as RSV at 30 µM, and a more effect at 100 µg/mL (Figure 5a). These results suggested that polyphenolic compounds present into RWE at lower concentrations act in a synergistic manner to decrease VEGF expression. This is in agreement with what we previously found regarding the effect of RWE in other models such as macrophages or immune cells [7,8]. This decrease in VEGF protein expression by RWE should normally be accompanied by a decrease in VEGF secretion by retinal cells. In order to verify this hypothesis, we quantified using an ELISA method, the levels of VEGF released into the culture medium. As assumed, 24 h of treatment, RWE decreased the levels of VEGF in a very significant manner for the concentrations of 50 and 100 µg/mL (Figure 5b). Surprisingly, the RSV at the concentrations of 30 µM after 24 h of treatment failed to decrease the production of VEGF in retinal cells.

2.3. RWE Prevents VEGF-A Secretion from ARPE-19 Cells and Its Protein Expression

Secretion of VEGF-A by retinal cells results from the activation of the signaling pathway involving VEGF-specific tyrosine kinase receptors whose activation loop results from a phosphorylation cascade through the induction of successive kinases [18]. Indeed, the binding of VEGF-A occurs mainly on the VEGF-R2 receptor, which induces its phosphorylation and the intracytoplasmic signaling cascade, passing through the phosphorylation of the mitogen-activated protein kinase kinase (MEK) protein, and with the ultimate activation of the phosphorylation of the extracellular regulated kinase 1/2 (ERK 1/2) protein. The latter once phosphorylated could then activate various nuclear transcription factors making it possible to activate the gene coding for VEGF. We observed by immunoblotting that RWE since low concentration at 30 µg/mL was able to strongly inhibit VEGF-R2 protein expression and its phosphorylated form (Figure 6). This disruption in VGEF-R2 activation through its intracytoplasmic phosphorylation leads to a decrease of activation of the MEK and ER $\frac{1}{2}$ pathway. As shown by the immunoblotting 24 h of treatment with RWE decreased significantly the phosphorylation of MEK and ERK 1/2 in ARPE-19 cells (Figure 6). Although RSV decreased significantly the expression of VEGF-R2, the polyphenol failed to prevent the phosphorylation of VEGF-R2 and subsequently then allowed the phosphorylation cascade to take place.

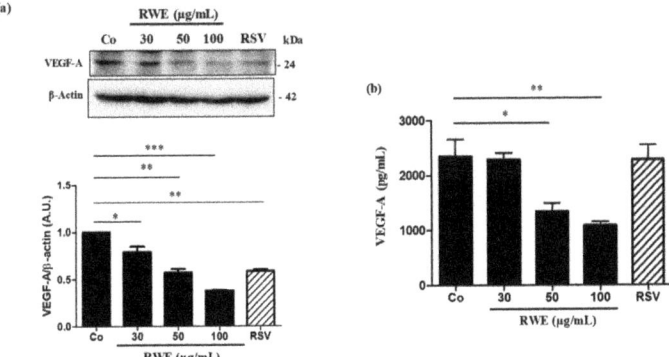

Figure 5. RWE decreases VEGF-A protein expression and its secretion from ARPE-19 cells. (**a**) Upper panel: representative immunoblot of VEGF6A protein expression from three independent experiments in human retinal ARPE-19 cells after 24 h of treatment without (Co) or with 30, 50 and 100 µg/mL of RWE or with RSV 20 µM. β-actin was used as a loading control. Down panel: densitometry quantification of Western blotting. Data are expressed as the mean folds' induction ± SEM of three independent experiments. p values were determined by a one-way ANOVA followed by Tukey's multiple comparison test. * $p < 0.05$, ** $p < 0.01$ and *** $p < 0.001$. (**b**) As in (a) VEGF-A secretion was measured in the cell medium by ELISA. The data are the mean ± S.D. of four independent experiments with $n = 10$. p values were determined by a one-way ANOVA followed by Tukey's multiple comparison test. * = $p < 0.05$; ** = $p < 0.01$; *** = $p < 0.001$.

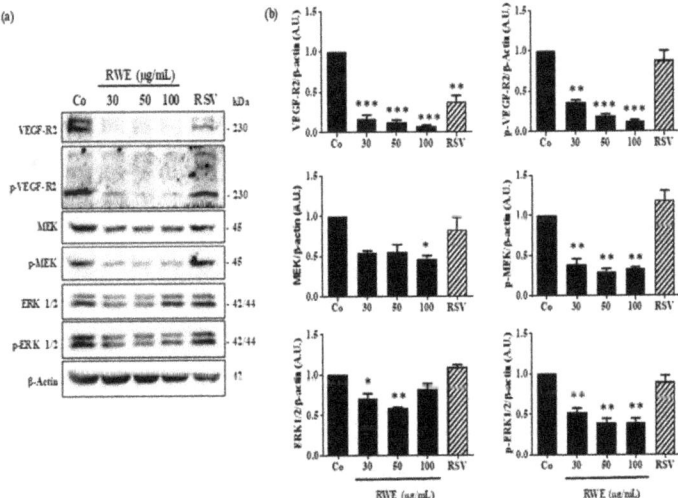

Figure 6. RWE disrupts VEGF-R2 kinase activation pathways. (**a**) Immunoblotting analysis of VEGF-R2, phospho VEGF-R2 (p-VEGF-R2), MEK, phospho MEK (p-MEK), ERK 1/2 and phospho-ERK 1/2 (p ERK 1/2)

in RWE-treated ARPE-19 cells with increasing concentration (30, 50 and 100 µg/mL) or with RSV (20 µM) for 24 h. β-actin was used as a loading control. (**b**) Densitometry quantification of Western blotting. Data are expressed as the mean folds induction ± SEM of three independent experiments. *p* values were determined by a one-way ANOVA followed by Tukey's multiple comparison test. * $p < 0.05$, ** $p < 0.01$ and *** $p < 0.001$.

3. Discussion

AMD is a multifactorial degenerative pathology, which results from the conjunction of several risk factors. The most important of these is age, with a sharp increase after the sixth decade, but there are also genetic, ethnic or environmental factors. Indeed, smoking, obesity and diet are linked to this disease [19]. Studies have shown that in developed countries, AMD is the leading cause of visual impairment and blindness affecting people over 65 years [20]. The molecular mechanism of AMD involved a growth factor, namely VEGF-A, for which the secretion induces the appearance of new immature and poor quality blood vessels that invade the different histological layers that make up the retina. This results in the destruction of the thin membrane separating the retina from the bloodstream [21]. This invasion combined with the fact that these vessels, of poor quality, allow serum to diffuse causes a progressive loss of vision by the destruction of the underlying cells. It therefore appears essential to control the secretion of VEGF in order to limit the phenomenon of neoangiogenesis and thus limits the disappearance of retinal cells. To overcome this VEGF-A secretion by retinal cells affected by AMD, there is a growing research interest to develop various antibodies against VEGF-A [22], but this strategy failed in one form of AMD, the dry form for which there is no treatment at present apart from recommendations in particular in terms of nutrition or supplementation [23]. Moreover, some resistance to anti-VEGF-A antibodies is highlighted in patients with an exudative form [24]. Thus some studies have tried to demonstrate the action of nutrition or supplementation against VEGF-A secretion from retinal cells such as oral nutritional supplementation in patients with intermediate or advanced AMD, where the risk of vision loss of three or more line was reduced by 19% with this supplementation [11]. In this way, we tested the ability of a polyphenol-enriched extract (RWE) from a red wine to act on the VEGF-A pathway in human retinal cells, which is an AMD phenotype. The present study highlights that RWE was able to prevent secretion of VEGF-A from ARPE-19 cells in a dose-dependent manner, which is associated with a decrease of VEGF-A protein expression. Usually, its activity is linked to its binding to the surface of tyrosine kinase receptors (VEGF-R or vascular endothelial growth factor receptor). The binding is done on the extracellular part of the transmembrane receptors. There are three isoforms of receptors that bind VEGFs with different affinities: VEGF-R1, VEGF-R2 and VEGF-R3. Each of them activates different signaling channels resulting in different effects. It has thus been possible to demonstrate the role of VEGF-R1 and VEGF-R2 in the process of angiogenesis, while that of VEGF-R3 is more linked to lymphangiogenesis [25]. More generally, VEGF-A binds to VEGF-R1 and VEGF-R2. These have 44% homology in their sequence, but their affinity for their ligand differs, and they induce different cellular and biological effects. The receptor with the strongest affinity for VEGF-A is VEGF-R1, but the receptor predominantly present on the surface of epithelial cells is VEGF-R2, so it is the latter that appears to be the main mediator of angiogenic activity. In addition, VEGF-R1 has been shown to have lower activity due to the presence of an inhibitory sequence, the absence of which in VEGF-R2 leads to an improvement in tyrosine kinase activity. VEGF binding to its receptor leads to phosphorylation of its intracytoplasmic domain for engaging the mitogen-activated protein kinase (MAP kinase) activation cascade including MEK and ERK (Figure 7).

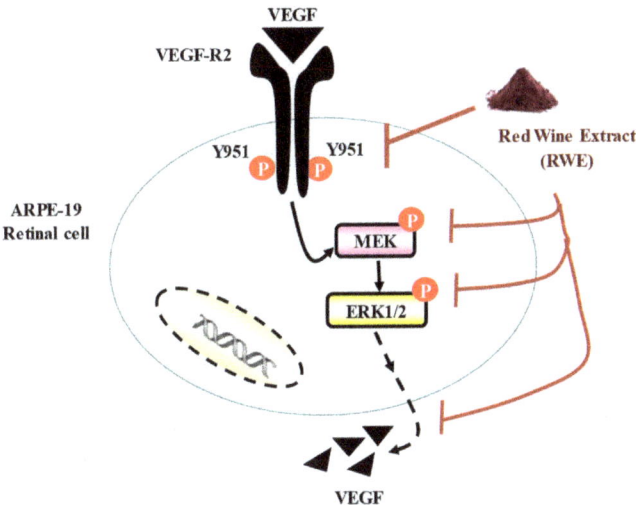

Figure 7. RWE prevents VEGF production by disruption of VEGF-R2 activation. RWE decreases the phosphorylation of VEGF-R2 (P-VEGF-R2) and subsequently prevents the phosphorylation of MEK (P-MEK) and ERK 1/2 (P-ERK 1/2) in human retinal cells ARPE-19.

We show in the present report that RWE was able to alter the phosphorylation of intracytoplasmic domain of VEGF-R2 leading a disrupting in kinase pathway (Figure 7). By disrupting the phosphorylation of MEK and ERK in retinal cells, RWE could alter the pathway inducing the VEGF production.

It is very surprising that the polyphenol RSV alone was not able to prevent this pathway at 20 µM. This absence of effect on VEGF secretion by retinal cells was with a lack of effect on the MAPK activation pathway. This could be explained by the fact that RWE contains many polyphenolic compounds that, even at very low concentrations, could act in synergy in order to exert an action against the activation of the VEGF-R2 pathway. Analysis of polyphenolic composition revealed a high content of phenolic acid (49%) and flavan 3-ols (36%). These compounds were particularly important since separately they were shown to exert an action on VEGF-A production. For example, among phenolic acids, gallic acid exerted an antiangiogenic effect in ovarian cancer cells [26] or in vascular smooth muscle cells [27], and caffeic acid reduces the VEGF secretion in human retinal pigment epithelial cells under hypoxic conditions [28]. Similarly, delphinidin has been shown to inhibit angiogenesis through the suppression of VEGF expression in lung cancer cells [29]. The presence of quercetin could explain a potential mechanism of synergism. Indeed, resveratrol + quercetin association increases resveratrol uptake by colon carcinoma cells, and in combination with RWE this combination increases the influx of resveratrol [9,30,31]. In a similar manner, the presence of quercetin in RWE could increase the uptake of some polyphenols and favors the synergism between the bioactive compounds to potentiate their action against neoangiogenesis in AMD.

4. Materials and Methods

4.1. Cell Lines and Cell Culture

The human retinal pigmented epithelial cell line ARPE-19, purchased from the American Type Culture Collection (Manassas, VA, USA), were maintained in Dulbecco's modified Eagle's F12 medium (DMEM/F12) supplemented with 10% fetal bovine serum (Dutscher, Brumath, France), 1% penicillin/streptomycin in a humidified atmosphere of 5% CO_2 at 37 °C. Cells were seeded and grown to a subconfluence of 60–70% in normoxia. Twenty four hours after seeding, the medium was removed and the cells were washed once with Hank's Balanced Salt Solution (HBSS, Dutscher, Brumath, France) before reincubating in DMEMF12 with 1% FBS and 1% penicillin/streptomycin. The following day, cells were treated with DMSO, RWE with indicated concentrations or resveratrol 20 µM.

4.2. Chemical Reagents and Antibodies

Resveratrol (RSV) was purchased from Sigma-Aldrich (St. Quentin Fallavier, France) and dissolved in ethanol 70%. VEGFR2 (sc-2479, 1:1000); p-VEGFR2 TYR951 (sc-4991, 1:1000); ERK1/2 (sc-4695, 1:1000); p-ERK1/2 (sc-9101, 1:1000); MEK1/2 (sc-91226, 1:1000) and p-MEK1/2 (Ser221; sc-2338, 1:1000) were obtained from Santa Cruz Biotechnology (Nanterre, France) and p-VEGFR2 (TYR 1054; 267,398, 1:1000) was obtained from EMD Millipore Corporation. B-Actin (A1978, 1:5000) was obtained from Abcam. (Paris, France). (+)-Catechin (>99%), (−)-epicatechin (>99%), procyanidin B1 (>90%), procyanidin B2 (>90%) and quercetin as a dihydrate (>99%) were obtained from Extrasynthese (Genay, France). Gallic acid (>97.5%) and caffeic acid (>98%) were obtained from Sigma-Aldrich (St Quentin Favrallier, France). Caftaric acid (>98%) was purchased from Carl Roth (Karslruhe, Germany). E-resveratrol, hopeaphenol and malvidin 3-glucoside were purified as standards in the MIB laboratory using a Varian Pro Star preparative HPLC. Purity was assessed to be over 90% by HPLC.

4.3. Preparation of the Red Wine Extract

The red wine extract (RWE) was obtained from French red wine, Santenay 1er cru Les Gravières 2012 (EARL Capuano-Ferreri Santenay, Côte-d'Or, France) selected by BIVB (Bureau Interprofessionnel des Vins de Bourgogne, Beaune, France) and provided by CTIVV (Centre Technique Interprofessionnel de la Vigne et du Vin, Beaune, France). Red wine extract dry powder was prepared and analyzed as previously described [7,8]. Briefly, the phenolic compounds contained in the wine were separated from the liquid using an absorption column and solubilized in alcohol. After evaporation of the alcoholic eluent using a rotary evaporator, the concentrated residue was deposited on the column (Diainon® HP-20, Supelco, Germany). For the retention phase, the column reservoir was filled with distilled water, and the flow rate was adjusted to approximately 20 drops/min. Then the polyphenol fraction retained was eluted using a solution of ethanol and 0.1% glacial citric acid, and the flow rate was adjusted to about 40 drops/min. The fractions collected after elution were concentrated to dryness with a rotary evaporator. In this way, we obtained, from 1 L of red wine, 104 g of phenolic extract in powder form, containing 5.04 mg g^{-1} of total phenolic compounds expressed as the gallic acid equivalent.

4.4. High-Performance Liquid Chromatography Analysis

Triplicates of 5 mg freeze-dried extract was dissolved with 200 µL of a mixture water:methanol (1:1) and centrifuged for 5 min at 10,000× g before anthocyanins and polyphenols analysis. Anthocyanins were analyzed with a Thermo Scientific Vanquish UHPLC equipped with a Thermo Scientific MWL detector operating at 520 nm. Of the sample 1 µL was injected in Agilent Zorbax SB-C18 (100 mm × 2.1 mm × 1.8 µm) column at 35° using the following conditions of separation: solvent A (5% formic acid in MilliQ water) and solvent B (5% formic acid in acetonitrile); flow: 0.35 mL/mi and gradient: 2.5% B (0–1 min), 17% B (5–7 min), 45% B (10–11 min), 95% B (11–12.5 min) and 2.5% B (13–15 min). A calibration curve in the range of 6.25–80 mg/L was built with malvidin 3-glucoside previously purified in our laboratory. The 5 quantified anthocyanins (delphinidin 3-glucoside, cyanidin 3-glucoside, petunidin 3-glucoside, peonidin 3-glucoside and malvidin 3-glucoside) were quantified as malvidin 3-glucoside. The rest of the polyphenols was analyzed by HPLC–MS/MS methodology previously published [32] with slight modifications. The compounds were separated with an Agilent 1260 HPLC instrument. Of samples 4 µL were eluted on an Agilent Zorbax SB-C18 (100 mm × 2.1 mm × 1.8 µm) column at 40 °C with a binary solvent system of solvent A (0.1% formic acid in water) and solvent B (0.1% formic acid in acetonitrile). The chromatographic separation was conducted with a flow rate of 0.4 mL/min and the following gradient: 10–18% B (0–1 min), 18–33% B (1–6.5 min), 33% B (6.5–9.5 min), 33–40% B (9.5–15 min), 40–90% B (15–16 min), 90% B (16–19 min) and 90–10% B (19–20 min). The HPLC was coupled to an Agilent 6430 Triple Quadrupole mass spectrometer, which operated under the following parameters: alternate positive/negative mode; drying gas (nitrogen), 11 L/min; nebulizer pressure, 15 psi; temperature, 350 °C and capillary voltage, 3000 V. Specific MRM transitions were used for the detection and quantification of each compound. Calibration curves were established with pure standards in the range of 0.03–15.00 mg/L except for catechin, gallic acid and caftaric acid (range 0.03–100 mg/L). All compounds were quantified as their corresponding standard except flavan 3-ol dimers B3 and B4, which were expressed as dimer B1 and B2 respectively, and isomers c-resveratrol and c-piceid, which were determined as their respective t-isomer.

4.5. Cell Viability Assays

The viability assays were assessed by crystal violet staining (Sigma Aldrich, St. Quentin Fallavier, France). Retinal ARPE-19 cells were seeded into 96-well plates after 24 h, the medium was replaced by new medium containing different concentrations of RWE or RSV and incubated for 24, 48 and 72 h. Then, cells were washed with phosphate-buffered saline (PBS) and fixed with ethanol for 10 min at 4 °C. Finally, cells were stained with a crystal violet solution (0.5% (w/v) crystal violet in 25% (v/v) methanol) for 15 min at room temperature, then the absorbance was measured at 590 nm using a Biochrom Assays UVM 340 microplate reader, following extraction of the dye using an acetic acid 33% solution.

4.6. Measurement of VEGF Secretion

Cell culture media were saved from the final 24 h of treatment of ARP-19 with RWE (30, 50 or 100 $\mu g \cdot mL^{-1}$) or RSV (20 μM). VEFG levels in cell culture conditioned medium were measured using the enzyme-linked immunosorbant assay (ELISA; BMS277-2 eBioscience) with antibodies mainly specific to VEGF-121; VEGF-165 and VEGF-189.

4.7. Immunoblotting Analysis

ARPE-19 cells were treated as described above. Next, cells were collected and lysed in radioimmunoprecipitation assay (RIPA) buffer (50 mM Tris-HCl, 150 mM sodium chloride, 0.1% sodium dodecyl sulfate, 0.5% sodium deoxycholate, 1% NP40 and pH 8) containing a protease inhibitor, phenylmethylsulfonyl fluoride (PMSF; 100 μM, Sigma-Aldrich, St. Quentin Fallavier, France), phosphatase inhibitor, sodium fluoride (50 mM) and a protease inhibitor cocktail (Roche, Boulogne-Billancourt, France). Protein concentrations were measured using the QuantiPro™ BCA (Bicinchoninic Acid; Sigma Aldrich, St. Louis, MO, USA; bovine serum albumin (BSA) was used as a standard). Fifty micrograms of proteins were prepared in the Laemmli gel loading buffer (50 mM Tris-HCl, 10% glycerol, 5% 2-mercaptoethanol, 2% sodium dodecyl sulfate, pH 6.8 and 0.1% bromophenol blue). After being boiled 5 min at 95 °C, samples were loaded and separated on sodium dodecyl sulfate–polyacrylamide gel electrophoresis (SDS-PAGE). Protein size markers (Thermo Fisher Scientific, Illkirch-Graffenstaden, France) were loaded without heating. Then, proteins were separated on sodium dodecyl sulfate–polyacrylamide gel electrophoresis (SDS-PAGE). Proteins separated on gels were transferred to nitrocellulose membrane (Amersham, Les Ulis, France). Membranes were blocked for 1 h at room temperature in either 5% of bovine serum albumin (BSA) or 5% of skimmed milk powder dissolved in PBS-T (PBS containing 0.1% Tween 20) and incubated with the primary antibody on a rocker platform at 4 °C overnight. Primary antibodies for Western blot listed in chemical reagents and antibodies were diluted with 5% w/v non-fat milk or 5% BS PBS-T After three 10 min in PBS-T, primary antibodies were detected using appropriate horseradish peroxidase (HRP)-conjugated secondary antibodies (Jackson ImmunoResearch, Interchim, Montlucon, France) for 1 h at room temperature, followed by exposure to enhanced chemiluminescence (ECL; Bio-Rad, Marnes-la-Coquette, France). Detection of immunoreactive bands was performed by ChemiDoc™ XRS + imaging system (Bio-Rad, Marnes-la-Coquette, France), and blots were analyzed with Image Lab™ version 6.0.1 software (Bio-Rad).

4.8. Statistical Analysis

Statistical analysis was conducted using the GraphPad6.0 Prism software (GraphPad Software, La Jolla, San Diego, CA, USA). Data are represented as means ± standard deviation (SD) for triplicate assay samples (otherwise mentioned), of at least three independent experiments. The difference between mean values was determined by the multiple Student's *t* test or by Mann–Whitney *U* test. All p values are two-tailed; $p < 0.05$ was considered significant (* $p < 0.05$, ** $p < 0.01$ and *** $p < 0.001$).

5. Conclusions

Increasing life expectancy will continue to increase the prevalence of age-related eye diseases in economically developed countries. Its chronic course is currently impossible to cure, but it can be delayed. In this, the search for new bioactive molecules of low toxicity could represent a major interest for the prevention or for delaying the progression of AMD. In this study we showed for the first time that a polyphenol-enriched extract, RWE, could decrease VEGF-A secretion for human retinal ARPE-19 cells mimicking the AMD phenotype. This disturbing of VEGF-A production is associated with a decrease of its protein expression. Very interestingly, RWE affects the MAP kinase pathway through downregulation of phosphorylated forms of MAK and ERK1/2 proteins. Thus the use of polyphenolic cocktails could represent a potential interest in a therapeutic strategy. Nonetheless, further studies should better clarify the role of each of the polyphenols present, but also to specify more precisely the molecular mechanisms involved and their effects in preclinical models of AMD.

Author Contributions: C.C., F.C. and M.T.-C. performed the experiments and analyzed the data; J.V.-F. and T.R. investigated the qualitative and quantitative polyphenols composition, D.M. helped for RWE extract methods; V.A. Methodology Project administration, D.D.; Supervision, D.D.; Writing—original draft, D.D. All authors have read and agreed to the published version of the manuscript.

Funding: This work was supported by grants from the ANRT N°2016/0003, by a French Government grant managed by the French National Research Agency under the program "Investissements d'Avenir", reference ANR-11-LABX-0021, the Conseil Régional Bourgogne, Franche-Comte (PARI grant) and the FEDER (European Funding for Regional Economic Development), the "Bureau Interprofessionnel des Vins de Bourgogne" (BIVB), and by the Bordeaux Metabolome Facility and MetaboHUB (ANR-11-INBS-0010) project.

Acknowledgments: The authors thank Ruth Hornedo Ortega for supplying the malvidin 3-glcuoside standard.

Conflicts of Interest: The authors declare no conflict of interest.

References

1. Renaud, S.C.; Gueguen, R.; Schenker, J.; d'Houtaud, A. Alcohol and mortality in middle-aged men from eastern France. *Epidemiology* **1998**, *9*, 184–188. [CrossRef] [PubMed]
2. Goldberg, D.M.; Soleas, G.J.; Levesque, M. Moderate alcohol consumption: The gentle face of Janus. *Clin. Biochem.* **1999**, *32*, 505–518. [CrossRef]
3. St Leger, A.S.; Cochrane, A.L.; Moore, F. Ischaemic heart-disease and wine. *Lancet* **1979**, *1*, 1294. [CrossRef]
4. Parodi, P.W. The French paradox unmasked: The role of folate. *Med. Hypotheses* **1997**, *49*, 313–318. [CrossRef]
5. Criqui, M.H.; Ringel, B.L. Does diet or alcohol explain the French paradox? *Lancet* **1994**, *344*, 1719–1723. [CrossRef]
6. Rifler, J.P.; Lorcerie, F.; Durand, P.; Delmas, D.; Ragot, K.; Limagne, E.; Mazue, F.; Riedinger, J.M.; d'Athis, P.; Hudelot, B.; et al. A moderate red wine intake improves blood lipid parameters and erythrocytes membrane fluidity in post myocardial infarct patients. *Mol. Nutr. Food Res.* **2012**, *56*, 345–351. [CrossRef]
7. Chalons, P.; Courtaut, F.; Limagne, E.; Chalmin, F.; Cantos-Villar, E.; Richard, T.; Auger, C.; Chabert, P.; Schini-Kerth, V.; Ghiringhelli, F.; et al. Red Wine Extract Disrupts Th17 Lymphocyte Differentiation in a Colorectal Cancer Context. *Mol. Nutr. Food Res.* **2020**, e1901286. [CrossRef]
8. Chalons, P.; Amor, S.; Courtaut, F.; Cantos-Villar, E.; Richard, T.; Auger, C.; Chabert, P.; Schni-Kerth, V.; Aires, V.; Delmas, D. Study of Potential Anti-Inflammatory Effects of Red Wine Extract and Resveratrol through a Modulation of Interleukin-1-Beta in Macrophages. *Nutrients* **2018**, *10*, 1856. [CrossRef]
9. Mazue, F.; Delmas, D.; Murillo, G.; Saleiro, D.; Limagne, E.; Latruffe, N. Differential protective effects of red wine polyphenol extracts (RWEs) on colon carcinogenesis. *Food Funct.* **2014**, *5*, 663–670. [CrossRef]

10. Walter, A.; Etienne-Selloum, N.; Brasse, D.; Khallouf, H.; Bronner, C.; Rio, M.C.; Beretz, A.; Schini-Kerth, V.B. Intake of grape-derived polyphenols reduces C26 tumor growth by inhibiting angiogenesis and inducing apoptosis. *FASEB J.* **2010**, *24*, 3360–3369. [CrossRef]
11. Marshall, L.L.; Roach, J.M. Prevention and treatment of age-related macular degeneration: An update for pharmacists. *Consult. Pharm.* **2013**, *28*, 723–737. [CrossRef] [PubMed]
12. Querques, G.; Benlian, P.; Chanu, B.; Portal, C.; Coscas, G.; Soubrane, G.; Souied, E.H. Nutritional AMD treatment phase I (NAT-1): Feasibility of oral DHA supplementation in age-related macular degeneration. *Eur. J. Ophthalmol.* **2009**, *19*, 100–106. [CrossRef] [PubMed]
13. Mendes, D.; Oliveira, M.M.; Moreira, P.I.; Coutinho, J.; Nunes, F.M.; Pereira, D.M.; Valentao, P.; Andrade, P.B.; Videira, R.A. Beneficial effects of white wine polyphenols-enriched diet on Alzheimer's disease-like pathology. *J. Nutr. Biochem.* **2018**, *55*, 165–177. [CrossRef] [PubMed]
14. Kang, J.H.; Choung, S.Y. Protective effects of resveratrol and its analogs on age-related macular degeneration in vitro. *Arch. Pharm. Res.* **2016**, *39*, 1703–1715. [CrossRef] [PubMed]
15. Dugas, B.; Charbonnier, S.; Baarine, M.; Ragot, K.; Delmas, D.; Menetrier, F.; Lherminier, J.; Malvitte, L.; Khalfaoui, T.; Bron, A.; et al. Effects of oxysterols on cell viability, inflammatory cytokines, VEGF, and reactive oxygen species production on human retinal cells: Cytoprotective effects and prevention of VEGF secretion by resveratrol. *Eur. J. Nutr.* **2010**, *49*, 435–446. [CrossRef]
16. Sheu, S.J.; Liu, N.C.; Chen, J.L. Resveratrol protects human retinal pigment epithelial cells from acrolein-induced damage. *J. Ocul. Pharmacol. Ther.* **2010**, *26*, 231–236. [CrossRef]
17. Ablonczy, Z.; Dahrouj, M.; Tang, P.H.; Liu, Y.; Sambamurti, K.; Marmorstein, A.D.; Crosson, C.E. Human retinal pigment epithelium cells as functional models for the RPE in vivo. *Investig. Ophthalmol. Vis. Sci.* **2011**, *52*, 8614–8620. [CrossRef] [PubMed]
18. Koch, S.; Tugues, S.; Li, X.; Gualandi, L.; Claesson-Welsh, L. Signal transduction by vascular endothelial growth factor receptors. *Biochem. J.* **2011**, *437*, 169–183. [CrossRef]
19. Clemons, T.E.; Milton, R.C.; Klein, R.; Seddon, J.M.; Ferris, F.L.; Age-Related Eye Disease Study Research Group. Risk factors for the incidence of Advanced Age-Related Macular Degeneration in the Age-Related Eye Disease Study (AREDS) AREDS report no. 19. *Ophthalmology* **2005**, *112*, 533–539.
20. Tranos, P.; Vacalis, A.; Asteriadis, S.; Koukoula, S.; Vachtsevanos, A.; Perganta, G.; Georgalas, I. Resistance to antivascular endothelial growth factor treatment in age-related macular degeneration. *Drug Des. Dev. Ther.* **2013**, *7*, 485–490.
21. Siemerink, M.J.; Augustin, A.J.; Schlingemann, R.O. Mechanisms of ocular angiogenesis and its molecular mediators. *Dev. Ophthalmol.* **2010**, *46*, 4–20. [PubMed]
22. Kovach, J.L.; Schwartz, S.G.; Flynn, H.W., Jr.; Scott, I.U. Anti-VEGF Treatment Strategies for Wet AMD. *J. Ophthalmol.* **2012**, *2012*, 786870. [CrossRef] [PubMed]
23. Krishnadev, N.; Meleth, A.D.; Chew, E.Y. Nutritional supplements for age-related macular degeneration. *Curr. Opin. Ophthalmol.* **2010**, *21*, 184–189. [CrossRef] [PubMed]
24. Yang, S.; Zhao, J.; Sun, X. Resistance to anti-VEGF therapy in neovascular age-related macular degeneration: A comprehensive review. *Drug Des. Dev. Ther.* **2016**, *10*, 1857–1867.
25. Kaipainen, A.; Korhonen, J.; Mustonen, T.; van Hinsbergh, V.W.; Fang, G.H.; Dumont, D.; Breitman, M.; Alitalo, K. Expression of the fms-like tyrosine kinase 4 gene becomes restricted to lymphatic endothelium during development. *Proc. Natl. Acad. Sci. USA* **1995**, *92*, 3566–3570. [CrossRef]
26. He, Z.; Chen, A.Y.; Rojanasakul, Y.; Rankin, G.O.; Chen, Y.C. Gallic acid, a phenolic compound, exerts anti-angiogenic effects via the PTEN/AKT/HIF-1alpha/VEGF signaling pathway in ovarian cancer cells. *Oncol. Rep.* **2016**, *35*, 291–297. [CrossRef]
27. Yang, H.L.; Huang, P.J.; Liu, Y.R.; Kumar, K.J.; Hsu, L.S.; Lu, T.L.; Chia, Y.C.; Takajo, T.; Kazunori, A.; Hseu, Y.C. Toona sinensis inhibits LPS-induced inflammation and migration in vascular smooth muscle cells via suppression of reactive oxygen species and NF-kappaB signaling pathway. *Oxidative Med. Cell. Longev.* **2014**, *901315*.
28. Paeng, S.H.; Jung, W.K.; Park, W.S.; Lee, D.S.; Kim, G.Y.; Choi, Y.H.; Seo, S.K.; Jang, W.H.; Choi, J.S.; Lee, Y.M.; et al. Caffeic acid phenethyl ester reduces the secretion of vascular endothelial growth factor through the inhibition of the ROS, PI3K and HIF-1alpha signaling pathways in human retinal pigment epithelial cells under hypoxic conditions. *Int. J. Mol. Med.* **2015**, *35*, 1419–1426. [CrossRef]

29. Kim, M.H.; Jeong, Y.J.; Cho, H.J.; Hoe, H.S.; Park, K.K.; Park, Y.Y.; Choi, Y.H.; Kim, C.H.; Chang, H.W.; Park, Y.J.; et al. Delphinidin inhibits angiogenesis through the suppression of HIF-1alpha and VEGF expression in A549 lung cancer cells. *Oncol. Rep.* **2017**, *37*, 777–784. [CrossRef]
30. Delmas, D.; Aires, V.; Limagne, E.; Dutartre, P.; Mazue, F.; Ghiringhelli, F.; Latruffe, N. Transport, stability, and biological activity of resveratrol. *Ann. N. Y. Acad. Sci.* **2011**, *1215*, 48–59. [CrossRef]
31. Delmas, D.; Lin, H.Y. Role of membrane dynamics processes and exogenous molecules in cellular resveratrol uptake: Consequences in bioavailability and activities. *Mol. Nutr. Food Res.* **2011**, *55*, 1142–1153. [CrossRef] [PubMed]
32. Loupit, G.; Prigent, S.; Franc, C.; De Revel, G.; Richard, T.; Cookson, S.J.; Fonayet, J.V. Polyphenol Profiles of Just Pruned Grapevine Canes from Wild Vitis Accessions and Vitis vinifera Cultivars. *J. Agric. Food Chem.* **2020**. [CrossRef] [PubMed]

Sample Availability: Samples of the compounds are not available from the authors.

Publisher's Note: MDPI stays neutral with regard to jurisdictional claims in published maps and institutional affiliations.

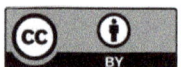

© 2020 by the authors. Licensee MDPI, Basel, Switzerland. This article is an open access article distributed under the terms and conditions of the Creative Commons Attribution (CC BY) license (http://creativecommons.org/licenses/by/4.0/).

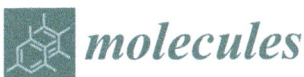

Article

Synthesis and Characterization of Novel Resveratrol Butyrate Esters That Have the Ability to Prevent Fat Accumulation in a Liver Cell Culture Model

You-Lin Tain [1,2], Li-Cheng Jheng [3], Sam K. C. Chang [4,5], Yu-Wei Chen [6], Li-Tung Huang [1,6], Jin-Xian Liao [7] and Chih-Yao Hou [7,*]

1. Department of Pediatrics, Kaohsiung Chang Gung Memorial Hospital and Chang Gung University College of Medicine, Kaohsiung 833, Taiwan; tainyl@hotmail.com (Y.-L.T.); litung.huang@gmail.com (L.-T.H.)
2. Institute for Translational Research in Biomedicine, Kaohsiung Chang Gung Memorial Hospital and Chang Gung University College of Medicine, Kaohsiung 833, Taiwan
3. Department of Chemical and Materials Engineering, National Kaohsiung University of Science and Technology, Kaohsiung 811, Taiwan; lcjheng@nkust.edu.tw
4. Experimental Seafood Processing Laboratory, Costal Research and Extension Center, Mississippi State University, Pascagoula, MS 39567, USA; schang@fsnhp.msstate.edu
5. Department of Food Science, Nutrition and Health Promotion, Mississippi State University, Starkville, MS 39762, USA
6. Department of Medicine, Chang Gung University, Linkow 333, Taiwan; naosa720928@gmail.com
7. Department of Seafood Science, National Kaohsiung University of Science and Technology, Kaohsiung 811, Taiwan; j0920181@gmail.com
* Correspondence: chihyaohou@gmail.com; Tel.: +886-985-300-345; Fax: +886-7-364-0364

Academic Editors: Paula Silva and Norbert Latruffe
Received: 3 August 2020; Accepted: 12 September 2020; Published: 14 September 2020

Abstract: To facilitate broad applications and enhance bioactivity, resveratrol was esterified to resveratrol butyrate esters (RBE). Esterification with butyric acid was conducted by the Steglich esterification method at room temperature with N-ethyl-N′-(3-dimethylaminopropyl) carbodiimide (EDC) and 4-dimethyl aminopyridine (DMAP). Our experiments demonstrated the synthesis of RBE through EDC- and DMAP-facilitated esterification was successful and that the FTIR spectra of RBE revealed absorption (1751 cm^{-1}) in the ester region. ^{13}C-NMR spectrum of RBE showed a peak at 171 ppm corresponding to the ester group and peaks between 1700 and 1600 cm^{-1} in the FTIR spectra. RBE treatment (25 or 50 µM) decreased oleic acid-induced lipid accumulation in HepG2 cells. This effect was stronger than that of resveratrol and mediated through the downregulation of p-ACC and SREBP-2 expression. This is the first study demonstrating RBE could be synthesized by the Steglich method and that resulting RBE could inhibit lipid accumulation in HepG2 cells. These results suggest that RBE could potentially serve as functional food ingredients and supplements for health promotion.

Keywords: resveratrol butyrate ester; resveratrol; butyric acid; Steglich esterification; prevent fat accumulation

1. Introduction

Resveratrol (RE) (trans-3,5,4′-trihydroxystilbene) is a phenolic stilbenoid compound with a C6–C2–C6 structure with three hydroxyl groups. It has been found in over 70 types of plants, including grape skin, grape seeds, giant knotweed, peanut, cassia seed, passion fruit, white tea, plums, and peanuts. It has powerful antioxidant activity and plays a role in the defense against pathogen infection, injury, and abiotic stress [1–7]. RE has been used in medicines, dietary supplements, and functional foods, and the excellent health benefits of RE have also been confirmed by several studies. It has preventive effects on oxidative stress, inflammation, and cardiovascular disease, and shows anti-carcinogenic activity [3,8–10]. Furthermore, RE has been proven to reduce the risk of developing diseases by inhibiting advanced glycation end product formation [11].

Based on its beneficial health effects, several studies focused on the use of RE in medicines, dietary supplements, and functional foods [12]. However, some studies have failed to confirm these beneficial effects, possibly due to RE's high absorption but low bioavailability in vivo [8,13,14], which limits its development for therapeutic applications. Therefore, research is needed to improve the bioavailability of RE. The effects of RE depend on the microenvironment; the presence of copper ions can promote DNA damage and have anti-tumor effects [15]. To improve its biological activity, RE has been esterified using 12 different fatty acids, and derivatives of varying chain lengths and degrees of unsaturation were produced (C3:0–C22:6). RE esters with long-chain fatty acids (C18:0 and C18:1) show higher antioxidant activity in the DPPH radical scavenging assay [16], whereas those with short-chain fatty acids (SCFAs; C3:0, C4:0, and C6:0) show higher antioxidant activity in the ABTS radical cation scavenging assay. Therefore, esterification of RE may improve its functional performance, and the effect of esterification depends on the position and number of esterification substitutions. However, the effect of esterification on the bioactivity of RE is still unclear and requires further research. Furthermore, SCFAs have recently become popular targets of scientific research aiming to link gut microbiota to pathological conditions and potential health-beneficial effects in humans [17,18]. SCFAs are primarily produced through carbohydrate fermentation and also through protein and amino acid decomposition. The majority of SCFAs (95%) are represented by acetic acid (C2), propionic acid (C3), and butyric acid (C4) [19]. There is increasing evidence that SCFAs play an important role in effective absorption from the colonic lumen, and they represent 10% of the human daily energy intake [20]. Unlike acetic and propionic acid, which are mainly absorbed into the blood stream, butyric acid serves as a principal energy source for colonocytes, and its derivatives have many applications in chemical, food, pharmaceutical, perfume, and animal feed industries. Therefore, supplementation with SCFAs such as butyrate may increase microbiota metabolism [20,21].

RE is limited due to its low bioavailability in vivo, and it has been demonstrated that esterification may increase bioactivity [22,23]. Therefore, it is imperative to develop fast and simple esterification methods to synthesize RE butyrate esters. Traditional esterification methods, such as Fischer esterification, require the treatment of a carboxylic acid with an alcohol in the presence of a dehydrating agent. The equilibrium constant for such reactions is approximately five for typical esters, for example, ethyl acetate. Sulfuric acid is a typical catalyst for this otherwise slow reaction. Many other acids are also used as catalysts such as polymeric sulfonic acids. Since esterification is highly reversible, the yield of the ester can be improved using alcohol in large excess, using a dehydrating agent, or by removing the water by physical means. This method is useful in specialized organic synthetic operations but is considered too hazardous and expensive for large-scale applications. Furthermore, because of the limitations in the preparation of large amounts of resveratrol ester derivatives using conventional plant extraction procedures, chemical synthesis is one of the best methods for large-scale production. Therefore, Steglich esterification, which is a method of forming esters under mild conditions, may be a good method. This method is popular in peptide synthesis, where the substrates are sensitive to harsh conditions such as high heat. In this study, RE esters made with butyrate were produced using Steglich esterification techniques. The chemical structure of resveratrol butyrate esters (RBE) after esterification was characterized by mass spectrometry (MS), Fourier-transform infrared spectroscopy (FTIR), and nuclear magnetic resonance (NMR) analysis. In addition, the mechanism by which RBE inhibits fat accumulation was also evaluated using the HepG2 cell model, which might be interesting for potential health promotion and disease risk reduction.

2. Results and Discussion

As shown in Figure 1, resveratrol butyrate esters (RBE) were synthesized from RE and butyl acid by Steglich esterification using *N*-ethyl-*N'*-(3-dimethylaminopropyl) carbodiimide (EDC) and

4-dimethylaminopyridine (DMAP). Compared to the traditional esterification reactions, this ester coupling reaction that is carried out at room temperature (about 28–30 °C) may prevent RE deactivation or degradation. N,N′–dicyclohexylcarbodiimide (DCC) is one of the most widely used activating and dehydrating agents in Steglich esterification, which was developed in 1978 by Neises and Steglich [24]. However, in preliminary experiments, we found that it was difficult to completely remove DCC from the resulting RE esters using either gravity filtration or gel column chromatography methods because during the coupling reaction, DCC dicyclohexylurea (DCU) is formed as a byproduct, which is insoluble in most organic solvents [25] but not soluble in water. Therefore, after esterification, it was difficult to separate RE and DCU from water. It has been reported that water-soluble EDC, an alternative to DCC, can be used for the esterification of phenol derivatives [26] and can be removed after esterification because it is water-soluble [25]. Hence, we replaced DCC with EDC for the esterification in the present study. Because EDC, DMAP, and the urea byproduct can be dissolved in water, we found that they did not significantly contaminate our RE butyrate esters after a simple purification by precipitating the product from deionized water.

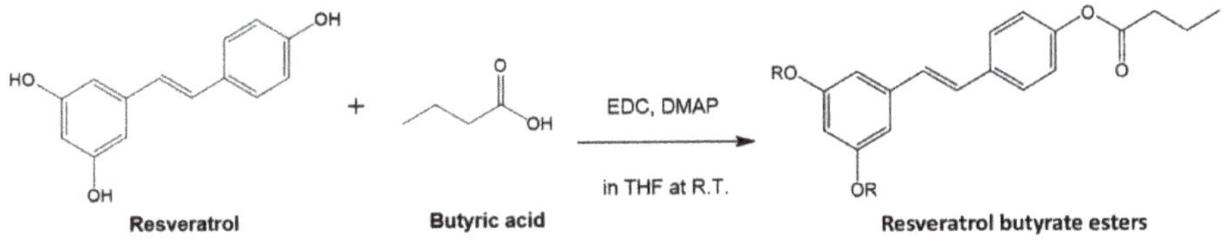

Figure 1. Synthesis of resveratrol butyrate esters. EDC, (1-ethyl-3-(3-dimethylaminopropyl) carbodiimide; DMAP, 4-N, N-dimethyl amino pyridine; THF, tetrahydrofuran; R.T., room temperature.

The Fourier-transform infrared spectroscopy (FTIR) spectra of RE and RBE are compared in Figure 2. The FTIR spectra of RE matches that reported by Porto I. et al. [27]. We found that a broad band in the region of 3400–3200 cm^{-1}, assigned to the O–H stretching, disappeared and a new absorption band at 1751 cm^{-1}, ascribed to the C=O stretching of the ester, appeared in the spectrum of RBE. This comparative finding proved that the esterification of RE occurred via the coupling reaction with EDC. The assignments of the other characteristic bands associated with RE and its ester derivatives are shown in Figure 2. For example, three bands at around 1600 cm^{-1}, 1510 cm^{-1}, and 1442 cm^{-1}, attributed to the C=C stretching in the aromatic ring of RE, can be seen in both spectra. In addition, a tiny band at about 3020 cm^{-1} associated with the C–H vibration of the alkene and the aromatic ring as well as a band at 1662 cm^{-1} related to the C=C stretching of the alkene were observed.

The esterification of RE and butyric acid would likely yield three types of resveratrol ester derivatives, including monoesters, diesters, and triesters. In the present work, LC-mass spectrometry analysis was employed to identify the composition of pristine RE and RBE in the resulting product. As seen in Figure 3a, the LC chromatogram in the negative ionization mode exhibited two separated peaks. Peak 1 was detected at approximately 10.3 min, which is identical to the retention time of the pristine RE compound. The mass spectrum of peak 1, as presented in Figure 3b, had only a single signal at m/z 227.1, which was assigned to the pristine RE. These results are in agreement with those of Liu et al., who sequentially detected trans-resveratrol metabolites by LC-ESI-MS/MS [28]. The peak 2 was detected at a retention time between 15.7 min and 16.3 min and was found to exhibit several signals in its mass spectrum as shown in Figure 3c. The m/z values of resveratrol's monoesters, diesters, and triesters were expected to be 299.1, 369.1, and 439.1, respectively. Two major signals at m/z 227.1 and 299.1, attributed to RE and its monoesters, can be found. In addition, the signals related to the diesters and triesters of resveratrol were insignificant (less than 1%). These LC-Mass spectrometry results revealed that the final product synthesized in this work was a mixture of pristine RE (approximately 26.63%) and RBE (approximately 73.37%). In addition, most of the RBE appear to be monoesters, but this result was somewhat different from the NMR analysis, therefore, it suggests RBE need further chromatographic purification in the future.

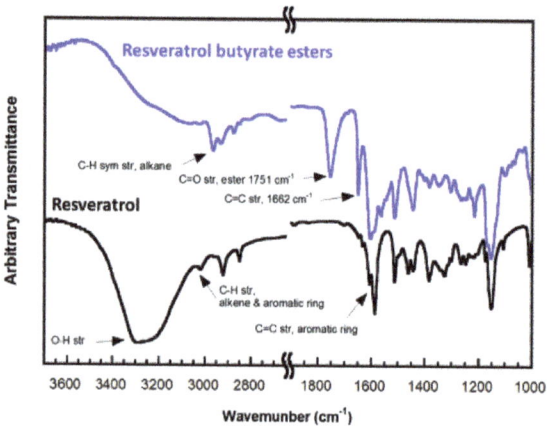

Figure 2. FTIR spectra of resveratrol and resveratrol butyrate esters.

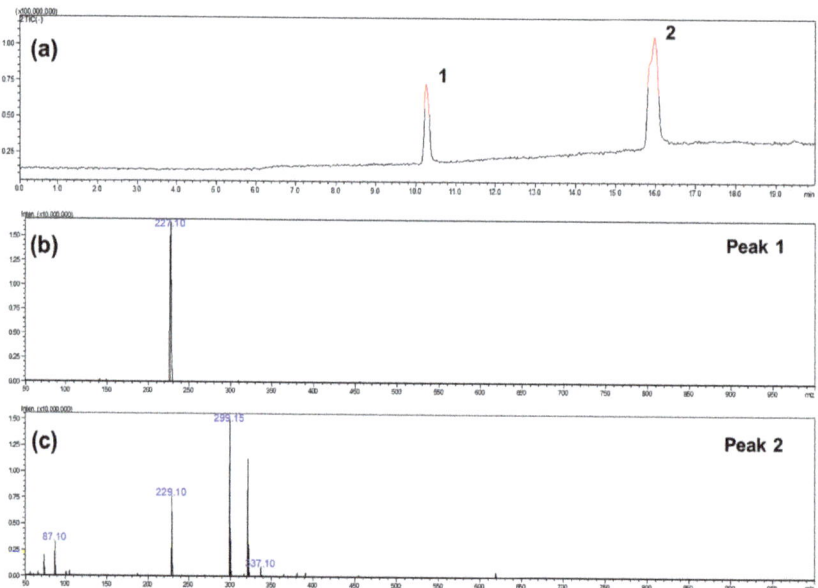

Figure 3. (a) LC chromatogram of resveratrol butyrate esters (RBE) as well as (b,c) mass spectra of peak 1 and peak 2. $^{1-2}$ peak of LC chromatogram.

The NMR technique was applied to confirm the chemical structure and RBE content. Figure 4 shows the ^{1}H NMR spectra of RE and RBE. The NMR spectral data of RE matches that reported by Lu et al. [29], which showed that several additional signals appeared in the chemical shift range between 6 and 10 ppm after esterification.

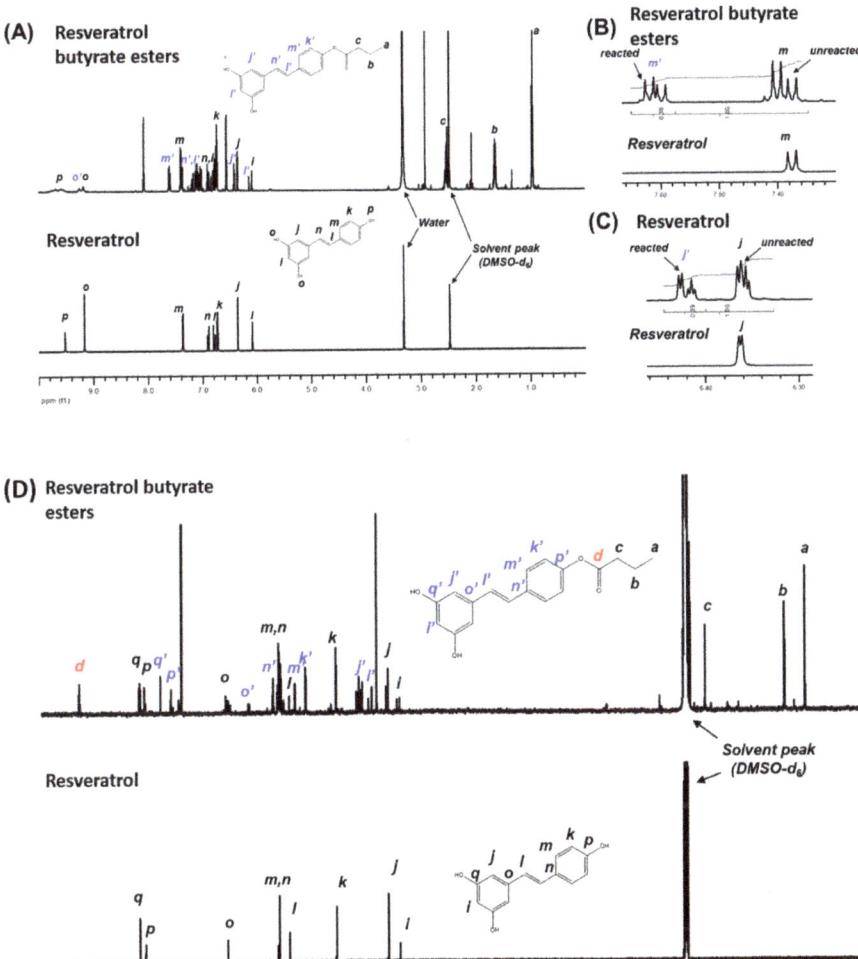

Figure 4. NMR spectra of resveratrol and RBE (**A**) ¹H NMR spectra of resveratrol and RBE. (**B**) ¹H NMR spectra of resveratrol and RBE reacted and unreacted segmentation from 7.32 to 7.66 ppm (t1). (**C**) ¹H NMR spectra of resveratrol and RBE reacted and unreacted segmentation from 6.46 to 6.30 ppm (t1). (**D**) ¹³C NMR spectra of resveratrol and RBE.

These signals are associated with the resveratrol ester with butyric acid. However, not all the original signals of pristine RE shifted and disappeared in the spectrum of the resveratrol ester. These findings suggested that the resulting product was a mixture, and the esterification was not complete, which is consistent with the LC-Mass spectrometry results. By comparing the integrated areas of the selected peaks, the ratio of the reacted and unreacted RE within the resulting product could be determined.

We found that the ratio was approximately 0.38/0.62 for the signals corresponding to one of the aromatic ring protons (e.g., m and m') at $\delta = 7.38$ ppm and $\delta = 7.52$ ppm. This finding indicates that the resulting product still contains 62% of pristine RE. When we considered the other signals assigned to another aromatic ring proton (e.g., j and j') at $\delta = 6.36$ ppm and $\delta = 6.42$ ppm, a similar ratio of the reacted and unreacted RE (0.39/0.61) was obtained. The ^{13}C NMR spectra of RE and RBE are shown in Figure 4. A signal at δ = 171.4 ppm corresponding to the carbons on the carbonyl group of the ester was found, indicating that esterification had occurred. As expected, additional peaks related to the original signals of pristine RE were detected.

Previous studies have reported that specific characteristics of the chemical structure of resveratrol determine its biological activities. It has been shown that the position of the hydroxyl groups is directly involved in its antioxidant properties, [30] and the presence of 4′-OH together with the trans stereochemistry are involved in its inhibitory effect on cell proliferation [31]. In addition, the biological properties of resveratrol are expanded through several modifications, including hydroxylation, methylation, isoprenylation, and by the formation of dimers, trimers, and oligomers [32]. Accordingly, the applications of resveratrol and its derivatives are also expanded, including the development of new anticancer agents. Oh and Shahidi [8] reported the production of twelve RE derivatives acyl chlorides of different chain lengths (C3:0–C22:6). The derivatives (RC6:0, RC8:0, RC10:0, RC12:0, RC16:0) showed better antioxidant activity in a bulk oil system. However, the resveratrol esters RC20:5n–3 (REPA) and RC22:6n–3 (RDHA) showed the highest antioxidant activity when added to ground meat. All these reports indicated that resveratrol derivatives or esterification had higher antioxidant activity in the oil system and their activities depend on the esterification position, the number of esterification substitutions, and the polymer structure.

The thermal gravimetric analysis (TGA) is the method of thermal analysis in which the mass of the sample is measured over time as the temperature changes, which can be used to evaluate the thermal stability of the sample, and it has been applied for investigation of the material properties in various fields such as pharmaceutical, food, and petrochemical applications [33]. TGA analysis results in Figure 5 showed that the thermal stability of RE was better than that of RBE. Both thermograms exhibited a major weight loss between 270 °C and 400 °C. This weight loss might be a result of the thermal decomposition of the phenol groups. In addition, a considerable weight loss between 140 °C and 270 °C was found only in the thermogram of RBE. This weight loss could be attributed to the degradation of the butyrate group, suggesting that the RBE was less thermally stable than RE.

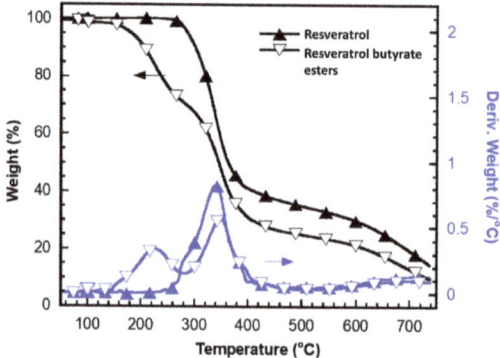

Figure 5. Thermograms of resveratrol and resveratrol butyrate esters under nitrogen from 50 °C to 750 °C.

Furthermore, we used HepG2 cells to compare the effects of RBE and RE on lipid metabolism and the underlying mechanisms. HepG2 cells were cultured with oleic acid for 48 h to induce excessive lipid accumulation. As shown in Figure 6, Nile red oil staining showed that administration of oleic acid increased lipid accumulation compared with the control group. RE, at the dose of 50 μM, reduced the levels of intracellular lipid droplets, whereas RBE showed a similar fat accumulation inhibition rate at a lower dose of 12.5 μM. At 50 μM, RBE displayed a greater inhibition on fat accumulation in a dose-dependent manner. A previous study reported that RE treatment attenuated hepatic steatosis and lowered the levels of intracellular triacylglycerides (TG) [34]. Furthermore, Western blot analysis showed that RE enhanced the phosphorylation of AMP-activated protein kinase (AMPK) and acetyl-CoA carboxylase (ACC) and downregulated the expression of sterol regulatory element-binding protein 1c (SREBP-1c) and lipin1 [34]. RE also had been shown to effectively regulate Sirt-1 and PPAR-γ and to inhibit fat accumulation [35]. Figure 6C shows that 50 µM of RE inhibited fat accumulation during Nile red staining and DAPI staining, and these results are similar to the results obtained in a previous study [36]. Here, we also found that RBE is more effective at the same concentrations, which may be associated with the change in the structure and lipophilic properties of RBE. Previous studies reported that RE derivatives also had better biological properties such as antioxidant activity and inhibition of LDL oxidation [8]. Our experiments substantiated the literature that esterification of RE could improve its biological activities.

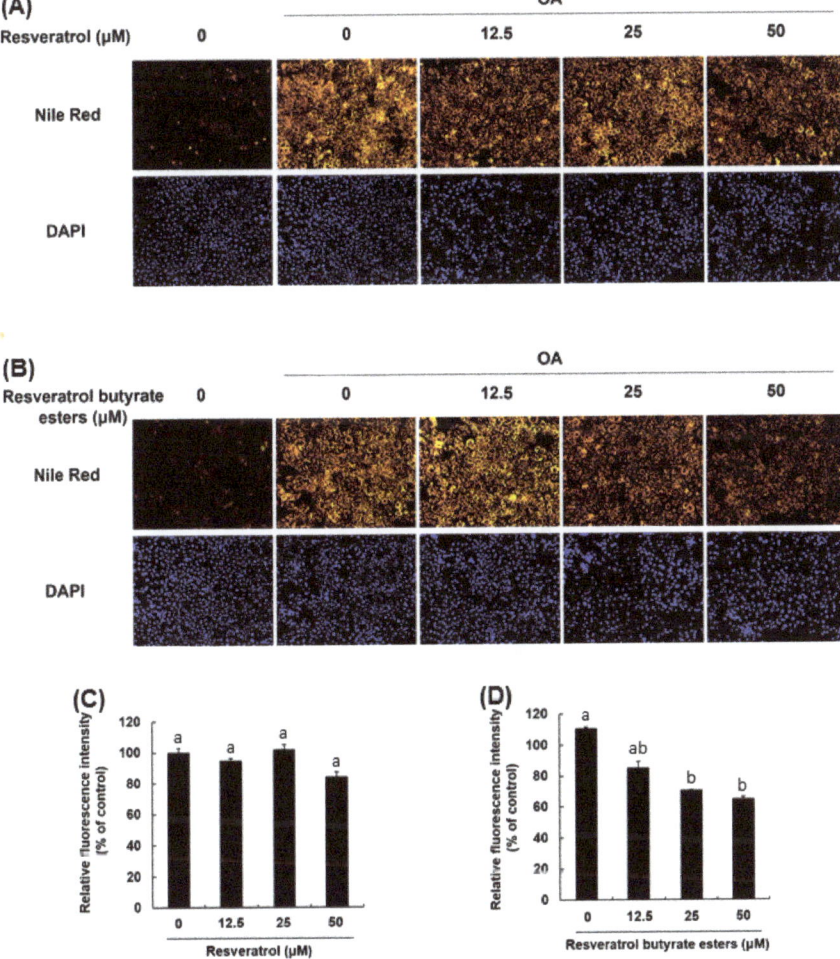

Figure 6. Effect of resveratrol and RBE on fat accumulation in HepG2 cells induced by treatment with 400 µM oleic acid. Nile red and DAPI stained cells treated with resveratrol (RE) (**A**) or RBE (**B**). Relative fluorescence intensity (% of control) at different RE concentrations (**C**). Relative fluorescence intensity (% of control) at different RBE concentrations (**D**). $n = 3$ per group. $^{a-b}$ $p < 0.05$ compared to the control.

RE affects host metabolism by targeting adipose tissue, skeletal muscle, liver, and intestinal microbiota [37]. These effects of RE may be partially due to the regulation of the transcription of genes involved in energy storage management or inflammation [38]. A previous study demonstrated that obese mice treated with RE had reduced levels of mRNA of genes related to the lipogenic pathway and triacylglycerol accumulation in adipose tissue [39]. Similarly, it was shown in cultured pre-adipose cells that the transcriptional effects of RE limited adipogenesis through increased mitochondrial function [40,41]. It is well known the AMPK and SREBP play an important inhibitory role in the lipogenic pathway and fat accumulation, and AMPK has emerged as a critical factor mediating the beneficial effects of polyphenols on lipid metabolic disorders [42] and energy metabolism by regulating downstream ACC and SREBP-1. Thus, these protein levels could be used as an index of cardiovascular disease and obesity [43]. The SREBP-1 targets lipogenic genes, whereas SREBP-2 is more specific to cholesterolemia gene expression, which plays an important role in controlling lipid and cholesterol metabolism [44]. Activation of SREBPs in response to a decrease in cellular sterol levels results in the acceleration of the synthesis of fatty acids, triacylglycerides, and cholesterol. Aberrant SREBP activity has been linked to metabolic diseases, such as obesity, fatty liver, insulin resistance, hyperlipidemia, and atherosclerosis. Thus, inhibition of SREBP activation might be a potential approach to mitigate metabolic disorders [45]. Numerous studies unanimously reported that the mechanism of the action of RE was associated with sirtuin 1 activation and AMPK phosphorylation. Activation of AMPK downregulates the activity of ACC by phosphorylation, resulting in inhibition of lipogenesis and increased energy metabolism [46,47]. As shown in Figure 7, RBE had no significant effects on AMPK, but could still effectively inhibit oleic acid-induced ACC phosphorylation. This finding showed that RBE could effectively increase the oxidation of fatty acids to reduce the accumulation of fatty acids. Furthermore, RBE significantly affected SREBP-1 and effectively reduced the synthesis of fatty acids (Figure 7). Therefore, this study indicates that the production through Steglich esterification of RE could enhance RE's biological activities, and that RBE could decrease fatty acid accumulation by 34.48% through the regulation of ACC and SREBP-1.

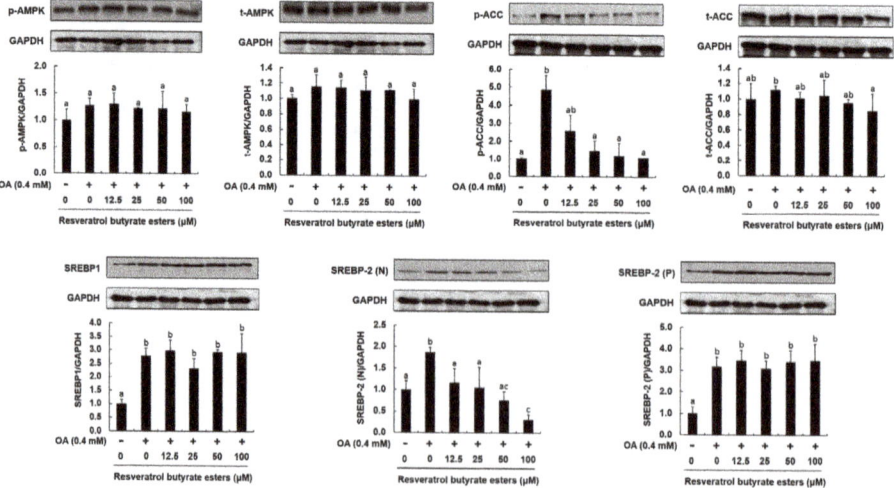

Figure 7. Effect of RBE on protein levels of p-AMPK, t-AMPK, p-ACC, t-ACC, SREBP-1, SREBP-2(N), and SREBP-2(p) in HepG2 cells. Histograms represent densitometric measurements of the specific bands of t-AMPK, p-ACC, t-ACC, SREBP-2(N), and SREBP-2(p) normalized for the expression levels of GAPDH, used as a control. Results are expressed as mean ± SD, $n = 3$ per group. Statistical significance was expressed as $^{a-c} p < 0.05$ compared to the control.

3. Materials and Methods

3.1. Materials

Trans-resveratrol was purchased from TCI Development Co., Ltd. (Shanghai, China). n-Butyric acid was procured from ACROS (Morris Plains, NJ, USA). N,N'-dicyclohexylcarbodiimide, EDAC, and 4-dimethylaminopyridine, DMAP, were supplied by Sigma-Aldrich (St. Louis, MO, USA). Dulbecco's modified Eagle's medium (DMEM) was supplied by Invitrogen Life Technologies (Carlsbad, MD, USA); fetal bovine serum, by Gibco-BRL (New York, NY, USA); and Bio-Rad protein assay kit, by Biorad (Hercules, CA, USA). The primary antibodies against p-AMPK, AMPK, and GAPDH were from GeneTex (Irvine, CA, USA). The primary antibodies against p-ACC, ACC, and SREPB-2 were from Cell Signaling Technology Inc. (Danvers, MA, USA).

3.2. Synthesis of RBE

RBE were synthesized according to a modified method by Neises and Steglich (1978) [24]. A mixture of *trans*-resveratrol (2.282 g, 10 mmol) and n-butyric acid (0.969 g, 11 mmol) was added to anhydrous tetrahydrofuran (THF) (Morris Plains, NJ, USA) (about 12 mL) in a three-neck flask with a magnetic stirrer. To perform the reaction in the dark, the flask was wrapped with aluminum foil. After all reactants were completely dissolved, predetermined amounts of EDC (1.708 g, 11 mmol) and DMPA (0.672 g, 5.5 mmol) were added into the solution. The esterification reaction was carried out by stirring the solution at room temperature under a nitrogen atmosphere for 60 h. Subsequently, the solution was poured into an excess amount of deionized water. Then, a viscous substance was precipitated. The viscous product was re-dissolved in acetone and collected, then the solvent was removed with a rotary vacuum concentrator. The concentrate of RBE was frozen at −80 °C and freeze-dried. Following freeze-drying, the light-yellow powder of RBE was obtained and stored in an opaque vial in a refrigerator at 4 °C.

3.3. Characterization of RE and RBE (FTIR, NMR, LC/MS, TGA)

FTIR was performed with the JASCO FTIR 460 spectrometer (Easton, MD USA). A transmission mode with 16 scans and a resolution of 2 cm^{-1} in the spectral range from 400 to 4000 cm^{-1} was applied to the analyses. In addition, we employed NMR spectroscopy to analyze the chemical structure of RE and RBE. Both ^{1}H NMR and ^{13}C NMR analyses were performed using the Bruker AVANCE 600 MHz NMR spectrometer, Bruker (Billerica, MA USA) with deuterated dimethyl sulfoxide (DMSO-d_6) as the solvent at 30 °C. RE and RBE were analyzed using a TA Q5000, TA Instruments (New Castle, DE, USA) thermogravimetric analyzer (TGA). Their thermograms were recorded at a heating rate of 10 °C/min from 50 °C to 750 °C in a nitrogen flow (20 mL/min). The compositions of RE and RBE were determined by high-performance liquid chromatography-mass spectrometry mass spectrometry (LC/MS/MS) using an Agilent 110 HPLC unit (Agilent Technologies, Palo Alto, CA, USA). A C18 column (4.6 mm × 250 mm × 5 μm with a guard column, Sigma-Aldrich, Oakville, ON, Canada) was used for separation. The mobile phase was methanol/5% acetonitrile in water at different ratios (60:40–95:5 *v/v*) varying from 0 to 70 min at 0.8 mL/min, and the compounds were detected at 306 nm.

3.4. Cell Viability

HepG2 cells were seeded in a 96-well plate at a density of 8×10^3 cells overnight. HepG2 cells were treated with RE or RBE at 1, 5, 25, 50, 75, and 100 μM for 24 h. Cell viability was determined using CellTiter-Glo® One Solution Assay (Promega, Madison, WI, USA) according to the manufacturer's instructions [48].

3.5. Cell Culture and Cell Treatment

HepG2 cells were cultured in DMEM (Invitrogen Life Technologies) supplemented with 10% fetal bovine serum (Gibco-BRL), 1% non-essential amino acids, and 1% antibiotic-antimycotic and incubated at 37 °C with 5% CO_2 [48].

3.6. Induction of Lipid Droplet Accumulation and Staining

HepG2 cells were seeded in a 96-well plate at a density of 8×10^3 cells per well and incubated overnight at 37 °C. The cells were treated with 400 µM oleic acid to stimulate lipid droplet accumulation and with vehicle or the compounds at 12.5, 25, and 50 µM for 24 h. The cells were fixed with 4% paraformaldehyde for 30 min and then stained with 1 µg/mL Nile red and 0.1 µg/mL DAPI for 15 min. The fluorescence of each sample was measured using a 550 Bio-Rad plate-reader (Bio-Rad) [49].

3.7. Western Blot Analysis

HepG2 cells were seeded in a 24-well plate (5×10^4 cells/well) and incubated overnight at 37 °C. The cells were treated with 400 µM oleic acid and vehicle or the compounds at 12.5, 25, 50, and 100 µM for 24 h. The cells were lysed for 30 min in a radio immunoprecipitation assay (RIPA) buffer containing 1 mM phenylmethanesulfonyl fluoride. The concentration of soluble protein was determined using a DC (detergent compatible) protein assay kit (Bio-Rad). An equal amount of protein was transferred onto a polyvinylidene difluoride membrane following separation on a 12% SDS-polyacrylamide gel. Next, the membrane was blocked with 5% non-fat dry milk in Tris-buffered saline, 0.1% Tween (TBST) and shaken continuously for 2 h at room temperature. The membrane was washed once with TBST for 5 min and incubated with specific primary antibodies against p-AMPK (1:5000), AMPK (1:5000), p-ACC (1:3000), ACC (1:3000), SREPB-2 (1:2000), and GAPDH (1:8000) overnight at 4 °C. GAPDH was used as a loading control. Finally, the membrane was incubated with horseradish peroxidase-conjugated secondary antibodies (1:5000) at room temperature for 1 h. After three washes, the chemiluminescence signals were developed using an ECL (Enhanced Chemiluminescent) detection kit (PerkinElmer, Shelton, CT, USA), and the density of bands was counted using ImageJ gel analysis software [50].

3.8. Statistical Analyses

All experiments were conducted at least twice, and triplicate samples were used for each test. Data were collected and analyzed using one-way ANOVA and Duncan's test. Significant differences were set at $p < 0.05$. All statistical analyses were performed using the SPSS program (version 12.0, St. Armonk, NY, USA).

4. Conclusions

Our study demonstrates that resveratrol butyrate esters can be produced from resveratrol and butyric acid using EDC and DMAP. FTIR, NMR, and LC/MS/MS analyses confirmed the structure of RBE, which was found to be more thermosensitive than RE. RBE reduced fat accumulation in HepG2 cells through the regulation of ACC and SREBP-1, and this effect was stronger than that of resveratrol at the same concentration. These results suggest that esterification of resveratrol improves its biological activities. The result clearly demonstrated that RBE might serve as potential anti-fat accumulation agents in functional food ingredients or additives and supplements for health promotion. Further studies are required to improve purification and confirm the effects of RBE in vivo using animal models.

Author Contributions: Conceptualization, Y.-L.T., Y.-W.C., L.-T.H., and C.-Y.H.; Data curation, L.-C.J. and J.-X.L.; Formal analysis, L.-C.J. and J.-X.L.; Funding acquisition, L.-C.J.; Investigation, L.-T.H.; Methodology, L.-C.J., Y.-W.C., and L.-T.H.; Project administration, Y.-L.T., J.-X.L., and C.-Y.H.; Resources, C.-Y.H.; Software, L.-C.J. and Y.-W.C.; Supervision, Y.-L.T. and Y.-W.C.; Validation, S.K.C.C. and C.-Y.H.; Visualization, S.K.C.C. and C.-Y.H.; Writing—original draft, Y.-L.T., S.K.C.C., and C.-Y.H.; Writing—review and editing, S.K.C.C. and C.-Y.H. All authors have read and agreed to the published version of the manuscript.

Funding: This research was funded by the Ministry of Science and Technology, Republic of China (grant no. 108-2221-E-992 -046; 109-2221-E-992-051) and USDA-ARS SCA 5860667081.

Conflicts of Interest: The authors declare no conflict of interest. The authors alone are responsible for the content and writing of the manuscript.

Abbreviations

RE	resveratrol
RBE	resveratrol butyrate ester
DCC	N,N'-dicyclohexylcarbodiimide
EDC	n-ethyl-N'-(3-dimethylaminopropyl) carbodiimide
DMAP	4-Dimethylaminopyridine
R.T.	room temperature
LC-ESI-MS/MS	liquid chromatography electrospray ionization tandem mass spectrometer
AMPK	AMP-activated protein kinase
SREBP	sterol regulatory element binding protein
SREBP-1c	sterol regulatory element-binding protein 1c

References

1. Fremont, L. Biological effects of resveratrol. *Life Sci.* **2000**, *66*, 663–673. [CrossRef]
2. Piotrowska, H.; Kucińska, M.; Murias, M. Biological activity of piceatannol: Leaving the shadow of resveratrol. *Mutat. Res.* **2011**, *750*, 60–82. [CrossRef]
3. Chastang, T.; Pozzobon, V.; Taidi, B.; Courot, E.; Clément, C.; Pareau, D. Resveratrol production by grapevine cells in fed-batch bioreactor: Experiments and modelling. *Biochem. Eng. J.* **2018**, *131*, 9–16. [CrossRef]
4. Liu, D.; Li, B.; Liu, H.; Guo, X.; Yuan, Y. Profiling influences of gene overexpression on heterologous resveratrol production in Saccharomyces cerevisiae. *Front. Chem. Sci. Eng.* **2017**, *11*, 117–125. [CrossRef]
5. Mei, Y.-Z.; Liu, R.-X.; Wang, D.-P.; Wang, X.; Dai, C.-C. Biocatalysis and biotransformation of resveratrol in microorganisms. *Biotechnol. Lett.* **2015**, *37*, 9–18. [CrossRef]
6. Jeandet, P.; Douillet-Breuil, A.-C.; Bessis, R.; Debord, S.; Sbaghi, M.; Adrian, M. Phytoalexins from the Vitaceae: Biosynthesis, phytoalexin gene expression in transgenic plants, antifungal activity, and metabolism. *J. Agric. Food Chem.* **2002**, *50*, 2731–2741. [CrossRef]
7. Jeandet, P.; Delaunois, B.; Conreux, A.; Donnez, D.; Nuzzo, V.; Cordelier, S.; Clément, C.; Courot, E. Biosynthesis, metabolism, molecular engineering, and biological functions of stilbene phytoalexins in plants. *Biofactors* **2010**, *36*, 331–341. [CrossRef]
8. Oh, W.Y.; Shahidi, F. Antioxidant activity of resveratrol ester derivatives in food and biological model systems. *Food Chem.* **2018**, *261*, 267–273. [CrossRef]
9. Donnelly, L.E.; Newton, R.; Kennedy, G.E.; Fenwick, P.S.; Leung, R.H.F.; Ito, K.; Russell, R.E.K.; Barnes, P.J. Anti-inflammatory effects of resveratrol in lung epithelial cells: Molecular mechanisms. *Am. J. Physiol. Lung Cell. Mol. Physiol.* **2004**, *287*, L774–L783. [CrossRef]
10. Nivelle, L.; Hubert, J.; Courot, E.; Jeandet, P.; Aziz, A.; Nuzillard, J.-M.; Renault, J.-H.; Clément, C.; Martiny, L.; Delmas, D.; et al. Anti-Cancer Activity of Resveratrol and Derivatives Produced by Grapevine Cell Suspensions in a 14 L Stirred Bioreactor. *Molecules* **2017**, *22*, 474. [CrossRef]
11. Shen, Y.; Xu, Z.; Sheng, Z. Ability of resveratrol to inhibit advanced glycation end product formation and carbohydrate-hydrolyzing enzyme activity, and to conjugate methylglyoxal. *Food Chem.* **2017**, *216*, 153–160. [CrossRef]
12. Baur, J.A.; Sinclair, D.A. Therapeutic potential of resveratrol: The in vivo evidence. *Nat. Rev. Drug Discov.* **2006**, *5*, 493–506. [CrossRef]
13. Walle, T. Bioavailability of resveratrol. *Ann. N. Y. Acad. Sci.* **2011**, *1215*, 9–15. [CrossRef]
14. Jeandet, P.; Sobarzo-Sánchez, E.; Silva, A.S.; Clément, C.; Nabavi, S.F.; Battino, M.; Rasekhian, M.; Belwal, T.; Habtemariam, S.; Koffas, M.; et al. Whole-cell biocatalytic, enzymatic and green chemistry methods for the production of resveratrol and its derivatives. *Biotechnol. Adv.* **2020**, *39*, 107461. [CrossRef]

15. Muqbil, I.; Beck, F.W.J.; Bao, B.; Sarkar, F.H.; Mohammad, R.M.; Hadi, S.M.; Azmi, A.S. Old wine in a new bottle: The Warburg effect and anticancer mechanisms of resveratrol. *Curr. Pharm. Des.* **2012**, *18*, 1645–1654. [CrossRef]
16. Oh, W.Y.; Shahidi, F. Lipophilization of Resveratrol and Effects on Antioxidant Activities. *J. Agric. Food Chem.* **2017**, *65*, 8617–8625. [CrossRef]
17. Chambers, E.S.; Preston, T.; Frost, G.; Morrison, D.J. Role of Gut Microbiota-Generated Short-Chain Fatty Acids in Metabolic and Cardiovascular Health. *Curr. Nutr. Rep.* **2018**, *7*, 198–206. [CrossRef]
18. Dalile, B.; VanOudenhove, L.; Vervliet, B.; Verbeke, K. The role of short-chain fatty acids in microbiota–gut–brain communication. *Nat. Rev. Gastroenterol. Hepatol.* **2019**, *16*, 461–478. [CrossRef]
19. Cook, S.I.; Sellin, J.H. Review article: Short chain fatty acids in health and disease. *Aliment. Pharmacol. Ther.* **1998**, *12*, 499–507. [CrossRef]
20. denBesten, G.; vanEunen, K.; Groen, A.K.; Venema, K.; Reijngoud, D.-J.; Bakker, B.M. The role of short-chain fatty acids in the interplay between diet, gut microbiota, and host energy metabolism. *J. Lipid Res.* **2013**, *54*, 2325–2340. [CrossRef]
21. Ríos-Covián, D.; Ruas-Madiedo, P.; Margolles, A.; Gueimonde, M.; deLos Reyes-Gavilán, C.G.; Salazar, N. Intestinal Short Chain Fatty Acids and their Link with Diet and Human Health. *Front. Microbiol.* **2016**, *7*, 185. [CrossRef]
22. Urbaniak, A.J.; Kacprzak, K.; Senol, F.S.; Orhan, I.E.; Radominska-Pandya, A. Biological Activity of Resveratrol-Hydroxycinnamic Acid Ester Conjugates. *FASEB J.* **2017**, *31*, 666.8.
23. Intagliata, S.; Modica, M.N.; Santagati, L.M.; Montenegro, L. Strategies to Improve Resveratrol Systemic and Topical Bioavailability: An Update. *Antioxidants* **2019**, *8*, 244. [CrossRef]
24. Neises, B.; Steglich, W. Simple Method for the Esterification of Carboxylic Acids. *Angew. Chem.* **1978**, *17*, 522–524. [CrossRef]
25. Sheehan, J.; Cruickshank, P.; Boshart, G. Notes—A Convenient Synthesis of Water-Soluble Carbodiimides. *J. Org. Chem.* **1961**, *26*, 2525–2528. [CrossRef]
26. Shelkov, R.; Nahmany, M.; Melman, A. Selective esterifications of alcohols and phenols through carbodiimide couplings. *Org. Biomol. Chem.* **2004**, *2*, 397–401. [CrossRef]
27. Porto, I.; Nascimento, T.; Oliveira, J.M.; Freitas, P.; Haimeur, A.; França, R. Use of polyphenols as a strategy to prevent bond degradation in the dentin-resin interface. *Eur. J. Oral Sci.* **2018**, *126*. [CrossRef]
28. Liu, W.; Shiue, Y.-L.; Lin, Y.-R.; Lin, H.; Liang, S.-S. A Derivative Method with Free Radical Oxidation to Predict Resveratrol Metabolites by Tandem Mass Spectrometry. *Curr. Anal. Chem.* **2015**, *11*, 1. [CrossRef]
29. Lu, D.-L.; Ding, D.; Yan, W.; Li, R.-W.; Dai, F.; Wang, Q.; Yu, S.-S.; Li, Y.; Jin, X.-L.; Zhou, B. Influence of Glucuronidation and Reduction Modifications of Resveratrol on its Biological Activities. *ChemBioChem* **2013**, *14*, 1094–1104. [CrossRef]
30. Fang, J.-G.; Lu, M.; Chen, Z.-H.; Zhu, H.-H.; Li, Y.; Yang, L.; Wu, L.-M.; Liu, Z.-L. Antioxidant effects of resveratrol and its analogues against the free-radical-induced peroxidation of linoleic acid in micelles. *Chemistry* **2002**, *8*, 4191–4198. [CrossRef]
31. Stivala, L.A.; Savio, M.; Carafoli, F.; Perucca, P.; Bianchi, L.; Maga, G.; Forti, L.; Pagnoni, U.M.; Albini, A.; Prosperi, E.; et al. Specific structural determinants are responsible for the antioxidant activity and the cell cycle effects of resveratrol. *J. Biol. Chem.* **2001**, *276*, 22586–22594. [CrossRef]
32. Liu, W.B.; Hu, L.; Hu, Q.; Chen, N.N.; Yang, Q.S.; Wang, F.F. New resveratrol oligomer derivatives from the roots of rheum lhasaense. *Molecules* **2013**, *18*, 7093–7102. [CrossRef] [PubMed]
33. Monajjemzadeh, F.; Ghaderi, F. Thermal Analysis Methods in Pharmaceutical Quality Control. *J. Mol. Pharm. Org. Process Res.* **2015**, *3*, 1–2.
34. Tang, L.Y.; Chen, Y.; Rui, B.B.; Hu, C.M. Resveratrol ameliorates lipid accumulation in HepG2 cells, associated with down-regulation of lipin1 expression. *Can. J. Physiol. Pharmacol.* **2016**, *94*, 185–189. [CrossRef] [PubMed]
35. Imamura, H.; Nagayama, D.; Ishihara, N.; Tanaka, S.; Watanabe, R.; Watanabe, Y.; Sato, Y.; Yamaguchi, T.; Ban, N.; Kawana, H.; et al. Resveratrol attenuates triglyceride accumulation associated with upregulation of Sirt1 and lipoprotein lipase in 3T3-L1 adipocytes. *Mol. Genet. Metab. Rep.* **2017**, *12*, 44–50. [CrossRef]
36. Hou, X.; Xu, S.; Maitland-Toolan, K.A.; Sato, K.; Jiang, B.; Ido, Y.; Lan, F.; Walsh, K.; Wierzbicki, M.; Verbeuren, T.J.; et al. SIRT1 regulates hepatocyte lipid metabolism through activating AMP-activated protein kinase. *J. Biol. Chem.* **2008**, *283*, 20015–20026. [CrossRef]

37. Carpene, C.; Les, F.; Casedas, G.; Peiro, C.; Fontaine, J.; Chaplin, A.; Mercader, J.; Lopez, V. Resveratrol Anti-Obesity Effects: Rapid Inhibition of Adipocyte Glucose Utilization. *Antioxidants* **2019**, *8*, 74. [CrossRef]
38. Hou, C.-Y.; Tain, Y.-L.; Yu, H.-R.; Huang, L.-T. The Effects of Resveratrol in the Treatment of Metabolic Syndrome. *Int. J. Mol. Sci.* **2019**, *20*, 535. [CrossRef]
39. Salazar, N.; Neyrinck, A.M.; Bindels, L.B.; Druart, C.; Ruas-Madiedo, P.; Cani, P.D.; de Los Reyes-Gavilán, C.G.; Delzenne, N.M. Functional Effects of EPS-Producing Bifidobacterium Administration on Energy Metabolic Alterations of Diet-Induced Obese Mice. *Front. Microbiol.* **2019**, *10*, 1809. [CrossRef]
40. Kim, S.; Jin, Y.; Choi, Y.; Park, T. Resveratrol exerts anti-obesity effects via mechanisms involving down-regulation of adipogenic and inflammatory processes in mice. *Biochem. Pharmacol.* **2011**, *81*, 1343–1351. [CrossRef]
41. Mercader, J.; Palou, A.; Bonet, M.L. Resveratrol enhances fatty acid oxidation capacity and reduces resistin and Retinol-Binding Protein 4 expression in white adipocytes. *J. Nutr. Biochem.* **2011**, *22*, 828–834. [CrossRef] [PubMed]
42. Li, Y.; Xu, S.; Mihaylova, M.M.; Zheng, B.; Hou, X.; Jiang, B.; Park, O.; Luo, Z.; Lefai, E.; Shyy, J.Y.-J.; et al. AMPK phosphorylates and inhibits SREBP activity to attenuate hepatic steatosis and atherosclerosis in diet-induced insulin-resistant mice. *Cell Metab.* **2011**, *13*, 376–388. [CrossRef] [PubMed]
43. Beauloye, C.; Marsin, A.S.; Bertrand, L.; Krause, U.; Hardie, D.G.; Vanoverschelde, J.L.; Hue, L. Insulin antagonizes AMP-activated protein kinase activation by ischemia or anoxia in rat hearts, without affecting total adenine nucleotides. *FEBS Lett.* **2001**, *505*, 348–352. [CrossRef]
44. Amemiya-Kudo, M.; Shimano, H.; Hasty, A.H.; Yahagi, N.; Yoshikawa, T.; Matsuzaka, T.; Okazaki, H.; Tamura, Y.; Iizuka, Y.; Ohashi, K.; et al. Transcriptional activities of nuclear SREBP-1a, -1c, and -2 to different target promoters of lipogenic and cholesterogenic genes. *J. Lipid Res.* **2002**, *43*, 1220–1235. [CrossRef] [PubMed]
45. Watanabe, M.; Uesugi, M. Small-molecule inhibitors of SREBP activation—Potential for new treatment of metabolic disorders. *Medchemcomm* **2013**, *4*, 1422–1433. [CrossRef]
46. Price, N.L.; Gomes, A.P.; Ling, A.J.Y.; Duarte, F.V.; Martin-Montalvo, A.; North, B.J.; Agarwal, B.; Ye, L.; Ramadori, G.; Teodoro, J.S.; et al. SIRT1 is required for AMPK activation and the beneficial effects of resveratrol on mitochondrial function. *Cell Metab.* **2012**, *15*, 675–690. [CrossRef]
47. Park, S.H.; Gammon, S.R.; Knippers, J.D.; Paulsen, S.R.; Rubink, D.S.; Winder, W.W. Phosphorylation-activity relationships of AMPK and acetyl-CoA carboxylase in muscle. *J. Appl. Physiol.* **2002**, *92*, 2475–2482. [CrossRef]
48. Hosseini, H.; Teimouri, M.; Shabani, M.; Koushki, M.; Babaei Khorzoughi, R.; Namvarjah, F.; Izadi, P.; Meshkani, R. Resveratrol alleviates non-alcoholic fatty liver disease through epigenetic modification of the Nrf2 signaling pathway. *Int. J. Biochem. Cell Biol.* **2020**, *119*, 105667. [CrossRef] [PubMed]
49. Chung, M.-Y.; Shin, E.J.; Choi, H.-K.; Kim, S.H.; Sung, M.J.; Park, J.H.; Hwang, J.-T. Schisandra chinensis berry extract protects against steatosis by inhibiting histone acetylation in oleic acid-treated HepG2 cells and in the livers of diet-induced obese mice. *Nutr. Res.* **2017**, *46*, 1–10. [CrossRef]
50. Huang, W.-C.; Chen, Y.-L.; Liu, H.-C.; Wu, S.-J.; Liou, C.-J. Ginkgolide C reduced oleic acid-induced lipid accumulation in HepG2 cells. *Saudi Pharm. J.* **2018**, *26*, 1178–1184. [CrossRef]

Sample Availability: Samples of the compounds are available from the authors Chih-Yao Hou.

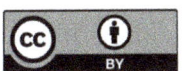

© 2020 by the authors. Licensee MDPI, Basel, Switzerland. This article is an open access article distributed under the terms and conditions of the Creative Commons Attribution (CC BY) license (http://creativecommons.org/licenses/by/4.0/).

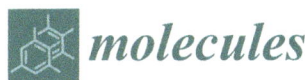

Article

Protective Effects of Some Grapevine Polyphenols against Naturally Occurring Neuronal Death

Laura Lossi [1],*, Adalberto Merighi [1], Vittorino Novello [2] and Alessandra Ferrandino [2],*

[1] Department of Veterinary Sciences (DSV), University of Turin, 10095 Grugliasco (TO), Italy; adalberto.merighi@unito.it
[2] Department of Agricultural, Forestry and Food Sciences (DISAFA), University of Turin, 10095 Grugliasco (TO), Italy; vittorino.novello@unito.it
* Correspondence: laura.lossi@unito.it (L.L.); alessandra.ferrandino@unito.it (A.F.); Tel.: +39-01-1670-9118 (L.L.); +39-01-1670-8755 (A.F.)

Academic Editors: Paula Silva, Norbert Latruffe and Derek J. McPhee
Received: 26 April 2020; Accepted: 22 June 2020; Published: 25 June 2020

Abstract: The interest in the biological properties of grapevine polyphenols (PPs) in neuroprotection is continuously growing in the hope of finding translational applications. However, there are several concerns about the specificity of action of these molecules that appear to act non-specifically on the permeability of cellular membranes. Naturally occurring neuronal death (NOND) during cerebellar maturation is a well characterized postnatal event that is very useful to investigate the death and rescue of neurons. We here aimed to establish a baseline comparative study of the potential to counteract NOND of certain grapevine PPs of interest for the oenology. To do so, we tested ex vivo the neuroprotective activity of peonidin- and malvidin-3-O-glucosides, resveratrol, polydatin, quercetin-3-O-glucoside, (+)-taxifolin, and (+)-catechin. The addition of these molecules (50 µM) to organotypic cultures of mouse cerebellum explanted at postnatal day 7, when NOND reaches a physiological peak, resulted in statistically significant (two-tailed Mann–Whitney test—$p < 0.001$) reductions of the density of dead cells (propidium iodide$^+$ cells/mm^2) except for malvidin-3-O-glucoside. The stilbenes were less effective in reducing cell death (to 51–60%) in comparison to flavanols, (+)-taxifolin and quercetin 3-O-glucoside (to 69–72%). Thus, molecules with a -OH group in ortho position (taxifolin, quercetin 3-O-glucoside, (+)-catechin, and peonidin 3-O-glucoside) have a higher capability to limit death of cerebellar neurons. As NOND is apoptotic, we speculate that PPs act by inhibiting executioner caspase 3.

Keywords: resveratrol; polydatin; peonidin 3-O-glucoside; malvidin 3-O-glucoside; quercetin 3-O-glucoside; (+)-catechin; (+)-taxifolin; apoptosis; neuronal death; cerebellum

1. Introduction

We know a great deal about the chemistry of grapevine polyphenols (PPs) because they are widely studied for their implications in wine production and biological role in the grapevine response to biotic and abiotic stress. Notably, there is also a huge body of preclinical evidence on the numerous cellular mechanisms targeted by these substances (resveratrol, in particular) in relation to several pathological conditions including neurological diseases [1,2], but results are often heterogeneous or inconsistent. There may be several reasons for the heterogeneity and lack of consistency of in vitro and/or animal studies on (grapevine) PPs. First, these studies have come under heavy criticism because they have used artificially high doses. However, an additional and even more important concern is that they are unreliable because many of the effects of polyhydroxylated natural phytochemicals, such as resveratrol and epigallocatechin gallate, were reported to be due to aspecific cell membrane perturbations, rather than specific protein binding [3]. Therefore, doubts arose that these molecules are pan-assay interference compounds that affect the accuracy of many assays [4,5]. Other more particular reasons for the divergences in the outcomes of animal experiments may be the following. First, researchers at times have tested the effects of pure molecules but, other times, those of crude plant extracts, with a substantial heterogeneity of results that have been difficult to compare because very often the concentrations of the individual PPs in extracts were unknown. Second, certain experiments used the PPs obtained from different grapevine organs, which contain very heterogeneous levels of these molecules, as it occurs, for example, for leaves compared to other organs of the grapevine [6,7]. Third, starting from different sources of PPs (wines) diverse extraction methods were reported to display very different degrees of efficiency, and to produce chemically heterogeneous extracts when the effects of three critical variables (sample volume, volume of each eluent, and solvent percentage in eluent) were evaluated for non-polymeric phenol and tannin recoveries from wine [8]. This is a very important issue to be considered when purifying PPs-containing samples for studying biological or health-related investigations as polymeric phenols are not absorbed by mammalian cells but are able to bind to and affect nearly any enzyme or receptor, producing irrelevant results [3]. Fourth, further complexity arose from the different results that researchers have reported in vivo or in vitro [6]. For instance, PPs displayed a very promising in vitro antioxidant capacity leading to the misconception that their cellular protection was mainly due to direct antioxidant scavenging [9]. Rather, studies with cellular and animal models demystified this concept, and now we know that the mode of action of PPs goes far beyond their antioxidant potential but also that their brain bioavailability is very limited [10]. Last, investigators have often focused their attention onto one single PP or group of chemically related molecules, thus making it quite difficult a sound comparison of the neuroprotective potential of individual PPs.

PPs of potential biomedical interest belong to several chemical families among which the most widely studied are stilbenes, anthocyanins, flavonols, and flavan-3-ols.

Stilbenes are a group of PPs that raised much interest in viticulture, as they are involved in the grapevine response to biotic stress, but also and even most in biology and health science. In preclinical neuroscience studies, resveratrol, the most widely investigated stilbene and the prototype of grapevine PPs studied so far, has been reported to have neuroprotective, antioxidant and anti-inflammatory, properties. Much of its purported benefits have been related to its ability to activate a family of proteins called sirtuins [11], but there is considerable conflict in the literature as regarding the true neuroprotective potential of these proteins [12]. The literature concerning the activation of sirtuin 1 (sirt1) by resveratrol is similarly controversial: the first studies indicated resveratrol as an activator of sirt1 [13], but subsequent experiments revealed that the stilbene-dependent activation of sirt1 was a technical artifact [14–16]. Resveratrol has also been touted as a treatment to slow physiological aging and age-related diseases including dementia and Alzheimer's disease (AD) to eventually extend healthy lifespan. However, although resveratrol significantly extended lifespan in yeast, worms, and fruit flies [13,17], most studies reported no effect in mammals [18,19] and, very recently, the molecule was reported to exhibit biphasic dose-dependent effects acting as an antioxidant or as a pro-oxidant at low and high concentrations, respectively [20].

In the present study, we tested the death-combating effects of *trans*-resveratrol and polydatin, the glucose derivative of resveratrol, also termed piceid. Polydatin is generally predominant in white wines, whereas in red wines Z- and E-resveratrol are both quantitatively important [21]. Resveratrol is accumulated also in grapevine leaves, where its concentration was found to be up to ten times higher in organically-managed vines, respect to conventionally grown vines, and in both cases extracts were effective in reducing the lipid and protein damages induced by hydrogen peroxide in the rat brain [22]. In addition, two very recent studies have shown that polydatin protected SH-SY5Y neurons after rotenone treatment to model Parkinson's disease [23] or from oxidative stress [24].

The efficacy of anthocyanins as potential therapeutic agents to combat neurodegeneration was tentatively linked to the different levels of hydroxylation in the B ring of the flavilyum ion, as it was suggested that the anthocyanins with a catechol moiety in their B ring could be more effective in neuroprotection compared to those devoid of catechol [25]. Specifically, the non-catechol pelargonidin 3-O-glucoside protected neurons from the oxidative stress elicited by glutamate but was ineffective against nitric oxide-induced apoptosis [26], whereas the catechol-structure cyanidin 3-O-glucoside (di-hydroxylated) was neuroprotective under both experimental conditions [27]. In addition, a combination of several anthocyanins was found to be protective against H_2O_2-induced oxidative stress in cultured human neuroblastoma cells [28] or C6 glial cells [29]. We here tested peonidin 3-O-glucoside (Pn-3OG) as the main representative of the anthocyanins in a few but locally very important varieties of *Vitis vinifera* [30] and malvidin 3-O-glucoside (Mv-3OG), quantitatively, without any doubt, the most important anthocyanin found in grape berries, musts and wines [31]. Another reason why we investigated the neuroprotective effect of Mv-3OG is that in vitro studies on SH-SY5Y human neuroblastoma cells [32] or C6 glial cells [29] have demonstrated protection against oxidative stress. However, the situation in vivo was quite different as the molecule overpassed the blood–brain barrier (BBB) in rats, but had no detectable effects in reducing the generation of the amyloid β (Aβ) peptides that are critical for the onset and progression of AD [33].

Flavonols are important PPs conferring to vegetal tissue high or very high antioxidant properties. They were protective in vitro against reactive oxygen species (ROS) challenge of SH-SY5Y neuroblastoma cells [32] and quercetin 3-O-glucuronide was capable to interfere with the generation of Aβ through the modulation of several different independent cellular mechanisms [33]. Moreover, quercetin 3-O-glucuronide significantly improved basal synaptic transmission in a hippocampal slice ex vivo preparation to model AD [33].

Based on these observations and on the fact that quercetin glycosides (glucoside + glucuronide) are, quantitatively, the most important flavonol in grape extracts and wines, we tested quercetin 3-O-glucoside as representative of the flavonols.

Monomeric grapevine flavan-3-ols include (+)-catechin with its diasteroisomer, (−)-epicatechin, and gallocatechin with its diasteroisomer epigallocatechin, differing for the level of hydroxylation in the B ring [34]. Monomeric flavan-3-ols were neuroprotective in a rat model of AD [35]. Therefore, we here have investigated (+)-catechin for its potential in limiting neuronal cell death.

Although at present not much is known about grapevine flavanonols, (+)-taxifolin (dihydroquercetin) has been very recently found to protect neurons against ischemic injury in vitro via the inhibition of excessive ROS production and of the irreversible increase of cytosolic Ca^{2+} concentration in GABAergic hippocampal neurons subjected to oxygen and glucose deprivation (OGD) to mimic ischemia [36].

Despite the notable amount of preclinical data on these four families of PPs, human clinical studies are occasional and thus the true translational potential of grapevine and other PPs in clinical neurology remains almost fully unexplored. For example, AD patients have lower cortical levels of sirt1, which indirectly correlated with greater levels of Aβ plaques and tau protein tangles [11,37]. Conversely, subjects with mild cognitive impairment (MCI) did not show reduced cortical sirt1 levels [11], indirectly suggesting that preventing sirt1 decreases at early stages of dementia may help delay or prevent the progression to AD. However, there is no evidence that treating humans with resveratrol can increase sirt1 in the brain [20]. In addition, clinical trials have up to now failed to show ameliorations of the clinical conditions in neurological patients under a resveratrol regimen [38,39] or epigallocatechin gallate [40] and a recent systematic review did not find sufficient evidence to confirm that PPs have beneficial effects against AD and other neurodegenerative conditions [41].

In the attempt to shed more light onto the neuroprotective potential of some grapevine PPs of shared interest for the viticulturists and the neuroscientists we have devised an initial study aiming to clarify the intervention of these molecules in protecting neurons from naturally occurring neuronal death (NOND) during the course of cerebellar maturation. Given the aforementioned limitations of much of the preclinical studies on the subject and the difficulty in translating these studies into the clinics, we have limited our work to a simplified and restricted experimental paradigm that: i. Exploits a well-known and widely characterized model of NOND [42]; ii. Compares the effects of commercially available purified PPs to overcome the problems that are inherent to the different extraction procedures; iii. Uses a slice culture approach to better mimic the in vivo situation; and iv. Uses a standardized concentration of PPs (50 µM) that is well below the highest doses (200 µM and above) employed in a wide number of studies in vitro [43]. We also discuss our results in relation to the information in the literature obtained from in vivo, ex vivo, and in vitro approaches.

2. Results

2.1. Effect of Ethanolic Media onto Naturally Occurring Neuronal Death (NOND) in Postnatal Cerebellum

During postnatal cerebellar development there is a well-characterized period of apoptotic cell death [42] currently referred to as naturally occurring neuronal death (NOND). NOND primarily affects the developing granule cells and is a massive phenomenon, so that it can be easily followed in slice cultures and is amenable to quantitative analysis (Figure 1A). As PPs are soluble in ethanolic solutions and ethanol itself induces death in neurons, we have devised a series of experiments in which cerebellar slices were maintained in vitro in the presence of progressively increasing concentrations of ethanol to assess the outcome on cerebellar NOND (Figure 1).

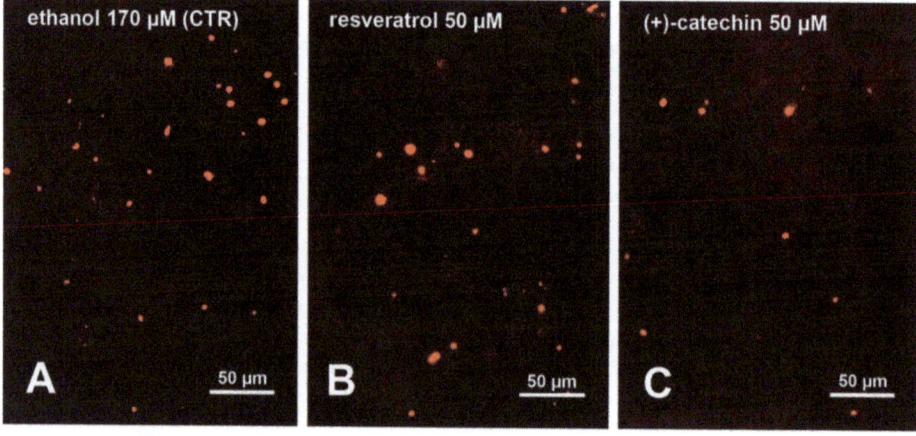

Figure 1. Limitation of naturally occurring neuronal death (NOND) in the postnatal cerebellum after ex vivo treatment with polyphenols (PPs). The nuclei of dead cells are strongly fluorescent in red after incubation with propidium iodide (PI). PI is a fluorescent intercalating DNA stain that is not membrane permeable. Thus, it only enters the nucleus of damaged cells and can therefore be used to differentiate dead cells (apoptotic, necrotic, etc.) from healthy cells based on membrane integrity. As 170 mM ethanol in which PPs are dissolved does not significantly alter cell death, it can be used as a baseline control (CTR) for the experiments to ascertain the effects of PPs onto NOND. The three panels are representative images of the experiments carried out with ethanol 170 mM (**A**) and with individual PPs, resveratrol 50 µM (**B**) and (+)-catechin 50 µM (**C**).

The graphs in Figure 2A,B show the effects of 1:100, 1:50, and 1:25 ethanol in medium (corresponding to 170, 340, and 680 mM, respectively) on the density of dead cells after PI staining (# cells stained with PI/mm^2). Notably, the density of dead cells (mean ± 95% CI) raised from 17.56 ± 17.73 in plain medium, to 23.47 ± 8.76 (170 mM ethanol), 34.24 ± 2.30 (340 mM ethanol), and 78.11 ± 22.41 (680 mM ethanol).

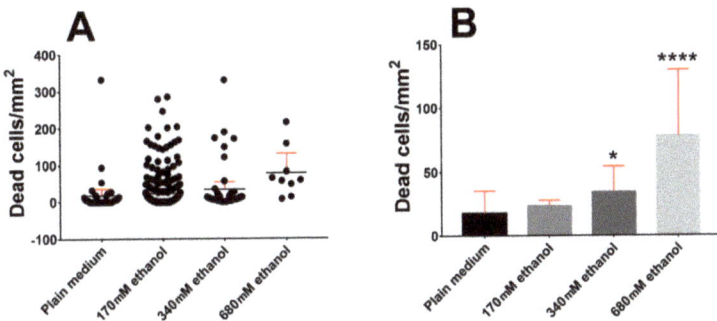

Figure 2. Descriptive exploratory statistics (**A**) and inferential statistics (**B**) of the effects of different ethanol concentrations in culture medium onto cerebellar naturally occurring neuronal death (NOND). Dead cells were stained with propidium iodide and results are expressed as means of dead cells/area. Two-tailed Kruskal–Wallis test and Dunn's multiple comparison test (plain medium vs ethanolic media) were applied, as data did not pass the D'Agostino and Pearson normality test. * $0.05 > p > 0.01$, **** $p < 0.0001$. Bars are 95% CI.

Dispersion of data in 680 mM ethanol was very likely due to the severe toxic effect of the alcohol onto slices that, differently from the two other experimental conditions in the study, displayed obvious morphological signs of tissue sufferance such as fragmentation, disaggregation, vacuolization, etc. It is worth noting that in vitro experiments onto cultured primary cerebellar granule cells demonstrated that 25 mM ethanol was already inducing death, but alcohol was generally used at much higher concentration (87–200 mM) to reach better statistical significance [44,45]. Thus, the concentration of ethanol in our PP control media is within the range of these in vitro experiments and compatible with that in organotypically cultured cortical neurons [46]. Yet our experiments show that 34 and 68 mM ethanol produced statistically significant increases in NOND, whereas there were no differences in the mean density of dead cells at 0 and 170 mM ethanol (mean ± 95% CI: 17.56 ±1 7.73 (no ethanol), 23.47 ± 8.76 (170 mM ethanol), adjusted P value = 0.0815). We have also done a linear regression analysis to model the relationship between ethanol concentration in medium and cell death and found that the two variables showed a very high goodness of fit ($R^2 = 0.9386$, Figure 3). The Pearson's correlation coefficient was r = 0.9688.

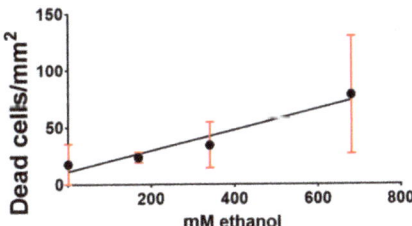

Figure 3. Linear regression curve of the density of dead cells related to different ethanol concentrations in culture media. Dead cells were stained with propidium iodide and results are expressed as means of dead cells/area. The curve demonstrates a positive correlation between the concentration of ethanol in medium and the density of dead cells. Slope was significantly non-zero: F = 30.55, p value = 0.0312. Equation: Y (dead cells/mm^2) = 0.09141 × (ethanol concentration) + 11.15. Bars indicate 95% CI.

Based on these observations, we hold those experiments with PPs in which control- and PPs-supplemented media contained 170 mM ethanol allowed us to monitor NOND appropriately and not ethanol-induced death.

2.2. Effects of PPs onto NOND and Ethanol-Induced Cell Death

Figure 1 shows, as an example, the results of incubating the organotypic cultures in the presence of 50 µM resveratrol (Figure 1B) or 50 µM (+)-catechin (Figure 1C).

We have statistically tested the effects of PPs onto cerebellar NOND using two-tailed Mann–Whitney tests (Figures 4 and 5). Statistics demonstrated that all PPs, except Mv-3OG (Figure 5G,H), were capable to reduce the density of dead cells in cerebellar cultures, with high significance.

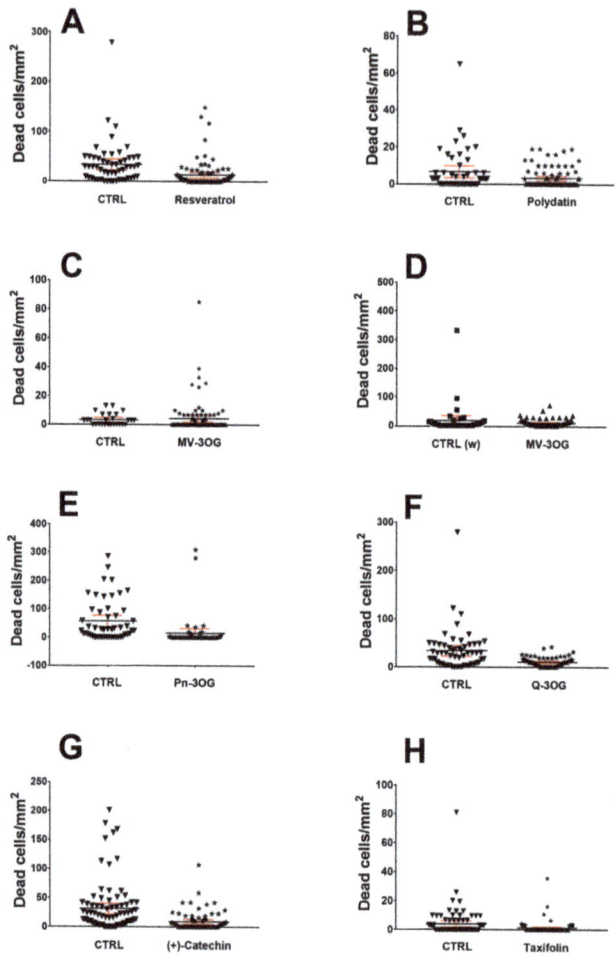

Figure 4. Descriptive exploratory statistics of the effect of different polyphenols ((**A**) = resveratrol; (**B**) = polydatin; (**C**) = Mv-3OG (malvidin 3-O-glucoside); (**D**) = aqueous medium-dissolved Mv-3OG; (**E**) =Pn-3OG (peonidin 3-O-glucoside); (**F**) = Q-3OG (quercetin 3-O-glucoside); (**G**) = (+)-catechin; (**H**) = taxifolin) on cerebellar naturally occurring neuronal death (NOND). Dead cells were stained with propidium iodide and results are expressed as means of dead cells/area with 95% CI. Scatter graphs show the dispersion and variability of data. Abbreviations: CTRL = control medium containing 170 mM ethanol; CTRL (w) = control medium (aqueous).

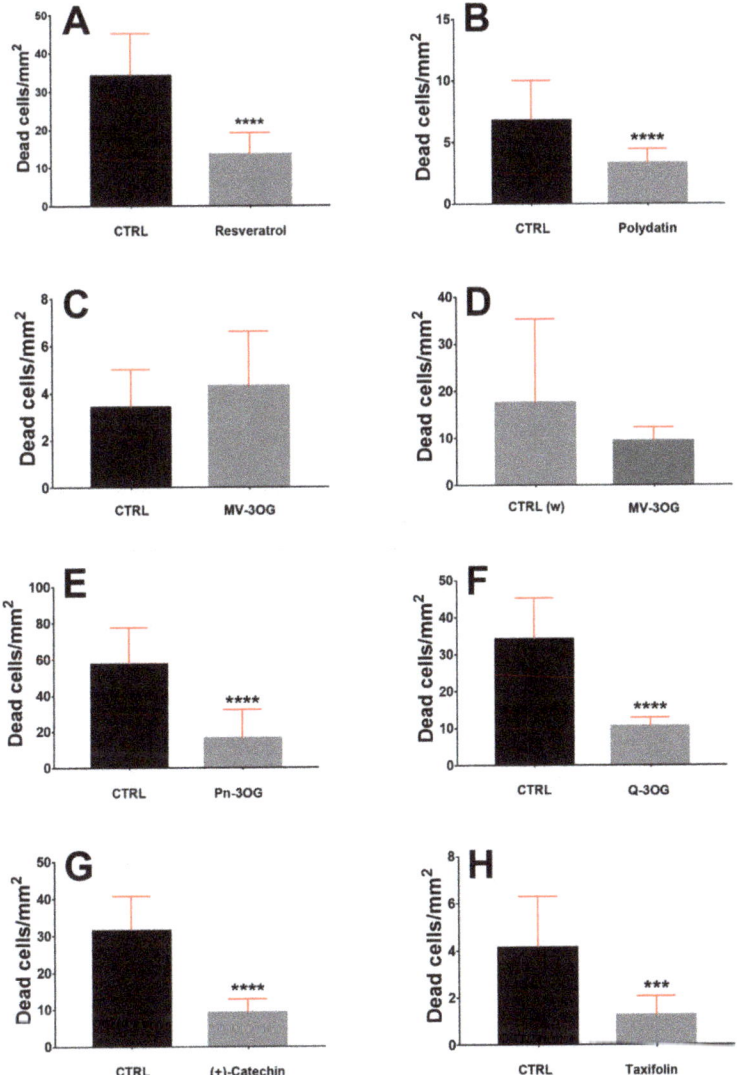

Figure 5. Inferential statistics of the effects of different polyphenols ((**A**) = resveratrol; (**B**) = polydatin; (**C**) = Mv-3OG (malvidin 3-O-glucoside); (**D**) = aqueous medium-dissolved Mv-3OG; (**E**) =Pn-3OG (peonidin 3-O-glucoside); (**F**) = Q-3OG (quercetin 3-O-glucoside), (**G**) = (+) catechin; (**H**) = taxifolin) on cerebellar naturally occurring neuronal death (NOND). Dead cells were stained with propidium iodide and results are expressed as means of dead cells/area. The two-tailed Mann-Whitney test was applied, as data did not pass the D'Agostino and Pearson normality test. *** $0.0001 > p > 0.001$, **** $p < 0.0001$. Bars are 95% CI. All PPs except Mv-3OG (C-D) reduced NOND in cerebellar slices. Abbreviations: CTRL = control medium containing 170 mM ethanol; CTRL (w) = control medium (aqueous).

We also observed that all PPs were as well effective in reducing ethanol-induced cell death (F = 15.11, p value < 0.0001) after Kruskal–Wallis test and Dunn's multiple comparison test (p values for all comparisons against 680 mM ethanol as a control < 0.0001). Specifically, the mean density of dead cells per mm^2 dropped from 78.11 (680 mM ethanol) to 16.20 (Pn-3OG), 13.59 (resveratrol), 10.53 (Q-3OG), 9.41 (Mv-3OG) 9.15 (Cat), 3.30 (polydatin), and 1.25 (taxifolin).

2.3. Comparison of the Effectiveness of PPs in Counteracting NOND

As we have related the effects of each PP against its own ethanolic (Figure 4A–C,E–H) or aqueous (Figure 4D) control, our experimental setup did not allow for correctly performing multiple comparison tests to make statistical inferences about the existence of possible differences in neuroprotective activities among the molecules used in this study. Nonetheless, we have calculated the ratios of the density of dead cells in controls and in the presence of each PPs (Figure 5A–C,E–H) and, thus, the per cent reduction of cell death for each molecule (Table 1). It is noteworthy that among the PPs here studied, the stilbenes (resveratrol and polydatin) appeared to be less effective in reducing cell death in comparison to Cat (a flavan-3-ol), Q-3OG (a flavonol), (+)-taxifolin (a flavanonol), and Pn-3OG (an anthocyanin). These four molecules, in fact, displayed very close percentages of reduction of cell death (69–72%) that were by far higher than those calculated for the stilbenes (51–60%). A remarkable observation was that, albeit in a statistically not significant way, aqueous Mv-3OG only reduced the density of death cells to 40% and even increased it to 127% in ethanolic solution.

Table 1. Percentages of reduction of the density of dead cells in controls (a) and after incubation in PPs (b) containing media.

PPs	Density of Dead Cells (PI$^+$ cells/mm^2)		Ratio (b/a)
	Control (a)	PP (b)	(c)
Pn-3OG	57.43	16.2	0.28
(+)-Catechin	31.32	9.15	0.29
Taxifolin	4.128	1.249	0.30
Q-3OG	34.04	10.53	0.31
Resveratrol	34.04	13.59	0.40
Polydatin	6.78	3.298	0.49
Mv-3OG (Water)	17.56	9.41	0.54

3. Discussion

In this study, we have analyzed the neuroprotective effects of seven different PPs among those known to be present at higher concentration in grapevine.

Cell death in the postnatal cerebellum is a well-known physiological neurodevelopmental event mainly affecting the cerebellar granule cells that are the largest population of neurons in central nervous system (CNS). Being they so numerous, NOND of the granules is a massive phenomenon, and occurs in a quite restricted and tightly regulated temporal window [47]. Therefore, the use of postnatal cerebellar cortex organotypic cultures offers an adequate tool to study the neuroprotective potential of PPs in a controlled experimental setup [42].

Using this approach, we have demonstrated that all PPs studied here, except Mv-3OG, were capable to reduce NOND with statistical significance. We have also proved that all molecules without exceptions were also effective in counteracting the neurotoxic effects of 680 mM ethanol, a very high concentration in relation to studies on the toxic effects of alcohol.

We will first discuss our results in relation to the suitability of the ex vivo approach to investigate grapevine PPs neuroprotection, then we will briefly consider the PPs' chemical structure and antioxidant activities and finally take into consideration the biological relevance of our findings.

3.1. Suitability of the Ex Vivo Approach to Study the Neuroprotective Effects of Grapevine PPs

As summarized in the Introduction, preclinical works aiming to characterize the biological and protective activity of PPs in the frame of neurodegeneration/inflammation display several limitations to the point that there is a strong debate onto their real translational relevance. We here used an ex vivo method to get rid of some of these limitations. Yet the use of organotypic cultures is not free of problems and does not represent a situation without controversies. We are aware of the shortcomings of our approach that paves the way for future better-focused pharmacological studies in vivo. Still, we believe it useful to discuss here the main problems related to the (generally) scarce bioavailability of PPs after in vivo administration. Taking resveratrol (and the stilbenes in more general terms) as the paradigmatic PP, its quantity in red wines is usually around 0.6 mg/L [21] but stilbenes can be up to 35 mg/L in certain Piedmont's red wines and autochthonous Uvalino, in particular, contains up to 100 mg/L of resveratrol [48,49]. These figures correspond to concentrations of 2.6, 135, and 438 µM, respectively. Indeed, data are very dissimilar between studies and substantial differences exist in the reported concentrations of the several PPs that may be present in wines. It is thus remarkable that those of most PPs here studied (other than resveratrol) range in wines from 45 to above 750 µM [50,51]. To this, one must add that different wines have different profiles of PPs deriving from grape seeds, skins, and pulps [52]. However, one can reasonably conclude that in wine the molar contents of many of the PPs that we have studied, except for resveratrol but not in the autochthonous Piedmont Uvalino, are above those used ex vivo in our study.

Yet, the real issue is the bioavailability of PPs and, primarily, the brain concentration that they may reach in vivo. Indeed, Tomé-Carneiro et al. [43], in reviewing preclinical and clinical studies on resveratrol, evidenced that the former often used concentrations up to 200 µM but that resveratrol, quercetin, and catechin and their metabolites were scant in both plasma and urine (max 2 µM). Therefore, from these (and other) considerations they concluded that most studies in vitro were irrelevant.

Comparing our figures with those obtained from other preclinical surveys is not easy principally because, in most cases, results are expressed as the PP quantity in relation to brain weight, a very low quantity indeed, in the order of ng or even pg/mg of nervous tissue [53]. A more rigorous comparison takes into consideration the PPs concentration in the cerebrospinal fluid (CSF), which bathes the brain in vivo similarly to medium in our cultures. No resveratrol was detected in CSF after intravenous infusion in rat, but, after nasal delivery in chitosan-coated lipid microparticles, resveratrol reached a C_{max} after 60 min of 9.7 ± 1.9 µg/mL [54], corresponding to 34–51 µM.

Data onto the CSF content of PPs are scarce, but this paper strongly indicates that by choosing an appropriate pharmacological preparation as well as an efficient route of administration it is possible to achieve brain concentrations of resveratrol (and other PPs) comparable with those here used ex vivo. This is an important result supporting the relevance ex vivo approaches to study PPs neuroprotection.

3.2. The Relationship Between PPs Chemical Structure and Neuroprotective Effects

The increasing interest in PPs extracted from vegetal matrix in relation to neuroprotection is primarily due to their widely established antioxidant capacity (AOC) that, following several different cellular mechanisms and pathways, may be beneficial to neurons [6,9]. In turn, AOC depends on the chemical structure of individual PPs. In addition, the molecular composition influences the bioavailability of PPs, as different aglycones display distinct efficiencies in cellular transport/absorption [55]. In vivo, bioavailability refers to the fraction of a drug/molecule that, after absorption, reaches unchanged the systemic circulation. When dealing with CNS, drugs/molecules must be able to also cross the BBB for reaching the nervous tissue and thence exert their biological activities [56]. In a system ex vivo, BBB is not an issue, yet PPs need to be able to cross cell membranes to reach intracellular compartments and have some sort of efficacy. Other issues that are irrelevant to the present discussion, as we have at the moment tested each PP separately, is the possible synergy or antagonism among different families of PPs that are present in grapevine extracts [57] as well as the degree of polymerization of certain natural compounds, such as proanthocyanidins and copigments [58].

Among the PPs studied, we have here observed that the flavonoids were more effective than the stilbenes in protecting cells from death, except for Mv-3OG (see below).

Pn-3OG (anthocyanin) and Q-3OG (flavonol), both glucosides and di-substituted (Figure 6), showed a very high and statistically significant capacity to reduce NOND, of 72% and 69% respect to the corresponding control, and were among the most effective PPs in this study. We have here used these two PPs in glucoside form for three reasons. First, previous studies have reported that flavonoid glucosides can be absorbed as such without the need to be hydrolyzed to an aglycone [55]. Second, glucosides showed significantly higher transport efficiency than galactosides [55]. Third, they very likely enter the BBB as such, beside as glucuronide form, as demonstrated for anthocyanins [6]. Our results indicate that nor the glycosylation of the C ring of a di-substituted flavonoid form or its methylation (in 3' of the B ring like in Pn-3OG respect to Q-3OG) negatively influenced the capability to reduce NOND. The anthocyanin Pn-3OG appeared to be the most effective in limiting not only NOND but also to counteract the adverse effects of high concentrations of ethanol in media. Therefore, it might be postulated that the B ring level of hydroxylation not alone but together with the total unsaturation of the C ring, typical of the anthocyanin molecules [59,60], are the key elements for explaining the capacity of Pn-3OG to drastically limit neuronal cell death in our ex vivo paradigm.

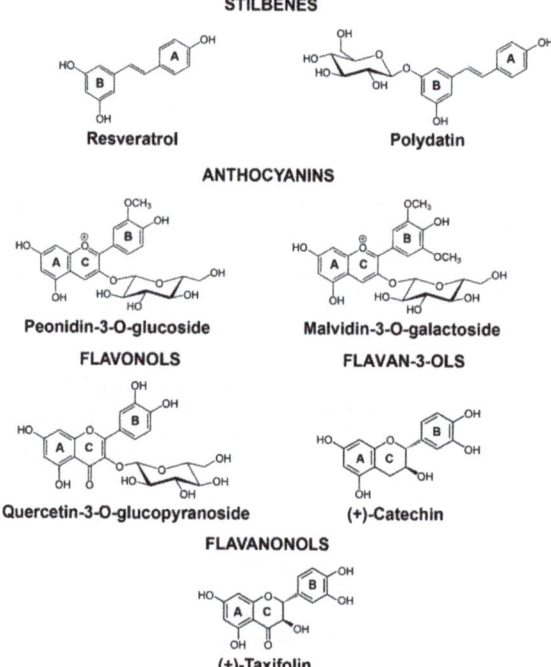

Figure 6. Chemical formulas of the PPs used to study neuroprotection in postnatal cerebellum.

The flavonoids (+)-catechin and (+)-taxifolin are also among the PPs demonstrating the highest efficacy in reducing NOND. They are aglycones, but, like Pn-3OG and Q-3OG, di-hydroxylated, in the B ring (Figure 6).

(+)-taxifolin (flavanonol) and Q-3OG displayed similar capacities to limit NOND, 69 and 70% respectively. The two molecules share identical hydroxylation of the B ring but two different unsaturations in C (Figure 6). In addition, (+)-catechin, (+)-taxifolin, and Q-3OG have an ortho-hydroxyl in B, which is usually the initial target of antioxidants [61].

The null effect exerted by Mv-3OG on NOND but not on ethanol-induced cell-death could be ascribed to several factors, among which is the tendency of tri-hydroxylated anthocyanins to degrade in vitro more rapidly than mono and di-hydroxylated anthocyanins [29] and the limited efficiency in cell transport of glucosides respect to galactosides [55].

Thus, there may be several chemical features of the different flavonoids that, in theory, contribute to the neuroprotective effects observed in this study, but additional observations will be required to substantiate a significant correlation with some or all of them.

The two stilbenes, resveratrol, and its glycoside (polydatin, also called piceid) were undoubtedly less effective in counteracting NOND. Yet, resveratrol capacity to limit cell death was higher respect to that of the corresponding glucoside. One of the main antioxidant mechanisms of resveratrol is based on the presence of two -OH groups in the ring B [62]. Besides, in the comparison vs quercetin, quercetin has a further reactive -OH in position 3′, which is absent in resveratrol. Thus, the resveratrol chemical structure may justify a lower AOC respect to that of other PPs, particularly some of the flavonoids that we have tested here.

3.3. Clues for In Vivo Neuroprotection

We have here tested PPs in a controlled environment ex vivo. In such a setup, advantages mainly derive from the possibility to manipulate carefully and specifically the system according to the experimenter's need, whereas disadvantages derive largely from the lack of information about bioavailability, metabolism and capability of crossing the BBB, i.e., the group of data that can be gathered only in vivo. Yet our approach permitted to provide an empirical demonstration that all PPs studied here were capable to cross cell membranes and to interfere with NOND. In addition, a great advantage in the specific use of postnatal cerebellar cultures is that cell death in this system is chiefly governed by the intracellular levels of caspase-3 (CASP3), one of the most important executioner caspases in apoptosis [47]. Although it is difficult to make direct comparisons due to the extreme variability of approaches, still one observes that all PPs that we have studied have been demonstrated to interact with CASP3 in vitro and/or in vivo not only in neurons but also in neuronal-like cells (Table 2). Remarkably, it should also be added that most of these molecules appeared to inhibit the activity of CASP3 after Aβ toxicity, a hallmark of AD [63].

Table 2. Experimental studies demonstrating an inhibition of caspase-3 (CASP3)-mediated apoptosis after treatment with plant PPs. Abbreviations: Aβ = amyloid-beta; APP = amyloid precursor protein; IRI = ischemia/reperfusion injury; OGD = oxygen/glucose deprivation; LPS = lipopolysaccharide; N/A = not/applicable; PS1 = presenilin 1.

PPs	Type of study	Organ/tissue/cell/Species	Death Inductor	Ref
Resveratrol	In vitro	PC12 cells/Rat	Aβ	[64]
		Primary cortical neurons/Rat	Aβ	[65]
		661W photoreceptor cells/Mouse	Blue light	[66]
		SH-SY5Y cells/human	Ethanol	[67]
	In vivo	Brain/Rat	Ethanol	[67]
Polydatin	In vitro	PC12 cells/Rat	Aβ	[64]
		Primary cortical neurons/rat	Aβ	[65]
	In vivo	Rat models of Parkinson's disease	Rotenone	[68]
Anthocyanins mix	In vitro	Hippocampal HT22 cells/Mouse	Aβ	[69]
		RGC-5/Mouse	H_2O_2 or Tunicamycin	[70]
		Primary hippocampal neurons/Rat	Ethanol	[71]
		APP/PS1 mouse model of AD	N/A	[69]
	In vivo	Brain/Rat	LPS	[72]
		Hippocampus/Rat	Ethanol	[73]

Table 2. Cont.

PPs	Type of study	Organ/tissue/cell/Species	Death Inductor	Ref
Peonidin	In vitro	RGC-5/Mouse	Tunicamycin	[70]
Malvidin	In vitro	661W photoreceptor cells/mouse	Blue light	[66]
	In vitro	Primary cortical neurons/Rat	Aβ	[74]
Quercetin		Primary hippocampal neurons/Rat	OGD	[75]
		Brain/Rat	IRI	[75]
	In vivo	Hippocampus/Mouse	IRI	[76]
		Brain/Rat	IRI	[77]
Epicatechin	In vivo	Brain/Rat	LPS	[78]
	In vitro	Auditory cells	Cisplatin	[79]
Epigallocatechin	In vitro	SH-SY5Y cells/human	Aβ	[80]
	In vivo	APP/PS1 mouse model of AD	Tunicamycin or Tapsigargin	[80]
Taxifolin	In vitro	PC12 cells/Rat	Proteasome inhibition	[81]

4. Materials and Methods

4.1. PPs

We tested seven different PPs belonging to five main groups present in wine and grapevine extracts (Figure 6): two anthocyanins, peonidin 3-O-glucoside (Pn-3OG) and malvidin 3-O-glucoside (Mv-3OG), two stilbenes, resveratrol (Res) and resveratrol-3-O-β-D-glucopyranoside (polydatin), one flavonol [quercetin 3-O-glucoside (Q-3OG), purchased as quercetin 3-O-glucopyranoside], one flavan-3-ol, (+)-catechin (Cat) and one flavanonol (2R,3R)-dihydroquercetin [(+)-taxifolin]. All PPs were purchased from Extrasynthèses (Genay, France). Stock solutions (5 mM) were prepared in absolute ethanol and/or water (for Mv-3OG only). Given the pilot nature of this work and the heterogeneity of results arising from the different wine PPs extraction procedures (see Introduction), we decided not to devise experiments using mixtures of PPs as these mix should more properly been produced once their (relative) concentrations in the territorial wines of interest will be fully established.

4.2. Animals

In this study, we used twenty-five 7-day-old mice. All animal procedures obtained authorization by Italian Ministry of Health and the Bioethics Committee of the University of Turin and were carried out according to the guidelines and recommendations of the European Union (Directive 2010/63/UE) as implemented by current Italian regulations on animal welfare (DL n. 26-04/03/2014). We kept the number of mice to the minimum necessary for statistical significance and we made all efforts to minimize animal suffering during sacrifice. We wanted to gather new information about the biological function(s) of grapevine PPs in a more complex system than primary neuronal cultures/cell lines, where interactions between different cell types are lost. Therefore, mice were employed; yet the use of an approach ex vivo permitted a reduction in their number according to the 3Rs principles.

4.3. Preparation of Cerebellar Cultures

Mice were euthanized with an overdose of intraperitoneal sodium pentobarbital. The brain was quickly removed and placed in ice cooled Gey's solution (Sigma Chemicals, St. Louis, MO, USA) supplemented with glucose and antioxidants (for 500 mL: 50% glucose 4.8 mL, ascorbic acid 0.05 g, sodium pyruvate 0.1 g). The cerebellum was then isolated and immediately sectioned in 350 µm parasagittal slices with a McIlwain tissue chopper (Brinkmann Instruments, Westbury, NY, USA), while submerged in a drop of cooled Gey's solution. Three cerebellar slices were plated onto Millicell-CM inserts (Millipore, Billerica, MA, USA). Each insert was subsequently placed inside a 35 mm Petri dish containing 1 mL of culture medium. Medium composition was 50% Eagle basal medium (BME, Sigma Chemicals, Merck, Darmstadt, Germany), 25% horse serum (Gibco®,

Life Technologies™, Carlsbad, CA, USA), 25% Hanks balanced salt solution (HBSS, Sigma Chemicals, Merck, Darmstadt, Germany), 0.5% glucose, 0.5% 200 mM L-glutamine, and 1% antibiotic/antimycotic solution. Cultures were incubated at 34 °C in 5% CO_2 for 4 days in vitro (DIV) before being treated with PPs.

4.4. Preparation of PPs-Containing Media, Incubation of Cultures with PPs and Staining of Dead Cells

Except for Mv-3OG that could also be directly dissolved in water, all other PPs were not soluble in water and were added to the culture medium from ethanolic stock solutions. Culture media containing 50 µM of each of the PPs were prepared by dissolving 10 µL 100% ethanol stock solutions in 1 mL medium. The same volume of ethanol was added to control media. In the case of Mv-3OG we prepared culture media both from ethanolic and aqueous stocks.

As alcohol is known to be toxic to neurons, we devised an ad hoc series of experiments to ascertain the effects of ethanol onto neuronal survival at the concentration necessary to prepare the PPs containing media (170 mM—corresponding to 10 µL ethanol/1 mL medium). In these experiments, we also incubated some cerebellar cultures in 340 mM or 680 mM ethanol (i.e., 20 or 40 µL ethanol/ 1 mL medium).

At DIV 5 cerebellar cultures were subdivided in five groups and incubated into: i. Fresh plain medium (control for ethanol toxicity at 170 mM); ii. medium with 170 mM ethanol (control medium for PPs experiments); iii. Medium with 340 mM ethanol; iv. medium with 680 mM ethanol; and v. Medium containing 50 µM of each PP dissolved in ethanol (at a 170 mM final concentration). After 24 h, cultures were incubated for 10 min in medium containing 1.5 mM propidium iodide (PI) to visualize the dead cells. We decided to employ PI, a general marker of cell death rather than focusing onto a more specific assay because there are severe concerns about the specificity of action of several plant PPs onto animal cells [3]. In addition, the number of cellular mechanisms that have been put into play for explaining the numerous purported actions of resveratrol and other vegetal PPs is so high that virtually all the major cell pathways appeared to be involved [82], at times with opposite effects [20]. In addition, PI is widely used to stain dead cells as it is extruded from live cells with an intact membrane irrespective of the mechanism and type of death [83] and PI-based experiments thus offered prompt and, very importantly, comparable readouts of the effect of each PP onto NOND, independently from its mechanism(s) of action.

After three washes in plain medium, cultures were fixed for 60 min in 4% paraformaldehyde dissolved in 0.1 M phosphate-buffered saline (PBS) pH 7.4–7.6. They were then washed in PBS (2 × 10 min) and double-distilled water (2 × 5 min) and finally mounted in fluorescence-free medium (Vectashield® Antifade Mounting Medium, Vector Laboratories, Burlingame, CA, USA). Slices were then photographed using a Leica DM6000 wide-field fluorescence microscope (Leica Microsystems, Wetzlar, Germany) with a 20 × lens. For each slice, three randomly selected microscope fields (0.3084 mm^2) were photographed at a resolution of 1392 × 1040 pixels and PI-stained nuclei were counted with the "Count Particles" function of the ImageJ software (NIH, Bethesda, MD, USA) in an interval of area size between 12.56 and 78.50 μm^2 (corresponding to a particle diameter of 4–10 µm). Results were expressed as the number of PI-stained cells (nuclei)/mm^2, i.e., density of PI-stained cells (nuclei).

4.5. Statistical Analysis

GraphPadPrism®7 (GraphPadSoftware, San Diego, CA, USA) was used for statistical analyses. These included I. Linear regression analysis and Pearson's correlation test on the effects of different ethanol concentrations on the density of dead cells in cultures. II. D'Agostino and Pearson omnibus normality test to check for normally distributed data. III. Unpaired two-tailed Mann–Whitney test to make comparisons between two groups (control and PP-treated cultures).

Multiple comparisons for control experiments with different ethanol concentrations were made using the non-parametric Kruskal–Wallis test followed by Dunn's multiple comparisons test.

5. Conclusions

In conclusion, we here demonstrate the usefulness of the ex vivo approach to study the neuroprotective potential of grapefruit PPs. Further studies will be required to confirm the relevance of our experiments in vivo considering the well-known problems regarding the bioavailability of these molecules following conventional pharmacological administration.

Author Contributions: Conceptualization, methodology, data curation, investigation, validation, formal analysis, visualization, writing-original draft, writing—review and editing L.L., A.M. and A.F.; resources, funding acquisition L.L. and A.F.; supervision, A.M. and V.N.; project administration, A.M. and V.N. All authors have read and agreed to the published version of the manuscript.

Funding: This research received no external funding.

Acknowledgments: We are greatly indebted with Prof. A. Granato for his critical reading of the manuscript and very useful suggestions.

Conflicts of Interest: The authors declare no conflict of interest.

References

1. Pervaiz, S. Resveratrol: From grapevines to mammalian biology. *FASEB J.* **2003**, *17*, 1975–1985. [CrossRef]
2. Nassiri-Asl, M.; Hosseinzadeh, H. Review of the Pharmacological Effects of Vitis vinifera (Grape) and its Bioactive Constituents: An Update. *Phytother. Res. PTR* **2016**, *30*, 1392–1403. [CrossRef]
3. Ingolfsson, H.I.; Thakur, P.; Herold, K.F.; Hobart, E.A.; Ramsey, N.B.; Periole, X.; de Jong, D.H.; Zwama, M.; Yilmaz, D.; Hall, K.; et al. Phytochemicals perturb membranes and promiscuously alter protein function. *ACS Chem. Biol.* **2014**, *9*, 1788–1798. [CrossRef]
4. Baell, J.; Walters, M.A. Chemistry: Chemical con artists foil drug discovery. *Nature* **2014**, *513*, 481–483. [CrossRef]
5. Visioli, F. The resveratrol fiasco. *Pharmacol. Res.* **2014**, *90*, 87. [CrossRef]
6. Kelly, E.; Vyas, P.; Weber, J.T. Biochemical Properties and Neuroprotective Effects of Compounds in Various Species of Berries. *Molecules* **2017**, *23*, 26. [CrossRef]
7. Kedrina-Okutan, O.; Novello, V.; Hoffmann, T.; Hadersdorfer, J.; Occhipinti, A.; Schwab, W.; Ferrandino, A. Constitutive Polyphenols in Blades and Veins of Grapevine (*Vitis vinifera* L.) Healthy Leaves. *J. Agric. Food Chem.* **2018**, *66*, 10977–10990. [CrossRef] [PubMed]
8. Pinelo, M.; Laurie, V.F.; Waterhouse, A.L. A simple method to separate red wine nonpolymeric and polymeric phenols by solid-phase extraction. *J. Agric. Food Chem.* **2006**, *54*, 2839–2844. [CrossRef] [PubMed]
9. Figueira, I.; Menezes, R.; Macedo, D.; Costa, I.; Dos Santos, C.N. Polyphenols Beyond Barriers: A Glimpse into the Brain. *Curr. Neuropharmacol.* **2017**, *15*, 562–594. [CrossRef] [PubMed]
10. Scheepens, A.; Tan, K.; Paxton, J.W. Improving the oral bioavailability of beneficial polyphenols through designed synergies. *Genes Nutr.* **2010**, *5*, 75–87. [CrossRef]
11. Hubbard, B.P.; Sinclair, D.A. Small molecule SIRT1 activators for the treatment of aging and age-related diseases. *Trends Pharm. Sci.* **2014**, *35*, 146–154. [CrossRef] [PubMed]
12. Sun, Y.; Dang, W. Chapter 17—The Controversy Around Sirtuins and Their Functions in Aging. In *Molecular Basis of Nutrition and Aging*; Malavolta, M., Mocchegiani, E., Eds.; Academic Press: San Diego, CA, USA, 2016; pp. 227–241.
13. Howitz, K.T.; Bitterman, K.J.; Cohen, H.Y.; Lamming, D.W.; Lavu, S.; Wood, J.G.; Zipkin, R.E.; Chung, P.; Kisielewski, A.; Zhang, L.L.; et al. Small molecule activators of sirtuins extend Saccharomyces cerevisiae lifespan. *Nature* **2003**, *425*, 191–196. [CrossRef] [PubMed]
14. Borra, M.T.; Smith, B.C.; Denu, J.M. Mechanism of human SIRT1 activation by resveratrol. *J. Biol. Chem.* **2005**, *280*, 17187–17195. [CrossRef]
15. Kaeberlein, M.; McDonagh, T.; Heltweg, B.; Hixon, J.; Westman, E.A.; Caldwell, S.D.; Napper, A.; Curtis, R.; DiStefano, P.S.; Fields, S.; et al. Substrate-specific activation of sirtuins by resveratrol. *J. Biol. Chem.* **2005**, *280*, 17038–17045. [CrossRef]
16. Beher, D.; Wu, J.; Cumine, S.; Kim, K.W.; Lu, S.C.; Atangan, L.; Wang, M. Resveratrol is not a direct activator of SIRT1 enzyme activity. *Chem. Biol. Drug Des.* **2009**, *74*, 619–624. [CrossRef] [PubMed]

17. Wood, J.G.; Rogina, B.; Lavu, S.; Howitz, K.; Helfand, S.L.; Tatar, M.; Sinclair, D. Sirtuin activators mimic caloric restriction and delay ageing in metazoans. *Nature* **2004**, *430*, 686–689. [CrossRef] [PubMed]
18. Miller, R.A.; Harrison, D.E.; Astle, C.M.; Baur, J.A.; Boyd, A.R.; de Cabo, R.; Fernandez, E.; Flurkey, K.; Javors, M.A.; Nelson, J.F.; et al. Rapamycin, but not resveratrol or simvastatin, extends life span of genetically heterogeneous mice. *J. Gerontol. Ser. A Biol. Sci. Med. Sci.* **2011**, *66*, 191–201. [CrossRef]
19. Strong, R.; Miller, R.A.; Astle, C.M.; Baur, J.A.; de Cabo, R.; Fernandez, E.; Guo, W.; Javors, M.; Kirkland, J.L.; Nelson, J.F.; et al. Evaluation of resveratrol, green tea extract, curcumin, oxaloacetic acid, and medium-chain triglyceride oil on life span of genetically heterogeneous mice. *J. Gerontol. Ser. A Biol. Sci. Med. Sci.* **2013**, *68*, 6–16. [CrossRef]
20. Shaito, A.; Posadino, A.M.; Younes, N.; Hasan, H.; Halabi, S.; Alhababi, D.; Al-Mohannadi, A.; Abdel-Rahman, W.M.; Eid, A.H.; Nasrallah, G.K.; et al. Potential Adverse Effects of Resveratrol: A Literature Review. *Int. J. Mol. Sci.* **2020**, *21*, 2084. [CrossRef]
21. Guerrero, R.F.; Garcia-Parrilla, M.C.; Puertas, B.; Cantos-Villar, E. Wine, resveratrol and health: A review. *Nat. Prod. Commun.* **2009**, *4*, 635–658. [CrossRef]
22. Dani, C.; Oliboni, L.S.; Agostini, F.; Funchal, C.; Serafini, L.; Henriques, J.A.; Salvador, M. Phenolic content of grapevine leaves (*Vitis labrusca* var. Bordo) and its neuroprotective effect against peroxide damage. *Toxicol. Vitr. Int. J. Publ. Assoc. BIBRA* **2010**, *24*, 148–153. [CrossRef] [PubMed]
23. Bai, H.; Ding, Y.; Li, X.; Kong, D.; Xin, C.; Yang, X.; Zhang, C.; Rong, Z.; Yao, C.; Lu, S.; et al. Polydatin protects SH-SY5Y in models of Parkinson's disease by promoting Atg5-mediated but parkin-independent autophagy. *Neurochem. Int.* **2020**, *134*, 104671. [CrossRef] [PubMed]
24. Potdar, S.; Parmar, M.S.; Ray, S.D.; Cavanaugh, J.E. Protective effects of the resveratrol analog piceid in dopaminergic SH-SY5Y cells. *Arch. Toxicol.* **2018**, *92*, 669–677. [CrossRef] [PubMed]
25. Winter, A.N.; Bickford, P.C. Anthocyanins and Their Metabolites as Therapeutic Agents for Neurodegenerative Disease. *Antioxidants* **2019**, *8*, 333. [CrossRef] [PubMed]
26. Sohanaki, H.; Baluchnejadmojarad, T.; Nikbakht, F.; Roghani, M. Pelargonidin improves memory deficit in amyloid beta25–35 rat model of Alzheimer's disease by inhibition of glial activation, cholinesterase, and oxidative stress. *Biomed. Pharmacother.* **2016**, *83*, 85–91. [CrossRef] [PubMed]
27. Winter, A.N.; Ross, E.K.; Khatter, S.; Miller, K.; Linseman, D.A. Chemical basis for the disparate neuroprotective effects of the anthocyanins, callistephin and kuromanin, against nitrosative stress. *Free Radic. Biol. Med.* **2017**, *103*, 23–34. [CrossRef]
28. Matias, A.A.; Rosado-Ramos, R.; Nunes, S.L.; Figueira, I.; Serra, A.T.; Bronze, M.R.; Santos, C.N.; Duarte, C.M. Protective Effect of a (Poly)phenol-Rich Extract Derived from Sweet Cherries Culls against Oxidative Cell Damage. *Molecules* **2016**, *21*, 406. [CrossRef]
29. Ereminas, G.; Majiene, D.; Sidlauskas, K.; Jakstas, V.; Ivanauskas, L.; Vaitiekaitis, G.; Liobikas, J. Neuroprotective properties of anthocyanidin glycosides against H2O2-induced glial cell death are modulated by their different stability and antioxidant activity in vitro. *Biomed. Pharmacother.* **2017**, *94*, 188–196. [CrossRef]
30. Ferrandino, A.; Carra, A.; Rolle, L.; Schneider, A.; Schubert, A. Profiling of hydroxycinnamoyl tartrates and acylated anthocyanins in the skin of 34 Vitis vinifera genotypes. *J. Agric. Food Chem.* **2012**, *60*, 4931–4945. [CrossRef]
31. Li, Y.; Li, L.; Cui, Y.; Zhang, S.; Sun, B. Separation and purification of polyphenols from red wine extracts using high speed counter current chromatography. *J. Chromatogr. B analytical Technol. Biomed. Life Sci.* **2017**, *1054*, 105–113. [CrossRef]
32. Rocha-Parra, D.; Chirife, J.; Zamora, C.; de Pascual-Teresa, S. Chemical Characterization of an Encapsulated Red Wine Powder and Its Effects on Neuronal Cells. *Molecules* **2018**, *23*, 842. [CrossRef] [PubMed]
33. Ho, L.; Ferruzzi, M.G.; Janle, E.M.; Wang, J.; Gong, B.; Chen, T.Y.; Lobo, J.; Cooper, B.; Wu, Q.L.; Talcott, S.T.; et al. Identification of brain-targeted bioactive dietary quercetin-3-O-glucuronide as a novel intervention for Alzheimer's disease. *FASEB J.* **2013**, *27*, 769–781. [CrossRef] [PubMed]
34. Csepregi, K.; Neugart, S.; Schreiner, M.; Hideg, E. Comparative Evaluation of Total Antioxidant Capacities of Plant Polyphenols. *Molecules* **2016**, *21*, 208. [CrossRef] [PubMed]
35. Schimidt, H.L.; Garcia, A.; Martins, A.; Mello-Carpes, P.B.; Carpes, F.P. Green tea supplementation produces better neuroprotective effects than red and black tea in Alzheimer-like rat model. *Food Res. Int.* **2017**, *100 Pt 1*, 442–448. [CrossRef]

36. Turovskaya, M.V.; Gaidin, S.G.; Mal'tseva, V.N.; Zinchenko, V.P.; Turovsky, E.A. Taxifolin protects neurons against ischemic injury in vitro via the activation of antioxidant systems and signal transduction pathways of GABAergic neurons. *Mol. Cell. Neurosci.* **2019**, *96*, 10–24. [CrossRef]
37. Baur, J.A.; Sinclair, D.A. Therapeutic potential of resveratrol: The in vivo evidence. *Nat. Rev. Drug Discov.* **2006**, *5*, 493–506. [CrossRef]
38. Turner, R.S.; Thomas, R.G.; Craft, S.; van Dyck, C.H.; Mintzer, J.; Reynolds, B.A.; Brewer, J.B.; Rissman, R.A.; Raman, R.; Aisen, P.S.; et al. A randomized, double-blind, placebo-controlled trial of resveratrol for Alzheimer disease. *Neurology* **2015**, *85*, 1383–1391. [CrossRef]
39. Moran, C.; Scotto di Palumbo, A.; Bramham, J.; Moran, A.; Rooney, B.; De Vito, G.; Egan, B. Effects of a Six-Month Multi-Ingredient Nutrition Supplement Intervention of Omega-3 Polyunsaturated Fatty Acids, vitamin D, Resveratrol, and Whey Protein on Cognitive Function in Older Adults: A Randomised, Double-Blind, Controlled Trial. *J. Prev. Alzheimer's Dis.* **2018**, *5*, 175–183.
40. Levin, J.; Maass, S.; Schuberth, M.; Giese, A.; Oertel, W.H.; Poewe, W.; Trenkwalder, C.; Wenning, G.K.; Mansmann, U.; Sudmeyer, M.; et al. Safety and efficacy of epigallocatechin gallate in multiple system atrophy (PROMESA): A randomised, double-blind, placebo-controlled trial. *Lancet Neurol.* **2019**, *18*, 724–735. [CrossRef]
41. Colizzi, C. The protective effects of polyphenols on Alzheimer's disease: A systematic review. *Alzheimer's Dement. (N. Y.)* **2019**, *5*, 184–196. [CrossRef]
42. Lossi, L.; Merighi, A. In vivo cellular and molecular mechanisms of neuronal apoptosis in the mammalian CNS. *Progr. Neurobiol.* **2003**, *69*, 287–312. [CrossRef]
43. Tomé-Carneiro, J.; Larrosa, M.; González-Sarrías, A.; Tomás-Barberán, F.A.; García-Conesa, M.T.; Espín, J.C. Resveratrol and clinical trials: The crossroad from in vitro studies to human evidence. *Curr. Pharm. Des.* **2013**, *19*, 6064–6093. [CrossRef] [PubMed]
44. Pantazis, N.J.; West, J.R.; Dai, D. The nitric oxide-cyclic GMP pathway plays an essential role in both promoting cell survival of cerebellar granule cells in culture and protecting the cells against ethanol neurotoxicity. *J. Neurochem.* **1998**, *70*, 1826–1838. [CrossRef] [PubMed]
45. Kouzoukas, D.E.; Bhalla, R.C.; Pantazis, N.J. Activation of cyclic GMP-dependent protein kinase blocks alcohol-mediated cell death and calcium disruption in cerebellar granule neurons. *Neurosci. Lett.* **2018**, *676*, 108–112. [CrossRef] [PubMed]
46. Mooney, S.M.; Miller, M.W. Ethanol-induced neuronal death in organotypic cultures of rat cerebral cortex. *Dev. Brain Res.* **2003**, *147*, 135–141. [CrossRef]
47. Lossi, L.; Cocito, C.; Alasia, S.; Merighi, A. Ex vivo imaging of active caspase 3 by a FRET-based molecular probe demonstrates the cellular dynamics and localization of the protease in cerebellar granule cells and its regulation by the apoptosis-inhibiting protein survivin. *Mol. Neurodegener.* **2016**, *11*, 34. [CrossRef]
48. Bertelli, A.; Falchi, M.; Lo Scalzo, R.; Morelli, R. EPR evaluation of the antiradical activity of wines containing high concentrations of resveratrol. *Drugs Exp. Clin. Res.* **2004**, *30*, 111–115.
49. Piano, F.; Bertolone, E.; Pes, D.; Asproudi, A.; Borsa, D. Focusing on bioactive compounds in grapes: Stilbenes in Uvalino cv. *Eur. Food Res. Technol.* **2013**, *237*, 897–904. [CrossRef]
50. Frankel, E.N.; Waterhouse, A.L.; Teissedre, P.L. Principal Phenolic Phytochemicals in Selected California Wines and Their Antioxidant Activity in Inhibiting Oxidation of Human Low-Density Lipoproteins. *J. Agric. Food Chem.* **1995**, *43*, 890–894. [CrossRef]
51. Caruana, M.; Cauchi, R.; Vassallo, N. Putative Role of Red Wine Polyphenols against Brain Pathology in Alzheimer's and Parkinson's Disease. *Front. Nutr.* **2016**, *3*, 31. [CrossRef]
52. Pantelić, M.M.; Dabić Zagorac, D.; Davidović, S.M.; Todić, S.R.; Bešlić, Z.S.; Gašić, U.M.; Tešić, Ž.; Natić, M.M. Identification and quantification of phenolic compounds in berry skin, pulp, and seeds in 13 grapevine varieties grown in Serbia. *Food Chem.* **2016**, *211*, 243–252. [CrossRef] [PubMed]
53. Passamonti, S.; Vrhovsek, U.; Vanzo, A.; Mattivi, F. Fast access of some grape pigments to the brain. *J. Agric. Food Chem.* **2005**, *53*, 7029–7034. [CrossRef] [PubMed]
54. Trotta, V.; Pavan, B.; Ferraro, L.; Beggiato, S.; Traini, D.; Des Reis, L.G.; Scalia, S.; Dalpiaz, A. Brain targeting of resveratrol by nasal administration of chitosan-coated lipid microparticles. *Eur. J. Pharm. Biopharm. J. Arb. Fur Pharm. Verfahr. E.V* **2018**, *127*, 250–259. [CrossRef] [PubMed]
55. Yi, W.; Akoh, C.C.; Fischer, J.; Krewer, G. Absorption of anthocyanins from blueberry extracts by caco-2 human intestinal cell monolayers. *J. Agric. Food Chem.* **2006**, *54*, 5651–5658. [CrossRef] [PubMed]

56. Zhao, D.; Simon, J.E.; Wu, Q. A critical review on grape polyphenols for neuroprotection: Strategies to enhance bioefficacy. *Crit. Rev. Food Sci. Nutr.* **2020**, *60*, 597–625. [CrossRef]
57. Di Majo, D.; La Guardia, M.; Giammanco, S.; La Neve, L.; Giammanco, M. The antioxidant capacity of red wine in relationship with its polyphenolic constituents. *Food Chem.* **2008**, *111*, 45–49. [CrossRef]
58. Xia, E.Q.; Deng, G.F.; Guo, Y.J.; Li, H.B. Biological activities of polyphenols from grapes. *Int. J. Mol. Sci.* **2010**, *11*, 622–646. [CrossRef]
59. Rice-Evans, C.A.; Miller, N.J.; Paganga, G. Structure-antioxidant activity relationships of flavonoids and phenolic acids. *Free Radic. Biol. Med.* **1996**, *20*, 933–956. [CrossRef]
60. Rice-Evans, C.A.; Miller, N.J. Antioxidant activities of flavonoids as bioactive components of food. *Biochem. Soc. Trans.* **1996**, *24*, 790–795. [CrossRef]
61. Kilmartin, P.A. Electrochemical detection of natural antioxidants: Principles and protocols. *Antioxid. Redox Signal.* **2001**, *3*, 941–955. [CrossRef]
62. Vo, Q.V.; Cam Nam, P.; Bay, M.V.; Minh Thong, N.; Hieu, L.T.; Mechler, A. A theoretical study of the radical scavenging activity of natural stilbenes. *RSC Adv.* **2019**, *9*, 42020–42028. [CrossRef]
63. Bastianetto, S.; Krantic, S.; Chabot, J.G.; Quirion, R. Possible involvement of programmed cell death pathways in the neuroprotective action of polyphenols. *Curr. Alzheimer Res.* **2011**, *8*, 445–451. [CrossRef] [PubMed]
64. Jang, M.H.; Piao, X.-L.; Kim, H.Y.; Cho, E.-J.; Baek, S.-H.; Kwon, S.W.; Park, J.H. Resveratrol oligomers from Vitis amurensis attenuate beta-amyloid-induced oxidative stress in PC12 cells. *Boil. Pharm. Bull.* **2007**, *30*, 1130–1134. [CrossRef]
65. Wen, H.; Fu, Z.; Wei, Y.; Zhang, X.; Ma, L.; Gu, L.; Li, J. Antioxidant Activity and Neuroprotective Activity of Stilbenoids in Rat Primary Cortex Neurons via the PI3K/Akt Signalling Pathway. *Mol.* **2018**, *23*, 2328. [CrossRef]
66. Ogawa, K.; Kuse, Y.; Tsuruma, K.; Kobayashi, S.; Shimazawa, M.; Hara, H. Protective effects of bilberry and lingonberry extracts against blue light-emitting diode light-induced retinal photoreceptor cell damage in vitro. *BMC Complement. Altern. Med.* **2014**, *14*, 120. [CrossRef]
67. Gu, X.; Cai, Z.; Cai, M.; Liu, K.; Liu, D.; Zhang, Q.; Tan, J.; Ma, Q. AMPK/SIRT1/p38 MAPK signaling pathway regulates alcohol induced neurodegeneration by resveratrol. *Mol. Med. Rep.* **2018**, *17*, 5402–5408. [CrossRef] [PubMed]
68. Chen, Y.; Zhang, D.-Q.; Liao, Z.; Wang, B.; Gong, S.; Wang, C.; Zhang, M.-Z.; Wang, G.-H.; Cai, H.; Liao, F.-F.; et al. Anti-oxidant polydatin (piceid) protects against substantia nigral motor degeneration in multiple rodent models of Parkinson's disease. *Mol. Neurodegener.* **2015**, *10*, 4. [CrossRef]
69. Ali, T.; Kim, T.; Rehman, S.U.; Khan, M.S.; Amin, F.U.; Khan, M.; Ikram, M.; Kim, M.O. Natural Dietary Supplementation of Anthocyanins via PI3K/Akt/Nrf2/HO-1 Pathways Mitigate Oxidative Stress, Neurodegeneration, and Memory Impairment in a Mouse Model of Alzheimer's Disease. *Mol Neurobiol.* **2018**, *55*, 6076–6093. [CrossRef] [PubMed]
70. Tanaka, J.; Nakanishi, T.; Shimoda, H.; Nakamura, S.; Tsuruma, K.; Shimazawa, M.; Matsuda, H.; Yoshikawa, M.; Hara, H. Purple rice extract and its constituents suppress endoplasmic reticulum stress-induced retinal damage in vitro and in vivo. *Life Sci.* **2013**, *92*, 17–25. [CrossRef] [PubMed]
71. Shah, S.A.; Ullah, I.; Lee, H.Y.; Kim, M.O. Anthocyanins Protect Against Ethanol-Induced Neuronal Apoptosis via GABAB1 Receptors Intracellular Signaling in Prenatal Rat Hippocampal Neurons. *Mol. Neurobiol.* **2013**, *48*, 257–269. [CrossRef] [PubMed]
72. Khan, M.S.; Ali, T.; Kim, M.W.; Jo, M.H.; Chung, J.I.; Kim, M.O. Anthocyanins Improve Hippocampus-Dependent Memory Function and Prevent Neurodegeneration via JNK/Akt/GSK3β Signaling in LPS-Treated Adult Mice. *Mol. Neurobiol.* **2018**, *56*, 671–687. [CrossRef] [PubMed]
73. Shah, S.A.; Yoon, G.H.; Kim, M.O. Protection of the Developing Brain with Anthocyanins against Ethanol-Induced Oxidative Stress and Neurodegeneration. *Mol. Neurobiol.* **2014**, *51*, 1278–1291. [CrossRef] [PubMed]
74. Wang, C.-N.; Chi, C.-W.; Lin, Y.-L.; Chen, C.-F.; Shiao, Y.-J. The Neuroprotective Effects of Phytoestrogens on Amyloid β Protein-induced Toxicity Are Mediated by Abrogating the Activation of Caspase Cascade in Rat Cortical Neurons. *J. Boil. Chem.* **2000**, *276*, 5287–5295. [CrossRef] [PubMed]
75. Dai, Y.; Zhang, H.; Zhang, J.; Yan, M. Isoquercetin attenuates oxidative stress and neuronal apoptosis after ischemia/reperfusion injury via Nrf2-mediated inhibition of the NOX4/ROS/NF-κB pathway. *Chem. Biol. Interact.* **2018**, *284*, 32–40. [CrossRef] [PubMed]

76. Pei, B.; Yang, M.; Qi, X.; Shen, X.; Chen, X.; Zhang, F. Quercetin ameliorates ischemia/reperfusion-induced cognitive deficits by inhibiting ASK1/JNK3/caspase-3 by enhancing the Akt signaling pathway. *Biochem. Biophys. Res. Commun.* **2016**, *478*, 199–205. [CrossRef] [PubMed]
77. Ghosh, A.; Sarkar, S.; Mandal, A.K.; Das, N. Neuroprotective Role of Nanoencapsulated Quercetin in Combating Ischemia-Reperfusion Induced Neuronal Damage in Young and Aged Rats. *PLoS ONE* **2013**, *8*, e57735. [CrossRef]
78. Schroeter, H.; Spencer, J.P.; Rice-Evans, C.; Williams, R.J. Flavonoids protect neurons from oxidized low-density-lipoprotein-induced apoptosis involving c-Jun N-terminal kinase (JNK), c-Jun and caspase-3. *Biochem. J.* **2001**, *358*, 547–557. [CrossRef]
79. Kim, C.-H.; Kang, S.U.; Pyun, J.; Lee, M.H.; Hwang, H.S.; Lee, H. Epicatechin protects auditory cells against cisplatin-induced death. *Apoptosis* **2008**, *13*, 1184–1194. [CrossRef]
80. Du, K.; Liu, M.; Zhong, X.; Yao, W.; Xiao, Q.; Wen, Q.; Yang, B.; Wei, Q. Epigallocatechin Gallate Reduces Amyloid β-Induced Neurotoxicity via Inhibiting Endoplasmic Reticulum Stress-Mediated Apoptosis. *Mol. Nutr. Food Res.* **2018**, *62*, 1700890. [CrossRef]
81. Nam, Y.J.; Lee, D.H.; Shin, Y.K.; Sohn, D.S.; Lee, C.S. Flavanonol Taxifolin Attenuates Proteasome Inhibition-Induced Apoptosis in Differentiated PC12 Cells by Suppressing Cell Death Process. *Neurochem. Res.* **2014**, *40*, 480–491. [CrossRef]
82. Bastianetto, S.; Menard, C.; Quirion, R. Neuroprotective action of resveratrol. *Biochim. Biophys. Acta* **2015**, *1852*, 1195–1201. [CrossRef] [PubMed]
83. Lossi, L.; Mioletti, S.; Aimar, P.; Bruno, R.; Merighi, A. In vivo analysis of cell proliferation and apoptosis in the CNS. In *Cellular and Molecular Methods in Neuroscience Research*; Merighi, A., Carmignoto, G., Eds.; Springer: New York, NY, USA, 2002; pp. 235–258.

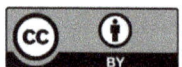

© 2020 by the authors. Licensee MDPI, Basel, Switzerland. This article is an open access article distributed under the terms and conditions of the Creative Commons Attribution (CC BY) license (http://creativecommons.org/licenses/by/4.0/).

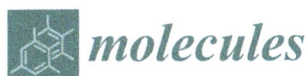

Article

Prevention of 7-Ketocholesterol-Induced Overproduction of Reactive Oxygen Species, Mitochondrial Dysfunction and Cell Death with Major Nutrients (Polyphenols, ω3 and ω9 Unsaturated Fatty Acids) of the Mediterranean Diet on N2a Neuronal Cells

Aline Yammine [1,2], Thomas Nury [1], Anne Vejux [1], Norbert Latruffe [1], Dominique Vervandier-Fasseur [3], Mohammad Samadi [4], Hélène Greige-Gerges [2], Lizette Auezova [2] and Gérard Lizard [1,*]

1. Team Bio-peroxIL, Biochemistry of the Peroxisome, Inflammation and Lipid Metabolism' EA 7270, University Bourgogne Franche-Comté, Inserm, 21000 Dijon, France; alineyammine5@gmail.com (A.Y.); thomas.nury@u-bourgogne.fr (T.N.); anne.vejux@u-bourgogne.fr (A.V.); norbert.latruffe@u-bourgogne.fr (N.L.)
2. Bioactive Molecules Research Laboratory, Doctoral School of Sciences and Technologies, Faculty of Sciences, Lebanese University, Fanar, P.O. Box 90656 Jdeidet, Lebanon; hgreige@ul.edu.lb (H.G.-G.); lauezova@ul.edu.lb (L.A.)
3. Team OCS, Institute of Molecular Chemistry of University of Burgundy (ICMUB UMR CNRS 6302), University Bourgogne Franche-Comté, 21000 Dijon, France; dominique.vervandier-fasseur@u-bourgogne.fr
4. LCPMC-A2, ICPM, Department of Chemistry, University Lorraine, Metz Technopôle, 57070 Metz, France; mohammad.samadi@univ-lorraine.fr
* Correspondence: gerard.lizard@u-bourgogne.fr; Tel.: +33-380-396-256; Fax: +33-380-396-250

Academic Editor: Francesca Giampieri
Received: 21 April 2020; Accepted: 12 May 2020; Published: 13 May 2020

Abstract: The brain, which is a cholesterol-rich organ, can be subject to oxidative stress in a variety of pathophysiological conditions, age-related diseases and some rare pathologies. This can lead to the formation of 7-ketocholesterol (7KC), a toxic derivative of cholesterol mainly produced by auto-oxidation. So, preventing the neuronal toxicity of 7KC is an important issue to avoid brain damage. As there are numerous data in favor of the prevention of neurodegeneration by the Mediterranean diet, this study aimed to evaluate the potential of a series of polyphenols (resveratrol, RSV; quercetin, QCT; and apigenin, API) as well as ω3 and ω9 unsaturated fatty acids (α-linolenic acid, ALA; eicosapentaenoic acid, EPA; docosahexaenoic acid, DHA, and oleic acid, OA) widely present in this diet, to prevent 7KC (50 µM)-induced dysfunction of N2a neuronal cells. When polyphenols and fatty acids were used at non-toxic concentrations (polyphenols: ≤6.25 µM; fatty acids: ≤25 µM) as defined by the fluorescein diacetate assay, they greatly reduce 7KC-induced toxicity. The cytoprotective effects observed with polyphenols and fatty acids were comparable to those of α-tocopherol (400 µM) used as a reference. These polyphenols and fatty acids attenuate the overproduction of reactive oxygen species and the 7KC-induced drop in mitochondrial transmembrane potential ($\Delta\Psi m$) measured by flow cytometry after dihydroethidium and $DiOC_6(3)$ staining, respectively. Moreover, the studied polyphenols and fatty acids reduced plasma membrane permeability considered as a criterion for cell death measured by flow cytometry after propidium iodide staining. Our data show that polyphenols (RSV, QCT and API) as well as ω3 and ω9 unsaturated fatty acids (ALA, EPA, DHA and OA) are potent cytoprotective agents against 7KC-induced neurotoxicity in N2a cells. Their cytoprotective effects could partly explain the benefits of the Mediterranean diet on human health, particularly in the prevention of neurodegenerative diseases.

Keywords: apigenin; docosahexaenoic acid; eicosapentaenoic acid; 7-ketocholesterol; α-linolenic acid; Mediterranean diet; N2a cells; oleic acid; oxidative stress; quercetin; resveratrol.

1. Introduction

In Parkinson's and Alzheimer's disease, protein aggregation and mitochondrial dysfunction are two factors that promote oxidative stress, which is considered a major element in the evolution of these diseases [1]. In Parkinson's disease, at the level of *substancia nigra pars compacta*, α-synuclein aggregates (Lewy bodies) induce a degeneration of dopaminergic neurons involving oxidative stress [1]. In Alzheimer's disease, the increase in oxidative stress mediated by β-amyloid protein aggregates (senile plaques) in the hippocampus and cortex promotes excitotoxicity (pathological process by which nerve cells are damaged or killed by excessive stimulation by neurotransmitters) and synaptic degeneration leading to neurodegeneration [1]. Identifying natural or synthetic molecules that could prevent oxidative stress is therefore a part of therapeutic strategies for treatment of Parkinson's and Alzheimer's diseases. Among the molecules already identified are neuropeptides and natural antioxidants which have both antioxidant and/or anti-aggregation properties [1–3]. Furthermore, one of the consequences of oxidative stress is to promote the formation of lipid derivatives, including oxidized cholesterol derivatives (oxysterols) such as 7-ketocholesterol (7KC, also named 7-oxocholesterol) and 7β-hydroxycholesterol [4–6], which contribute to amplifying the oxidative stress that promotes inflammation and cell death, two other important components of neurodegeneration [7]. Preventing the toxicity of these oxysterols, particularly the predominantly formed 7KC, is also part of the pharmacological options for preventing neurodegeneration and more specifically Alzheimer's disease [8]. Indeed, in post-mortem samples of the brain from Alzheimer's disease patients, significant increases in 7KC have been identified in different areas from the frontal and occipital cortex [9]. In Parkinson's disease, because of the oxidative stress present in the lesions, the contribution of 7KC is very probable [10]. Among the oxysterols associated with different diseases, 7KC is mainly increased in body fluids and lesions in age-related diseases (cardiovascular diseases, ocular diseases, Alzheimer's disease, some cancers), in inflammatory bowel diseases and in some rare diseases (Niemann Pick's disease, Smith Lemli Opitz syndrome and X-linked adrenoleukodystrophy (X-ALD)) [6,11]. Currently, various studies have shown a reduced risk of developing age-related diseases in people with a Mediterranean diet characterized by an important consumption in fruits and vegetables containing many polyphenols as well as fishes (sardines, mackerel, tuna) rich in ω3 and ω9 unsaturated fatty acids [12–14]. This suggests that nutrients present in the Mediterranean diet (polyphenols, fatty acids) could have cytoprotective effects against 7KC.

At the moment, only few data are available on the ability of polyphenols and fatty acids to prevent 7KC-induced cytotoxicity. The cytoprotective activities of polyphenols in the context of 7KC-induced toxicity involving oxidative stress that can lead to cell death, take into account their antioxidant activities linked to their chemical structures, but also their ability to act on the mitochondria by stimulating mitochondrial proliferation and activity [12,13]. Moreover, neurotrophic activities of several polyphenols are also described due to cytoprotective capacities (ability to prevent oxidative stress and cell death) associated with differentiating capacities on different types of cells [15]. Thus, on N2a cells, resveratrol (RSV) and apigenin (API) protect against hydrogen peroxide (H_2O_2)-induced cell death and also promote neuronal differentiation by stimulating the growth of neurites (dendrites and axons) [16,17]. Because of their neurotrophic properties, polyphenols such as RSV, QCT and API are therefore suitable molecules for counteracting neurodegeneration by preventing oxidative stress and stimulating neurogenesis [15,17]. When an oxysterols mixture containing 7α-hydroxycholesterol, 7β-hydroxycholesterol, 7-KC, cholesterol 5α,6α-epoxide, cholesterol 5β,6β-epoxide, cholestane-3β,5α,6β-triol and 25-hydroxycholesterol was used on human colon adenocarcinoma cells (Caco-2) [18] or human peripheral blood mononuclear cells [19], protective effects of cocoa bean shells containing a high level of epicatechin, and of olive oil polyphenols were observed, respectively. When differentiated murine PC12 cells and human neuroblastoma SH-SY5Y cells were treated with taxifolin (dihydroquercetin), it was also shown that 7KC-induced neuronal apoptosis was prevented [20]. On human retinal ARPE-19 cells, 7KC-induced cell death was also attenuated by RSV [21]. However, nothing is known on the ability of polyphenols to prevent 7KC-induced oxidative stress in murine N2a neuronal cells frequently used as pharmacological model in the context of neurodegenerative diseases [16,22]. So, we choose three polyphenols, which are widely represented in the Mediterrannean diet: RSV, QCT and API [12]. Among polyphenols, two classes are distinguished: Flavonoids and non-flavonoids [23]. Resveratrol (RSV; including trans-RSV which is biologically active) is a non-flavonoid; it is a member of the stilbenoid class of polyphenols; QCT (flavonol) and API (flavone) belong to the flavonoids class. RSV is mainly found in grapes, blackberries, peanuts and red wine. QCT and API are ubiquitously distributed in plant kingdom. QCT is present in lot of fruits and vegetables, and API in parsley, rosemary, celery and chamomile. Importantly, since polyphenols have the ability of interacting with the underlying pathomechanisms of several diseases associated with increased levels of 7KC, it was important to determine whether some of them (RSV, QCT and API) were able to prevent 7KC-induced cytotoxic effects, mainly reactive oxygen species (ROS) overproduction and mitochondrial dysfunction [8]. Although the ability of polyphenols to cross the blood-brain barrier is considered weak and remains still poorly understood [24,25], the intranasal administration of polyphenols (including RSV, QCT and API) has been proven effective to deliver these drugs to the brain while maintaining their activity [26].

As for fatty acids, the choice of these molecules to prevent the toxicity of 7KC takes into account their different and complementary properties from those of polyphenols. Compared to polyphenols, fatty acids do not by themselves have antioxidant properties. On the other hand, when they are added to cells on which oxidative stress is stimulated by some oxysterols, they can prevent oxidative stress as well as organelle dysfunction (mitochondria, lysosome and peroxisome) contributing to cell death [1]. Currently, only few lipids or lipid mixtures (oils) have been shown to be effective in preventing 7KC-induced ROS overproduction. These are α-tocopherol [27], ω3 and ω9 fatty acids (oleic acid (OA; C18:1 n-9) [28,29], and docosahexaenoic acid (DHA; C22:6 n-3)) [30,31]. In addition, several oils (argan oil, olive oil and milk thistle seed oil), which are rich in α-tocopherol and OA, have also shown cytoprotective effects against 7KC: they prevent organelle dysfunction, ROS overproduction and cell death [32]. While the cytoprotective mechanism of α-tocopherol can be explained at least in part by its ability to prevent the accumulation of 7KC in the lipid rafts [27,33], little is known on the cytoprotection of OA and DHA against 7KC. It can be assumed that they could both neutralize 7KC by esterification [34,35] and act by reducing oxidative stress and mitochondrial dysfunction leading to cell death [36,37]. Thus, in human U937 monocytic cells, while 7KC and 7β-OHC induce a type of death by apoptosis associated with oxidative stress and autophagic criteria, 7KC-oleate and 7β-OHC-oleate are not cytotoxic [35]. A major reason for the cytoprotective effects of fatty acids present in the Mediterranean diet could be the prevention of 7KC-induced plasma membrane destabilization which could lead to inactivation of the PDK1/Akt pathway resulting in the activation of GSK3 allowing the phosphorylation of Mcl-1 and the inhibition of sequestration in the cytoplasm of the pro-apoptotic molecules Bak and Bax; the latter could then interact with the mitochondrial membrane and contribute to inducing the drop in mitochondrial transmembrane potential ($\Delta\Psi m$) activating apoptosis [38]. Furthermore, it is well recognized that DHA present in phospholipids in the sn-2 position can lead to the formation of the highly anti-apoptotic neuroprotectin D1 (NPD1) [39]. Furthermore, it is known that 7KC modifies the fluidity of the plasma membrane by intercalating between phospholipids [40]. Preventing 7KC-induced plasma membrane disorganization by using fatty acids associated with the Mediterranean diet is therefore a promising avenue to counter 7KC toxicity. The interest of fatty acids comes from their ability to pass the blood-brain barrier and accumulate in the brain; for DHA, several mechanisms associated with crossing the blood-brain barrier have been described [41]. As OA and DHA, which are present in significant amounts in the Mediterranean diet, can be used in functional foods and dietary supplements, it is therefore important to have more information on these molecules, as well as on the precursors of DHA (α-linolenic acid (ALA/C18:3 n-3) and eicosapentaenoic acid (EPA/C20:5 n-3)) which are present in significant amount in several Mediterranean fishes and oils.

In the present study, we evaluated and compared for the first time the cytoprotective effects of polyphenols (RSV, QCT and API) and fatty acids (OA, ALA, EPA, and DHA) on 7KC-treated N2a neuronal cells which are considered as a relevant model to characterize the toxicity of different compounds and to identify natural or synthetic molecules with cytoprotective activities that could give rise to pharmacological applications. The effects of these compounds were compared with those of α-tocopherol (the main component of Vitamin E constituted of four tocopherols and four tocotrienols) as the reference cytoprotective molecule. Our data show that nutrients (polyphenols, ω3 and ω9 unsaturated fatty acids) present at high amount in the Mediterranean diet have the ability to attenuate 7KC-induced ROS overproduction and cell death reinforcing the interest of the Mediterranean diet and some of its compounds for the prevention of certain age-related diseases such as neurodegenerative diseases.

2. Results

2.1. Effects of Polyphenols (Resveratrol, Quercetin, Apigenin), ω3 and ω9 Unsaturated Fatty Acids (α-Linolenic Acid, Eicosapentaenoic Acid, Docosahexaenoic Acid, Oleic Acid) and 7-Ketocholesterol on Cell Viability Evaluated with the Fluorescein Diacetate Assay

Whereas the polyphenols are known for their anti-oxidant properties, it is also well established that some of them have cytotoxic properties [42]. It is also known that several fatty acids can be toxic for several tissues, especially liver [43]. So, before to simultaneously treat N2a cells for 48 h with 7KC associated with polyphenols (RSV, QCT or API) or ω3 and ω9 unsaturated fatty acids (ALA, EPA, DHA and OA), it was important to evaluate the toxicity of these different compounds. Therefore, first of all, it was necessary to evaluate the cytotoxicity of studied compounds on N2a cells. To this end, the widely used fluorescein diacetate (FDA) assay, based on the measurement of esterase activity, was chosen to determine the cell viability. Comparatively to untreated cells, in a range of concentrations from 1.5 to 50 µM, significant cytotoxic effects were observed with trans-resveratrol (RSV) at 12.5, 25 and 50 µM (Figure 1A) and with QCT at 25 and 50 µM (Figure 1B) whereas no cytotoxic effects were found with API (Figure 1C). With RSV used at 6.25 µM, FDA activity was also decreased but the difference is not significant (Figure 1A); however, no decrease in FDA activity was observed with QCT and API used at this concentration (Figure 1B,C). In addition, comparatively to untreated cells, in a range of concentrations from 1.5 to 200 µM, significant cytotoxic effects were observed with ALA at 200 µM (Figure 2A), with EPA at 100, 150 and 200 µM (Figure 2B), with DHA at 100, 150 and 200 µM (Figure 2C), and with OA at 150 µM (Figure 2D). On the other hand, stimulating effects of the esterase activity revealed by the FDA assay were observed with ALA (25 µM) (Figure 2A), EPA (6.25 and 12.5 µM) (Figure 2B) and OA (25 µM) (Figure 2D). With 7KC used in a range of concentrations from 1.5 to 100 µM for 48 h, the 50% inhibiting concentration (IC50) was around 50 µM (Supplementary Figure S1). Consequently, for further experiments, 7KC was therefore used at 50 µM, and among the concentrations of polyphenols and fatty acids chosen to assess cytoprotection, concentrations less than or equal to 6.25 µM, and 25 or 50 µM were used, respectively.

2.2. Evaluation with the Fluorescein Diacetate Assay of the Effects of Polyphenols (Resveratrol, Quercetin, Apigenin), ω3 and ω9 Unsaturated Fatty Acids (α-Linolenic Acid, Eicosapentaenoic Acid, Docosahexaenoic Acid, Oleic Acid) and α-Tocopherol on 7-Ketocholesterol-Induced Cytotoxicity

When 7KC (50 µM) was simultaneously incubated with the polyphenols (RSV, QCT or API; concentrations ≤6.25 µM, 48 h), the decrease of FDA positive cells observed under treatment with 7KC was strongly attenuated especially at 3.125 and 6.25 µM (Figure 1D–F). Similarly, when 7KC (50 µM) was simultaneously incubated with the ω9 and ω3 fatty acids (ALA, EPA, DHA and OA; concentrations ≤50 µM, 48 h), the decrease of FDA positive cells observed under treatment with 7KC was strongly attenuated especially at 12.5 and 25 µM whatever the fatty acid considered (Figure 2E–H). In the presence of α-tocopherol (400 µM), used as a reference to prevent 7KC-induced cell damages, cytoprotective effects were also found (Figure 1D–F; Figure 2E–H). Consequently, for further experiments, polyphenols have been used at 3.125 and 6.25 µM, and fatty acids at 12.5 and 25 µM.

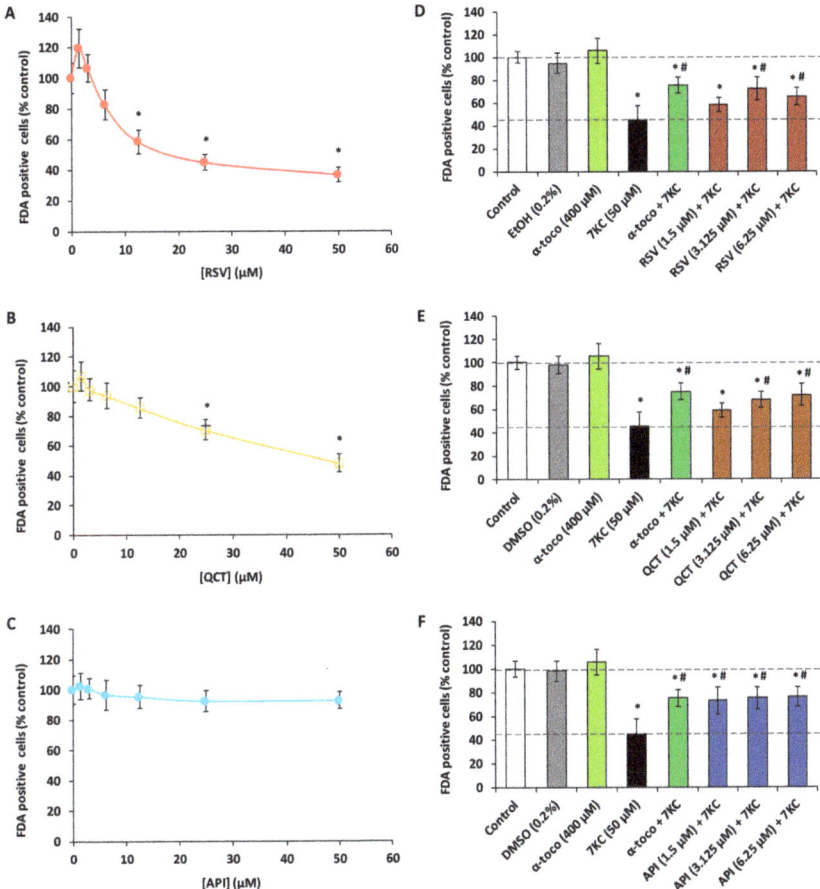

Figure 1. Evaluation with the fluorescein diacetate (FDA) assay of the effects of polyphenols (resveratrol, quercetin and apigenin) with and without 7-ketocholesterol on cell viability of N2a cells. Murine neuroblastoma N2a cells, previously cultured for 24 h, were further cultured for 48 h with or without resveratrol (RSV), quercetin (QCT), apigenin (API) in the presence or absence of 7-ketocholesterol (7KC; 50 µM). Polyphenols concentrations used alone range from 1.5 to 50 µM (**A–C**). Polyphenols were used at concentrations ≤6.25 µM when associated with 7KC (50 µM) (**D–F**). α-tocopherol (400 µM) was used as positive reference to prevent 7KC-induced cell death. The results are expressed in percentages relatively to the control (untreated cells). Data obtained with the FDA assay are shown. Data shown are expressed as mean ± standard deviation (SD) of four independent experiments performed in triplicate. Significance of the differences between control (untreated cells) and RSV-, QCT-, API-, α-toco or 7KC-treated cells; Mann Whitney test: * $P < 0.05$ or less. Significance of the differences between 7KC-treated cells and (7KC + (RSV, QCT, API or α-toco))-treated cells; Mann Whitney test: # $P < 0.05$ or less. No significant differences were found between control and vehicle-treated cells (ethanol (EtOH) and DMSO).

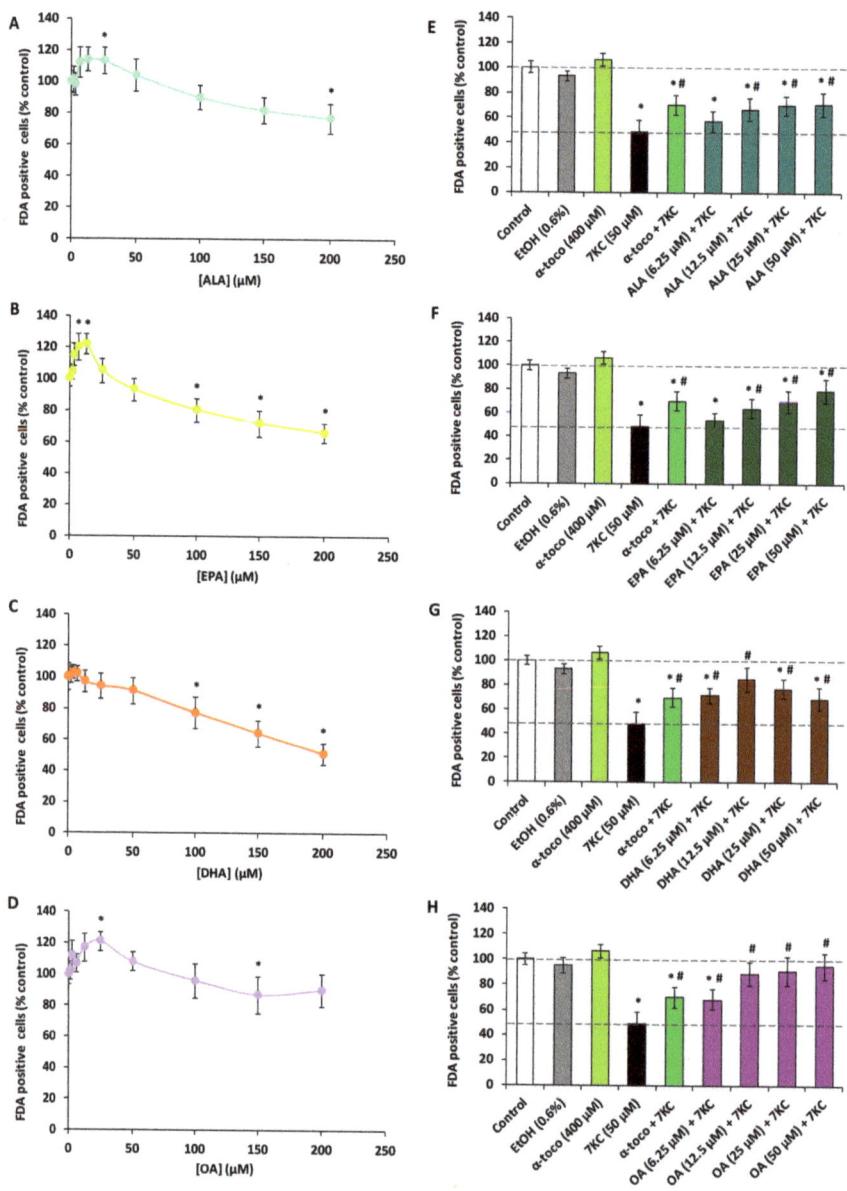

Figure 2. Evaluation with the fluorescein diacetate (FDA) assay of the effects of ω3 and ω9 unsaturated fatty acids (α-linolenic acid, eicosapentaenoic acid, docosahexaenoic acid and oleic acid) with and without 7-ketocholesterol on cell viability of N2a cells. Murine neuroblastoma N2a cells, previously cultured for 24 h, were further cultured for 48 h with or without α-linolenic acid (ALA), eicosapentaenoic acid (EPA), docosahexaenoic acid (DHA) or oleic acid (OA) in the presence or absence of 7-ketocholesterol (7KC; 50 μM). Fatty acids concentrations used alone range from 1.5 to 200 μM (**A–D**). Fatty acids were used at concentrations ≤50 μM when associated with 7KC (50 μM) (**E–H**). α-tocopherol (α-toco; 400 μM)

was used as positive reference to prevent 7KC-induced cell death. The results are expressed in percentages relatively to the control (untreated cells). Data obtained with the FDA assay are shown. Data shown are expressed as mean ± standard deviation (SD) of four independent experiments performed in triplicate. Significance of the differences between control (untreated cells) and ALA-, EPA-, DHA-, OA-, α-toco or 7KC-treated cells; Mann Whitney test: * $P < 0.05$ or less. Significance of the differences between 7KC-treated cells and (7KC + (ALA, EPA, DHA, OA or α-toco))-treated cells; Mann Whitney test: # $P < 0.05$ or less. No significant differences were found between control and vehicle-treated cells (Ethanol (EtOH)).

2.3. Evaluation of the Effects of Polyphenols (Resveratrol, Quercetin, Apigenin), ω3 and ω9 Unsaturated Fatty Acids (α-Linolenic Acid, Eicosapentaenoic Acid, Docosahexaenoic Acid, Oleic Acid) and α-Tocopherol on 7-Ketocholesterol-Induced Reactive Oxygen Species (ROS) Overproduction

In N2a cells, 7KC (50 µM, 48 h) induces an overproduction of ROS which results in an increase in HE positive cells (Figures 3 and 4). Since the most significant cytoprotective effects with the FDA assay were observed with polyphenols at 3.125 and 6.25 µM and with fatty acids at 12.5 and 25 µM, the ability of polyphenols and fatty acids to reduce 7KC-induced overproduction of ROS was investigated at these concentrations. By flow cytometry, after DHE staining, a strong increase in the percentage of HE positive cells (cells overproducing superoxide anions) was observed in the presence of 7KC (Figures 3 and 4). The percentage of HE positive cells was significantly reduced by α-tocopherol (400 µM) used as positive control (Figures 3 and 4). This percentage was also significantly reduced in the presence of polyphenols (RSV, QCT, API) (Figure 3) and fatty acids (ALA, EPA, DHA, OA) (Figure 4A,B) demonstrating that these compounds attenuate the oxidative stress induced by 7KC. When used singularly, polyphenols (QCT, API) and fatty acids (ALA, EPA, DHA, OA) as well as α-tocopherol have no effect on the production of ROS; on the other hand, comparatively to untreated (control) and vehicle-treated cells, RSV (6.25 µM) slightly but significantly increases this production (Figures 3 and 4).

2.4. Evaluation of the Effects of ω3 and ω9 Unsaturated Fatty Acids (α-Linolenic Acid, Eicosapentaenoic Acid, Docosahexaenoic Acid, Oleic Acid) and α-Tocopherol on 7-Ketocholesterol-Induced Loss of Transmembrane Mitochondrial Potential and Cell Death

In N2a cells, 7KC (50 µM, 48 h) induces a loss of transmembrane mitochondrial potential ($\Delta\Psi m$) as well as increased permeability of plasma membrane to PI which is considered to enter dead cells only (Figures 5 and 6). Since the most significant cytoprotective effects with the FDA assay were observed with polyphenols at 3.125 and 6.25 µM and with fatty acids at 12.5 and 25 µM, the ability of polyphenols and fatty acids to prevent 7KC-induced loss of $\Delta\Psi m$ and cell death was investigated at these concentrations (Figures 5 and 6). By flow cytometry, after $DiOC_6(3)$ staining, a strong increase in the percentage of $DiOC_6(3)$ negative cells (cells with low $\Delta\Psi m$) was observed in the presence of 7KC (Figures 5 and 6). In the presence of (QCT, API) and fatty acids (ALA, EPA, DHA and OA) as well as α-tocopherol no effect on $\Delta\Psi m$ was observed whereas with RSV (6.25 µM) a slight but significant increase in the percentage of $DiOC_6(3)$ negative cells (cells with low $\Delta\Psi m$) was found (Figures 5 and 6). The percentage of $DiOC_6(3)$ negative cells was significantly reduced by α-tocopherol (400 µM) used as positive control (Figures 5 and 6). This percentage of $DiOC_6(3)$ negative cells was also significantly reduced in the presence of polyphenols (RSV, QCT, API) (Figure 5A–C) and fatty acids (ALA, EPA, DHA and OA) (Figure 6A–D) demonstrating that these compounds attenuate the loss of $\Delta\Psi m$ induced by 7KC.

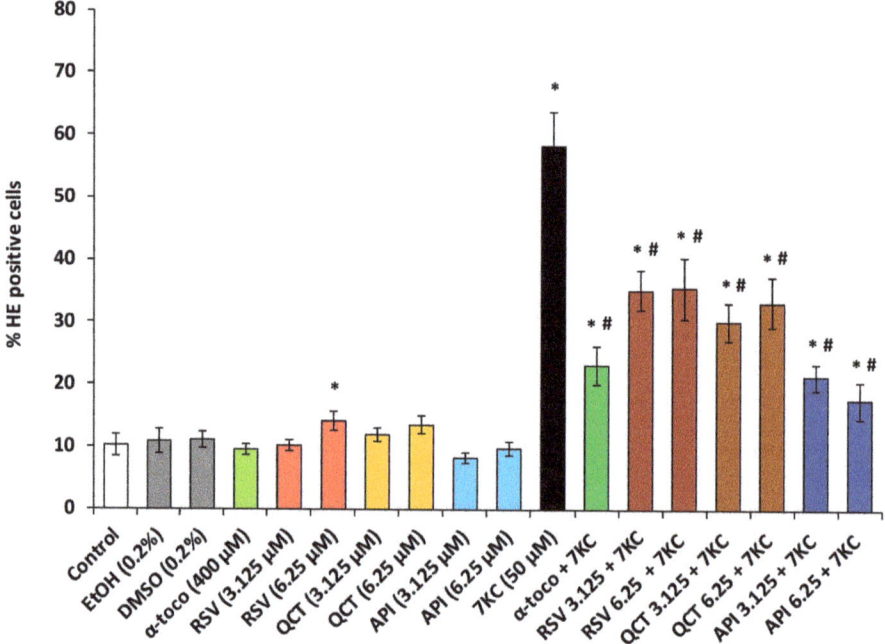

Figure 3. Effect of polyphenols (resveratrol, quercetin, apigenin) with and without 7-ketocholesterol on reactive oxygen species (ROS) overproduction. N2a cells, previously cultured for 24 h, were further cultured for 48 h with or without 7-ketocholesterol (7KC, 50 µM) in the presence or absence of polyphenols: resveratrol (RSV), quercetin (QCT) or apigenin (API) used at a concentration of 3.125 and/or 6.25 µM. α-tocopherol (α-toco; 400 µM) was used as positive reference to prevent 7KC-induced cell death. ROS overproduction was measured by flow cytometry after staining with dihydroethidine (DHE) and evaluated by the percentage of HE positive cells. Data shown are mean ± standard deviation (SD) of three independent experiments conducted in triplicate. Significance of the differences between control (untreated cells) and RSV-, QCT-, API-, α-toco- or 7KC-treated cells; Mann Whitney test: * $P < 0.05$ or less. Significance of the differences between 7KC-treated cells and (7KC + (RSV, QCT, API or α-toco))-treated cells; Mann Whitney test: # $P < 0.05$ or less. No significant differences were found between control and vehicle-treated cells (Ethanol (EtOH) and DMSO).

In addition, by flow cytometry, after PI staining, a strong increase in the percentage of PI positive cells (cells with a loss of plasma membrane integrity considered as dead cells) was observed in the presence of 7KC (Figures 5 and 6). The percentage of PI positive cells was also significantly reduced by α-tocopherol (400 µM) used as positive control (Figures 5 and 6). This percentage of PI positive cells was also significantly reduced in the presence of polyphenols (RSV, QCT and API) (Figure 5D–F) and fatty acids (ALA, EPA, DHA and OA) (Figure 6E–H) demonstrating that these dietary compounds attenuate 7KC-induced cell death which is associated with plasma membrane alterations. Noteworthy, when used singularly, API (3.125 and 6.25 µM) and fatty acids (ALA, EPA, DHA and OA) (12.5 and 25 µM) as well as α-tocopherol (400 µM) have no effect on plasma membrane integrity whereas RSV and QCT (6.25 µM) slightly but significantly increase the % of PI positive cells indicating an effect of these molecules on plasma membrane integrity (Figures 5 and 6).

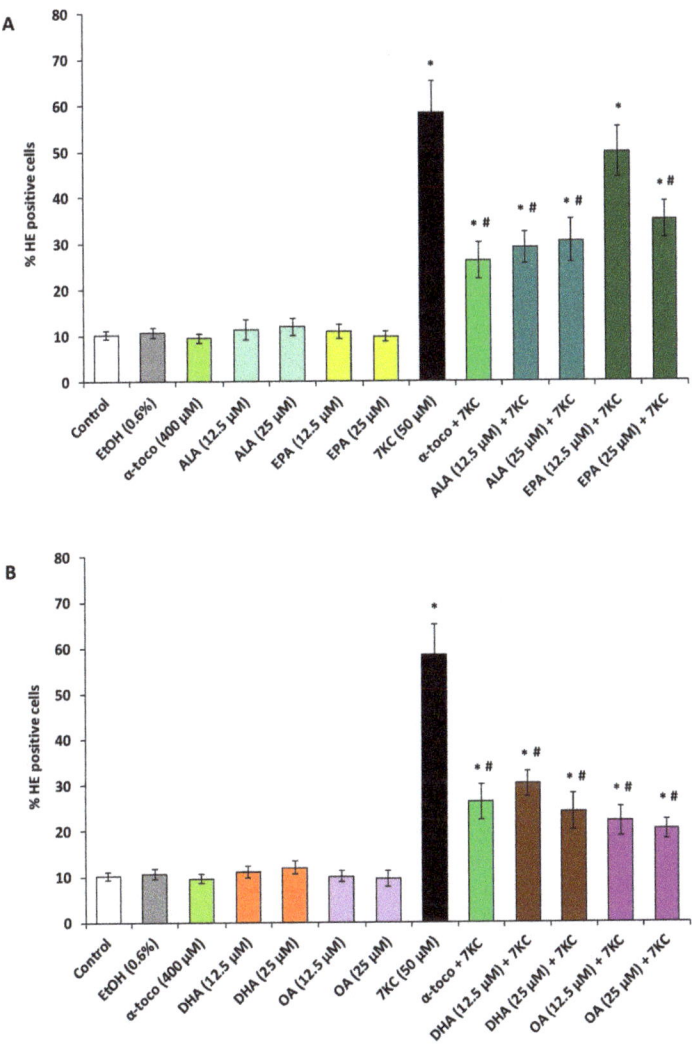

Figure 4. Effect of ω3 and ω9 unsaturated fatty acids (α-linolenic acid, eicosapentaenoic acid, docosahexaenoic acid and oleic acid) with and without 7-ketocholesterol on reactive oxygen species (ROS) overproduction. N2a cells, previously cultured for 24 h, were further cultured for 48 h with or without 7-ketocholesterol (7KC, 50 μM) in the presence or absence of α-linolenic acid (ALA), eicosapentaenoic acid (EPA), docosahexaenoic acid (DHA) or oleic acid (OA) used at a concentration of 12.5 and 25 μM. α-tocopherol (α-toco; 400 μM) was used as positive reference to prevent 7KC-induced cell death. ROS overproduction was measured by flow cytometry after staining with dihydroethidine (DHE) and evaluated by the percentage of HE positive cells (**A**): data obtained with ALA and EPA are shown; (**B**): data obtained with DHA and OA are shown). Data shown are mean ± standard deviation (SD) of three independent experiments conducted in triplicate. Significance of the differences between control (untreated cells) and ALA-, EPA-, DHA-, OA-, α-toco- or 7KC-treated cells; Mann Whitney test: * $P < 0.05$ or less. Significance of the differences between 7KC-treated cells and (7KC + (ALA, EPA, DHA, OA or α-toco))-treated cells; Mann Whitney test: # $P < 0.05$ or less. No significant differences were found between control and vehicle-treated cells (Ethanol (EtOH)).

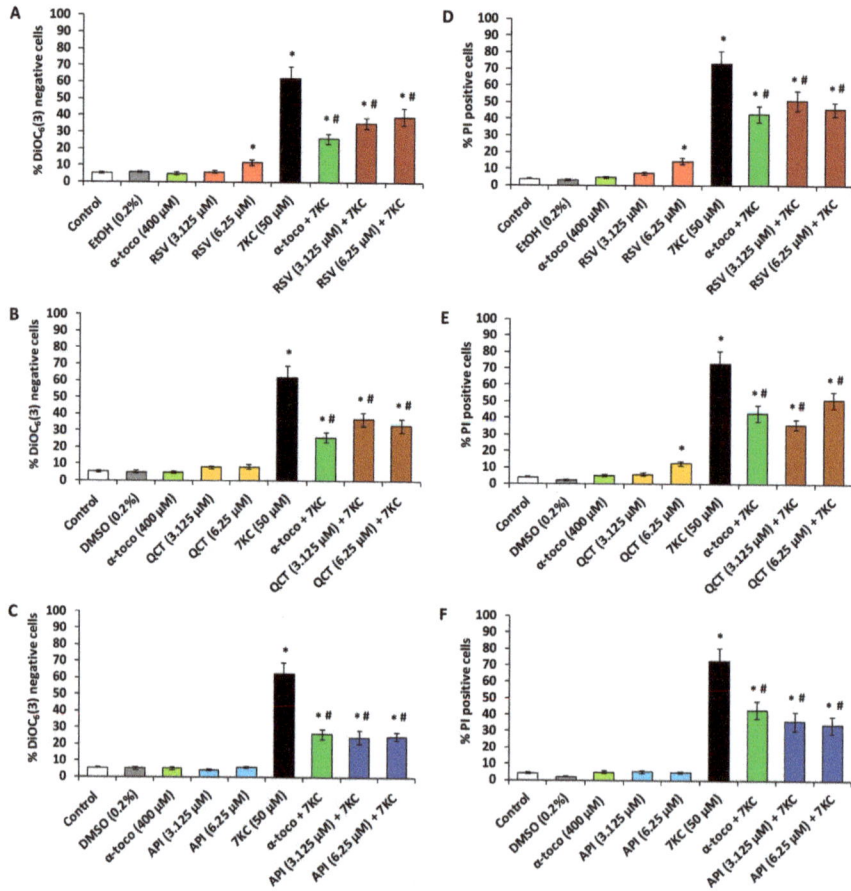

Figure 5. Effect of polyphenols (resveratrol, quercetin, apigenin) with and without 7-ketocholesterol on mitochondrial transmembrane potential (ΔΨm) and plasma membrane permeability. N2a cells, previously cultured for 24 h, were further cultured for 48 h with or without 7-ketocholesterol (7KC, 50 µM) in the presence or absence of polyphenols: resveratrol (RSV), quercetin (QCT) or apigenin (API) used at a concentration of 3.125 and/or 6.25 µM. α-tocopherol (α-toco; 400 µM) was used as positive reference to prevent 7KC-induced cell death. Loss of transmembrane mitochondrial potential (ΔΨm) was measured by flow cytometry after staining with $DiOC_6(3)$ and evaluated by the percentage of $DiOC_6(3)$ negative cells (**A–C**). Plasma membrane permeability was measured by flow cytometry after staining with propidium iodide (PI): for each assay, the percentage of PI positive cells was determined (**D–F**). Data shown are mean ± standard deviation (SD) of three independent experiments conducted in triplicate. Significance of the differences between control (untreated cells) and RSV-, QCT-, API-, α-toco- or 7KC-treated cells; Mann Whitney test: * $P < 0.05$ or less. Significance of the differences between 7KC-treated cells and (7KC + (RSV, QCT, API or α-toco))-treated cells; Mann Whitney test: # $P < 0.05$ or less. No significant differences were found between control and vehicle-treated cells (Ethanol (EtOH) and DMSO).

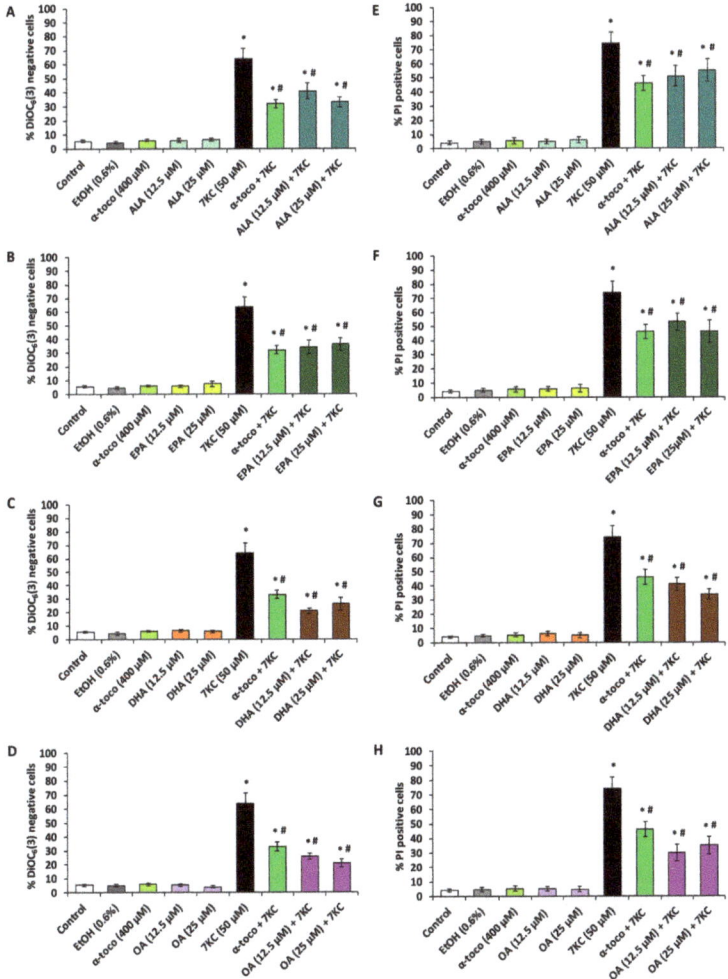

Figure 6. Effect of ω3 and ω9 unsaturated fatty acids (α-linolenic acid, eicosapentaenoic acid, docosahexaenoic acid and oleic acid) with and without 7-ketocholesterol on mitochondrial transmembrane potential (ΔΨm) and plasma membrane permeability. N2a cells, previously cultured for 24 h, were further cultured for 48 h with or without 7-ketocholesterol (7KC, 50 µM) in the presence or absence of α-linolenic acid (ALA), eicosapentaenoic acid (EPA), docosahexaenoic acid (DHA) or oleic acid (OA) used at a concentration of 12.5 and 25 µM. α-tocopherol (α-toco; 400 µM) was used as positive reference to prevent 7KC-induced cell death. Loss of transmembrane mitochondrial potential (ΔΨm) was measured by flow cytometry after staining with DiOC$_6$(3) and evaluated by the percentage of DiOC$_6$(3) negative cells (**A–D**). Plasma membrane permeability was measured by flow cytometry after staining with propidium iodide (PI): for each assay, the percentage of PI positive cells was determined (**E–H**). Data shown are mean ± standard deviation (SD) of three independent experiments conducted in triplicate. Significance of the differences between control (untreated cells) and ALA-, EPA-, DHA-, OA-, α-toco- or 7KC-treated cells; Mann Whitney test: * $P < 0.05$ or less. Significance of the differences between 7KC-treated cells and (7KC + (ALA, EPA, DHA, OA or α-toco))-treated cells; Mann Whitney test: # $P < 0.05$ or less. No significant differences were found between control and vehicle-treated cells (Ethanol (EtOH)).

3. Discussion

Preventing the 7KC cytotoxicity by means of nutrients present in the Mediterranean diet (polyphenols, fatty acids) could be a means to counteract several diseases associated with oxidative stress leading to increased levels of 7KC mainly formed by cholesterol auto-oxidation [6,44]. In the present study, we showed that 7KC-induced cytotoxicity on murine neuronal N2a cells is characterized by ROS overproduction, alteration of plasma membrane, and drop of transmembrane mitochondrial potential ($\Delta \Psi m$) leading to cell death. As the Mediterranean diet is rich in polyphenols, which are potent antioxidant molecules, we asked whether some of them such as RSV, QCT and API, could prevent the cytotoxic effects of 7KC. We also asked whether some fatty acids which are abundant in the Mediterranean diet (ALA, EPA, DHA and OA) and which are known to improve some brain functions, mainly cognition [45], were also able to prevent 7KC-induced cell death. Our results obtained with the polyphenols (RSV, QCT and API), and with $\omega 3$ and $\omega 9$ fatty acids (ALA, EPA, DHA and OA) on N2a cells show that these molecules are powerful cytoprotectors against 7KC-induced cytotoxicity: they strongly attenuate 7KC-induced ROS overproduction, alteration of plasma membrane, and loss of $\Delta \Psi m$ causing cell death.

As it was previously reported on microglial and glial cells (murine oligodendrocytes 158N and murine microglial BV-2 cells that 7KC triggers cell death [8,37], we asked whether similar effects were observed on N2a cells. In agreement with data obtained on 158N and BV-2 cells, our data demonstrate that 7KC (50 µM, 48 h of treatment) is a strong inducer of cell death on N2a cells. Whereas no significant cytotoxic effects were observed with 7KC used at 1.5625, 3.125, 6.25, 12.5 and 25 µM, significant cytotoxic effects were observed at 50 and 100 µM with the FDA assay (evaluating esterase activity). In those conditions, after 48 h of culture of N2a cells with 7KC, the IC50 value of this oxysterol was 50 µM. So, the cell characteristics of 7KC-induced cell death were determined at this concentration. Also, in agreement with the abovementioned study on 158N and BV-2 cells, adding 7KC induced alterations of plasma membrane (decreased esterase activity measured by FDA, and increased permeability to PI) which could be at least in part the consequence of ROS overproduction measured with DHE. ROS overproduction in 7KC-treated human aortic smooth muscle cells and on human red blood cells is mediated by an upregulation of Nox-4, a ROS-generating NAD(P)H oxidase homologue [46], and is considered as a consequence of NADPH oxidase activation through a signaling mechanism including Rac GTPase and PKCζ [47], respectively. This important oxidative stress could also favor the drop of $\Delta \Psi m$ observed under treatment with 7KC. Our data confirm that ROS overproduction and loss of $\Delta \Psi m$ are general features associated with 7KC-induced cell death whatever the cells considered [6,8,37]. Thus, it is likely, that molecules which are able to prevent 7KC-induced toxicity in one cell type will also be effective in other cell types.

In the presence of 7KC, the highly conserved cell death characteristics from one type of cell to another may have important consequences for preventing the diseases associated with 7KC. It can thus be assumed that molecules capable of opposing the cytotoxicity of 7KC on N2a cells would also be capable to counteract the cytotoxicity of 7KC on other brain cells (glial and microglial cells) and on other cell types which can be exposed to high levels of 7KC (retinal and vascular cells). This hypothesis is partly validated by the use of α-tocopherol (400 µM) as a positive cytoprotective control in this study, which strongly reduces the cytotoxicity of 7KC not only on N2a but also on 158N oligodendrocytes and BV-2 microglial cells as well as many other cell types [8,37]. It can therefore be assumed that the cytoprotection observed on N2a with polyphenols (RSV, QCT, API at concentrations ≤ 6.25 µM) and fatty acids (ALA, EPA, DHA, OA at concentrations ≤ 50 µM) associated with the Mediterranean diet would present similar characteristics on other brain cells as those observed on N2a cells.

In order to inhibit or reduce 7KC-induced cell death and based on the signaling pathways of which have been described by Vejux et al. [37], we have chosen to use synthetic and natural molecules as well as mixtures of molecules [8]. To date, only few molecules have proved effective in opposing the cytotoxic effects of 7KC on nerve cells defined as oxiapoptophagy (OXIdative stress + APOPTOsis + autoPHAGY) based on data obtained on 158N murine oligodendrocytes and murine microglial BV-2 cells [48–50]. Among the synthetic molecules are two activators of the Nrf2 pathway, dimethyl fumarate (DMF) and its major metabolite, monomethyl fumarate (MMF), which have shown cytoprotective effects on 158N cells [51]. Some lipids, such as α-tocopherol, OA and DHA have also cytoprotective activities against 7KC: they prevent oxidative stress, mitochondrial dysfunction (loss of $\Delta\Psi m$), peroxisomal changes, apoptosis and autophagy [8]. α-tocopherol, which prevents the accumulation of 7KC in the lipid rafts, inhibits the cascade of events leading to cell death [27,33].

Until now, there is no study on the effects of polyphenols (RSV, QCT and API) on 7KC-induced cell death on N2a neuronal cells. The present work demonstrates for the first time cytoprotective activities of some polyphenols (RSV, QCT and API) associated with the Mediterranean diet on 7KC-induced cell death and reinforces the interest of polyphenols to prevent 7KC-induced neurotoxicity. Indeed, on N2a cells, our data clearly show that RSV, QCT and API attenuate 7KC-induced ROS overproduction, plasma membrane alteration and drop of $\Delta\Psi m$ leading to cell death. The cytoprotective effects of RSV, QCT and API were studied at concentrations ≤6.25 µM because at higher concentrations a decrease of esterase activity was observed with RSV and QCT on N2a cells. These cytotoxic effects including decrease activity of esterase associated or not with ROS overproduction, loss of $\Delta\Psi m$ and/or increased plasma membrane permeability, which can affect cell viability, are probably related to the anti-tumor activities described with several polyphenols including RSV and QCT [52]. In contrast, API up to 50 µM does not induce cell death. Due to its lack of cytotoxicity on N2a cells, API therefore appears to be a better candidate than RSV and QCT to prevent 7KC-induced cell death. Despite these differences in toxicity, at concentrations of 3.125 and 6.25 µM, all the three polyphenols, RSV, QCT and API, have similar cytoprotective effects against 7KC and are as efficient as α-tocopherol used at 400 µM.

Currently, as it is the case with polyphenols, the cytoprotective activities of ω3 and ω9 fatty acids (ALA, EPA, DHA and OA), present in large amount in the Mediterranean diet, on the neurotoxicity of 7KC are still not well known. We however previously reported on 158N murine oligodendrocytes and murine microglial BV-2 cells that 7KC-induced oxidative stress, mitochondrial dysfunction and cell death by oxiapoptophagy were strongly attenuated with DHA and OA as well as with argan, olive and milk thistle seed oils which are rich in α-tocopherol and OA [32]. In the present study, our data clearly show that ALA, EPA, DHA and OA also attenuate 7KC-induced ROS overproduction, plasma membrane alteration and drop of $\Delta\Psi m$ leading to cell death on N2a neuronal cells, thus bringing new elements reinforcing the interest of using ω3 and ω9 unsaturated fatty acids to prevent the neurotoxicity of 7KC. These cytoprotective effects of ω3 and ω9 fatty acids were found at concentrations (≤50 µM) higher than those identified with polyphenols (≤6.25 µM) but nevertheless lower than that obtained with α-tocopherol (400 µM). However, it is important to underline that at these concentrations ω3 and ω9 fatty acids do not show toxicity: They have no effects on esterase activity, ROS production and mitochondrial transmembrane potential ($\Delta\Psi m$). Thus, in N2a cells, ω3 and ω9 unsaturated fatty acids (ALA, EPA, DHA, OA) but also polyphenols (RSV, QCT, API) are therefore more efficient natural molecules than α-tocopherol, considered until now as the best natural reference molecule to prevent 7KC toxicity. The ability of these polyphenols and fatty acids associated with the Mediterranean to prevent 7KC-induced cell damages reinforces the value of the Mediterranean diet and its associated nutrients in preventing neurodegeneration.

Since polyphenols (RSV, QCT, API) as well as ω3 and ω9 unsaturated fatty acids (ALA, EPA, DHA and OA) have similar cytoprotective effects on 7KC-induced toxicity and reduce plasma membrane alteration, ROS overproduction and drop in $\Delta\Psi m$, pharmacological targets that are otherwise common but lead to the same effects should be sought. Based on the cytoprotective effects observed with natural and synthetic molecules [8], RSV, QCT and API as well as ALA, EPA, DHA, and OA could reduce the overproduction of ROS via the Nrf2 pathway and by acting on the activation of NADPH-oxidase. Since (RSV, QCT, API), and ω3 and ω9 fatty acids can activate the nuclear Liver X Receptors (LXRs) [53] and Peroxisome Proliferator-Activated Receptors (PPARs) [54], respectively, cytoprotection resulting from gene activation, which could be evaluated by transcriptomic analysis, is also possible. In order to link the cytoprotective activity of polyphenols and fatty acids from the plasma membrane to the mitochondria, an action at the PI3-K/PDK1/Akt/GSK3 pathway is possible. Preserving the functionality of this pathway makes it possible to link plasma membrane signaling to mitochondrial activity. This hypothesis has moreover been validated on U937 cells treated with 7KC associated or not with α-tocopherol [27,38].

In conclusion, on N2a cells, 7KC induces cell damages (oxidative stress and mitochondrial dysfunction) associated with neurodegeneration on N2a cells which are strongly attenuated by polyphenols (RSV, QCT and API) and fatty acids (ALA, EPA, DHA and OA) present in large amounts in the Mediterranean diet. These data provide new evidence in favor of 7KC as a potential risk factor for neurodegeneration and shows the capacity of some nutrients (polyphenols, fatty acids) as well as α-tocopherol to prevent 7KC-induced cytotoxicity: ROS overproduction, loss of ΔΨm and cell death associated with enhanced plasma membrane permeability. This study also underlines the chemopreventive effects of phytochemicals against cell dysfunction caused by oxysterols [55]. On the other hand, in vitro, in order to enhance the cytoprotection, a combined use of these nutrients can be envisaged. In vivo, due to the likely and rapid degradation of these nutrients (elimination in the gastrointestinal tract, short plasma half-life) before reaching their target, various micro- and nano-encapsulation strategies protecting these nutrients without altering their cytoprotective activities could be considered for further studies [56,57]. Thus, when QCT is nanoencapsulated, it has been described to decrease the inflammation induced by various oxysterols on SH-SY5Y human neuronal cells [58]. As mitochondrial and ROS overproduction is a general feature of 7KC-induced cell death whatever the cells considered, it may be advisable to micro- or nano-encapsulate these nutrients in order to promote access to their therapeutic targets. In addition, the ability of polyphenols and fatty acids to strongly reduce the 7KC-induced drop in ΔΨm indicates that these nutrients are potentially suitable molecules for mitotherapy [59]. Associated a targeted mitotherapy using functionalized nanoparticles (Targeted Organel Nano-therapy: TORN therapy) [60,61] containing polyphenols as well as ω3 and/or ω9 unsaturated fatty acids could thus be envisaged to treat diseases associated with increased 7KC-levels.

4. Materials and Methods

4.1. Cell Culture and Treatments

The murine neuro-2a (N2a) neuroblastoma cell line (Ref: CCL-131; ATCC, Manassas, VA, USA) is maintained in Dulbecco's modified Eagle medium (DMEM, Lonza, Amboise, France) containing 10% (v/v) of heat-inactivated fetal bovine serum (FBS) (Pan Biotech, Aidenbach, Germany) (30 min, 56 °C) and 1% (v/v) of penicillin (100 U/mL) / streptomycin (100 mg/mL) (Pan Biotech). They were incubated at 37 °C in a humidified atmosphere (5% CO_2, 95% air) and passaged twice a week. The cells were seeded, for the different experimental conditions, at a density of 1.2×10^5 cells per well containing 1 mL of culture medium with 10% FBS in 6-well plates (FALCON, Becton Dickinson, Le Pont de Claix, France) or in Petri dishes at 30.000 cells/cm^2 (100 mm diameter) in order to assess the ability of polyphenols (trans-resveratrol (RSV), quercetin (QCT) and apigenin (API)) and fatty acids (α-linolenic acid (ALA/C18:3 n-3); eicosapentaenoic acid (EPA/C20:5 n-3); docosahexaenoic acid (DHA, C22:6 n-3); oleic acid (OA, C18:1 n-9)) to counteract the cytotoxicity induced by 7-ketocholesterol (7KC). 7KC (Ref: C2394), the polyphenols (RSV, QCT and API) and the fatty acids (ALA, DHA and OA) were from Sigma-Aldrich (St Quentin-Fallavier, France) whereas EPA was from Enzo Life Sciences (Villeurbanne, France). The stock solution of 7KC (800 µg/mL; 2 mM) was prepared in a mixture of absolute ethanol and culture medium (0.04, 0.96, v/v) as previously described [27]. The stock solutions of polyphenols were prepared as follows: RSV at 50 mM in absolute ethanol (EtOH; Carlo Erba Reagents, Val de Reuil, France), whereas dimethyl sulfoxide (DMSO; Sigma-Aldrich) was used as vehicle to dissolve QCT and API prepared at 50 mM. Fatty acids stock solutions were prepared at 50 mM (ALA, DHA, OA) or 200 mM (EPA) in absolute ethanol and stored at −20 °C. After 24 h of culture, the culture medium was removed and the cells were further incubated for an additional 48 h period of time with or without polyphenols or fatty acids associated or not with 7KC. Polyphenols (RSV, QCT and API) or fatty acids (ALA, EPA, DHA and OA) were used at concentrations ranging from 1.5 to 50 µM and from 1.5 to 200 µM, respectively, to determine their effects on cell viability. When associated with 7KC, polyphenols (RSV, QCT and API) and fatty acids (ALA, EPA, DHA and OA) were used at concentrations which have no impact on cell viability ranging from 1.5 to 6.25 µM and from 6.25 to 50 µM, respectively. The choice of the concentration of 7KC is based on the viability tests performed in this study which show that 50 µM is the 50% inhibiting concentration (IC50) for N2a cells (Supplementary Figure S1). α-tocopherol (Sigma-Aldrich) was used as a positive control for cytoprotection; the α-tocopherol solution was prepared at 80 mM in absolute ethanol and diluted in the culture medium to obtain a 400 µM final concentration. α-tocopherol was used at the highest non-cytotoxic concentration (400 µM) able to prevent 7KC-induced apoptosis [27].

4.2. Quantification of Cell Viability by the Fluorescein Diacetate (FDA) Assay

N2a cells viability was assessed using a lipophilic fluorochrome, fluorescein diacetate (FDA) (Sigma-Aldrich). In the presence of intracellular esterases of living cells, the non-fluorescent FDA is transformed into a green fluorescent metabolite "fluorescein" [16,22]. At the end of the treatment, cells were incubated in the dark with FDA (15 µg/mL, 5 min, 37 °C), washed twice with phosphate buffer saline (PBS 0.1 M, pH 7.4), and then lysed with 10 mM Tris-HCl solution containing 1% sodium dodecyl sulfate (SDS). Fluorescence intensity of fluorescein was measured with excitation at 485 nm and emission at 528 nm using a microplate reader (Sunrise spectrophotometer, TECAN, Lyon, France) in order to quantify living cells. All assays were performed in at least four independent experiments and realized in triplicate. The results were expressed as % of control: (Fluorescence (assay) × 100)/Fluorescence (control).

4.3. Flow Cytometric Evaluation of Reactive Oxygen Species (ROS) Production Using Dihydroethidium Staining

ROS overproduction, including the intracellular superoxide anion ($O_2^{\bullet-}$), was detected by dihydroethidium staining (DHE). DHE is a non-fluorescent probe capable of diffusing through the cell membranes; it is rapidly oxidized by ROS to fluorescent hydroethidium (HE) that exhibits an orange/red fluorescence (λ Ex max = 488 nm; λ Em max = 575nm). The HE intercalates at the DNA base level [62]. The stock solution of DHE (Invitrogen/Thermo Fisher Scientific, Courtaboeuf, France) was prepared in DMSO at a concentration of 10 mM and was subsequently used on the cells at a final concentration of 2 µM. N2a cells incubated for 48 h with or without 7KC in the presence or absence of polyphenols (RSV, QCT or API) or fatty acids (ALA, EPA, DHA, or OA) were trypsinized, washed and then suspended in 1 mL of 1X PBS containing DHE (2 µM). After 15 min of incubation at 37 °C, the analysis of stained cells was carried out by flow cytometry on a BD Accuri™ C6 flow cytometer. The fluorescence of HE was collected through a 580 nm band pass filter. Ten thousand cells were acquired per sample and the fluorescence was quantified on a logarithmic scale. The data were analyzed with FlowJo software v10.6.2 (Tree Star Inc., Ashland, OR, USA). The percentage of ROS producing cells corresponds to the percentage of HE positive cells. At least three independent experiments were realized.

4.4. Flow Cytometric Measurement of Transmembrane Mitochondrial Potential Using $DiOC_6(3)$

The measurement of transmembrane mitochondrial potential ($\Delta\Psi m$) is widely used to characterize mitochondrial metabolic state and cell death. The decrease in $\Delta\Psi m$ is a sign of a depolarized mitochondria with a poor ability to accumulate lipophilic cationic probes such as 3,3'-dihexyloxacarbocyanine iodide $DiOC_6(3)$ (λ Ex max = 484 nm; λ Em max = 501 nm) used in flow cytometry. $DiOC_6(3)$ accumulates in the mitochondrial matrix as a function of the potential difference: this probe accumulates all the more in the mitochondria with a normal $\Delta\Psi m$ (living cells) compared to the mitochondria with a low $\Delta\Psi m$ (dying and dead cells) which will cause a decrease in green fluorescence collected through a 520 ± 10 nm band pass filter. To evaluate the effect on $\Delta\Psi m$ of the different compounds tested at different concentrations, the adherent and non-adherent cells were pooled after 48 h of treatment, washed and stained with a solution of $DiOC_6(3)$ (Invitrogen/Thermo Fisher Scientific) at 40 nM for 15 min at 37 °C. At the end of the incubation time, the fluorescence associated with $DiOC_6(3)$ was immediately measured on a BD Accuri™ C6 flow cytometer. Ten thousand cells were acquired per sample and the fluorescence was quantified on a logarithmic scale. Data were analyzed with FlowJo software (Tree Star Inc.). The percentage of cells with depolarized mitochondria corresponds to the percentage of $DiOC_6(3)$ negative cells. At least three independent experiments were realized.

4.5. Flow Cytometric Evaluation of Plasma Membrane Permeability and Cell Death Using Propidium Iodide

Propidium iodide (PI) is a hydrophilic fluorescent agent intercalating nucleic acids (DNA; RNA) which produces a red/orange fluorescence when it is excited by a blue light (488 nm). It is used to quantify cell viability and plasma membrane permeability: it only stains the nucleic acids of dead cells that have lost their cytoplasmic membrane integrity [63,64]. The stock solution of PI was prepared in milliQ water at a concentration of 1 mg/mL. N2a cells (adherent and nonadherent cells) were stained with a PI solution at 1 µg/mL in 1X PBS for 5 min at 37 °C in order to assess their mortality after a treatment of 48 h with polyphenols (RSV, QCT or API) or with fatty acids (ALA, EPA, DHA, and OA) associated or not with 7KC. The cells were analyzed on a BD Accuri™ C6 flow cytometer and the fluorescence of PI was selected on a 630 nm long pass filter. Ten thousand cells were acquired per sample and the fluorescence was quantified on a logarithmic scale. Data were analyzed with FlowJo software (Tree Star Inc.). The percentage of dead cells corresponds to the percentage of PI positive cells. At least three independent experiments were realized.

4.6. Statistical Analysis

Statistical analyses were done using XLSTAT software 2020.1 (Microsoft, St. Redmond, WA, USA). Data were expressed as mean ± standard deviation (SD); data were considered statistically different (Mann-Whitney test) at a *P*-value of 0.05 or less.

Supplementary Materials: The following are available online. Figure S1: Evaluation with the fluorescein diacetate (FDA) assay of the effects of 7-ketocholesterol on the cell viability of N2a cells.

Author Contributions: Conceptualization: G.L; Investigation/Experimental work: A.Y., T.N. and G.L.; study management: G.L.; Writing original draft: A.Y. and G.L.; Discussion: A.Y., G.L., N.L., A.V., D.V.-F., M.S., H.G.-G. and L.A. All authors have read and agreed to the published version of the manuscript.

Funding: This work was funded by Université de Bourgogne (Dijon, France) and Université Libanaise (Beirut/Fanar, Lebanon; Research Funding Program at the Lebanese University (2020–2022)).

Acknowledgments: Aline Yammine received a financial support from Nutrition Méditerranéenne & Santé (NMS) and was awarded the NMS prize in 2019. The present work was presented as part of the annual NMS meeting held in Arbois (France) on June 1, 2019 (oral presentation) as well as at the 9th ENOR meeting in Edinburgh (UK) on September 19–20, 2019 (poster).

Conflicts of Interest: The authors declare no conflict of interest.

References

1. Nury, T.; Lizard, G.; Vejux, A. Lipids Nutrients in Parkinson and Alzheimer's Diseases: Cell Death and Cytoprotection. *Int. J. Mol. Sci.* **2020**, *21*, 2501. [CrossRef] [PubMed]
2. Albarracin, S.L.; Stab, B.; Casas, Z.; Sutachan, J.J.; Samudio, I.; Gonzalez, J.; Gonzalo, L.; Capani, F.; Morales, L.; Barreto, G.E. Effects of natural antioxidants in neurodegenerative disease. *Nutr. Neurosci.* **2012**, *15*, 1–9. [CrossRef]
3. Masmoudi-Kouki, O.; Hamdi, Y.; Ghouili, I.; Bahdoudi, S.; Kaddour, H.; Leprince, J.; Castel, H.; Vaudry, H.; Amri, M.; Vaudry, D.; et al. Neuroprotection with the Endozepine Octadecaneuropeptide, ODN. *Curr. Pharm. Des.* **2018**, *24*, 3918–3925. [CrossRef] [PubMed]

4. Mutemberezi, V.; Guillemot-Legris, O.; Muccioli, G.G. Oxysterols: From cholesterol metabolites to key mediators. *Prog. Lipid. Res.* **2016**, *64*, 152–169. [CrossRef]
5. Zerbinati, C.; Iuliano, L. Cholesterol and related sterols autoxidation. *Free. Radic. Biol. Med.* **2017**, *111*, 151–155. [CrossRef] [PubMed]
6. Anderson, A.; Campo, A.; Fulton, E.; Corwin, A.; Jerome, W.G., 3rd; O'Connor, M.S. 7 Ketocholesterol in disease and aging. *Redox. Biol.* **2020**, *29*, 101380. [CrossRef]
7. Testa, G.; Rossin, D.; Poli, G.; Biasi, F.; Leonarduzzi, G. Implication of oxysterols in chronic inflammatory human diseases. *Biochimie.* **2018**, *153*, 220–231. [CrossRef]
8. Brahmi, F.; Vejux, A.; Sghaier, R.; Zarrouk, A.; Nury, T.; Meddeb, W.; Rezig, L.; Namsi, A.; Sassi, K.; Yammine, A.; et al. Prevention of 7-ketocholesterol-induced side effects by natural compounds. *Crit. Rev. Food Sci. Nutr.* **2019**, *59*, 3179–3198. [CrossRef]
9. Testa, G.; Staurenghi, E.; Zerbinati, C.; Gargiulo, S.; Iuliano, L.; Giaccone, G.; Fantò, F.; Poli, G.; Leonarduzzi, G.; Gamba, P. Changes in brain oxysterols at different stages of Alzheimer's disease: Their involvement in neuroinflammation. *Redox. Biol.* **2016**, *10*, 24–33. [CrossRef]
10. Doria, M.; Maugest, L.; Moreau, T.; Lizard, G.; Vejux, A. Contribution of cholesterol and oxysterols to the pathophysiology of Parkinson's disease. *Free. Radic. Biol. Med.* **2016**, *101*, 393–400. [CrossRef]
11. Zarrouk, A.; Vejux, A.; Mackrill, J.; O'Callaghan, Y.; Hammami, M.; O'Brien, N.; Lizard, G. Involvement of oxysterols in age-related diseases and ageing processes. *Ageing Res. Rev.* **2014**, *18*, 148–162. [CrossRef] [PubMed]
12. Latruffe, N. *Vin, nutrition méditerranéenne et santé: Une association vertueuse*; Editions Universitaires de Dijon; Collection Sciences: Dijon France, 2017.
13. Tosti, V.; Bertozzi, B.; Fontana, L. Health Benefits of the Mediterranean Diet: Metabolic and Molecular Mechanisms. *J. Gerontol. A Biol. Sci. Med. Sci.* **2018**, *73*, 318–326. [CrossRef] [PubMed]
14. Román, G.C.; Jackson, R.E.; Gadhia, R.; Román, A.N.; Reis, J. Mediterranean diet: The role of long-chain ω-3 fatty acids in fish; polyphenols in fruits, vegetables, cereals, coffee, tea, cacao and wine; probiotics and vitamins in prevention of stroke, age-related cognitive decline, and Alzheimer disease. *Rev. Neurol. (Paris)* **2019**, *175*, 724–741. [CrossRef] [PubMed]
15. Moosavi, F.; Hosseini, R.; Saso, L.; Firuzi, O. Modulation of neurotrophic signaling pathways by polyphenols. *Drug Des. Devel. Ther.* **2015**, *10*, 23–42. [PubMed]
16. Namsi, A.; Nury, T.; Hamdouni, H.; Yammine, A.; Vejux, A.; Vervandier-Fasseur, D.; Latruffe, N.; Masmoudi-Kouki, O.; Lizard, G. Induction of Neuronal Differentiation of Murine N2a Cells by Two Polyphenols Present in the Mediterranean Diet Mimicking Neurotrophins Activities: Resveratrol and Apigenin. *Diseases* **2018**, *6*, 67. [CrossRef]
17. Namsi, A. Etude des mécanismes moléculaires associés aux effets neutrotrophiques de l'ODN et de polyphénols sur des cellules nerveuses. Ph.D. Thesis, Neurosciences & Biologie Moléculaire et Cellulaire, University Tunis El Manar & University Bourgogne Franche-Comté, Dijon, France, 2019.
18. Serra, G.; Incani, A.; Serreli, G.; Porru, L.; Melis, M.P.; Tuberoso, C.I.G.; Rossin, D.; Biasi, F.; Deiana, M. Olive oil polyphenols reduce oxysterols-induced redox imbalance and pro-inflammatory response in intestinal cells. *Redox. Biol.* **2018**, *17*, 348–354. [CrossRef]
19. Serra, G.; Deiana, M.; Spencer, J.P.E.; Corona, G. Olive Oil Phenolics Prevent Oxysterol-Induced Proinflammatory Cytokine Secretion and Reactive Oxygen Species Production in Human Peripheral Blood Mononuclear Cells, Through Modulation of p38 and JNK Pathways. *Mol Nutr Food Res.* **2017**, *61*, 1700283. [CrossRef]
20. Kim, A.; Nam, Y.J.; Lee, C.S. Taxifolin reduces the cholesterol oxidation product-induced neuronal apoptosis by suppressing the Akt and NF-κB activation-mediated cell death. *Brain Res. Bull.* **2017**, *134*, 63–71. [CrossRef]
21. Dugas, B.; Charbonnier, S.; Baarine, M.; Ragot, K.; Delmas, D.; Ménétrier, F.; Lherminier, J.; Malvitte, L.; Khalfaoui, T.; Bron, A.; et al. Effects of oxysterols on cell viability, inflammatory cytokines, VEGF, and reactive oxygen species production on human retinal cells: Cytoprotective effects and prevention of VEGF secretion by resveratrol. *Eur. J. Nutr.* **2010**, *49*, 435–446. [CrossRef]

22. Namsi, A.; Nury, T.; Khan, A.S.; Leprince, J.; Vaudry, D.; Caccia, C.; Leoni, V.; Atanasov, A.G.; Tonon, M.C.; Masmoudi-Kouki, O.; et al. Octadecaneuropeptide (ODN) Induces N2a Cells Differentiation through a PKA/PLC/PKC/MEK/ERK-Dependent Pathway: Incidence on Peroxisome, Mitochondria, and Lipid Profiles. *Molecules* **2019**, *24*, 3310. [CrossRef]

23. Singla, R.K.; Dubey, A.K.; Garg, A.; Sharma, R.K.; Fiorino, M.; Ameen, S.M.; Haddad, M.A.; Al-Hiary, M. Natural Polyphenols: Chemical Classification, Definition of Classes, Subcategories, and Structures. *J. AOAC Int.* **2019**, *102*, 1397–1400. [CrossRef] [PubMed]

24. Ferri, P.; Angelino, D.; Gennari, L.; Benedetti, S.; Ambrogini, P.; Del Grande, P.; Ninfali, P. Enhancement of flavonoid ability to cross the blood brain barrier of rats by co-administration with α-tocopherol. *Food Funct.* **2015**, *6*, 394–400. [CrossRef] [PubMed]

25. Figueira, I.; Garcia, G.; Pimpão, R.C.; Terrasso, A.P.; Costa, I.; Almeida, A.F.; Tavares, L.; Pais, T.F.; Pinto, P.; Ventura, M.R.; et al. Polyphenols journey through blood-brain barrier towards neuronal protection. *Sci. Rep.* **2017**, *7*, 11456. [CrossRef] [PubMed]

26. Long, Y.; Yang, Q.; Xiang, Y.; Zhang, Y.; Wan, J.; Liu, S.; Li, N.; Peng, W. Nose to brain drug delivery—A promising strategy for active components from herbal medicine for treating cerebral ischemia reperfusion. *Pharmacol. Res.* **2020**, 104795. [CrossRef]

27. Ragot, K.; Mackrill, J.J.; Zarrouk, A.; Nury, T.; Aires, V.; Jacquin, A.; Athias, A.; Pais de Barros, J.P.; Véjux, A.; Riedinger, J.M.; et al. Absence of correlation between oxysterol accumulation in lipid raft microdomains, calcium increase, and apoptosis induction on 158N murine oligodendrocytes. *Biochem. Pharmacol.* **2013**, *86*, 67–79. [CrossRef]

28. Debbabi, M.; Nury, T.; Zarrouk, A.; Mekahli, N.; Bezine, M.; Sghaier, R.; Grégoire, S.; Martine, L.; Durand, P.; Camus, E.; et al. Protective Effects of α-Tocopherol, γ-Tocopherol and Oleic Acid, Three Compounds of Olive Oils, and No Effect of Trolox, on 7-Ketocholesterol-Induced Mitochondrial and Peroxisomal Dysfunction in Microglial BV-2 Cells. *Int. J. Mol. Sci.* **2016**, *17*, 1973. [CrossRef]

29. Debbabi, M.; Zarrouk, A.; Bezine, M.; Meddeb, W.; Nury, T.; Badreddine, A.; Karym, E.M.; Sghaier, R.; Bretillon, L.; Guyot, S.; et al. Comparison of the effects of major fatty acids present in the Mediterranean diet (oleic acid, docosahexaenoic acid) and in hydrogenated oils (elaidic acid) on 7-ketocholesterol-induced oxiapoptophagy in microglial BV-2 cells. *Chem. Phys. Lipids* **2017**, *207*, 151–170. [CrossRef]

30. Nury, T.; Zarrouk, A.; Mackrill, J.J.; Samadi, M.; Durand, P.; Riedinger, J.M.; Doria, M.; Vejux, A.; Limagne, E.; Delmas, D.; et al. Induction of oxiapoptophagy on 158N murine oligodendrocytes treated by 7-ketocholesterol-, 7β-hydroxycholesterol-, or 24(S)-hydroxycholesterol: Protective effects of α-tocopherol and docosahexaenoic acid (DHA; C22:6 n-3). *Steroids* **2015**, *99*, 194–203. [CrossRef]

31. Zarrouk, A.; Nury, T.; Samadi, M.; O'Callaghan, Y.; Hammami, M.; O'Brien, N.M.; Lizard, G.; Mackrill, J.J. Effects of cholesterol oxides on cell death induction and calcium increase in human neuronal cells (SK-N-BE) and evaluation of the protective effects of docosahexaenoic acid (DHA; C22:6 n-3). *Steroids* **2015**, *99*, 238–247. [CrossRef]

32. Zarrouk, A.; Martine, L.; Grégoire, S.; Nury, T.; Meddeb, W.; Camus, E.; Badreddine, A.; Durand, P.; Namsi, A.; Yammine, A.; et al. Profile of fatty acids, tocopherols, phytosterols and polyphenols in mediterranean oils (argan oils, olive oils, milk thistle seed oils and nigella seed oil) and evaluation of their antioxidant and cytoprotective activities. *Curr. Pharm. Des.* **2019**, *25*, 1791–1805. [CrossRef]

33. Royer, M.C.; Lemaire-Ewing, S.; Desrumaux, C.; Monier, S.; Pais de Barros, J.P.; Athias, A.; Néel, D.; Lagrost, L. 7-ketocholesterol incorporation into sphingolipid/cholesterol-enriched (lipid raft) domains is impaired by vitamin E: A specific role for alpha-tocopherol with consequences on cell death. *J. Biol. Chem.* **2009**, *284*, 15826–15834. [CrossRef] [PubMed]

34. Tabas, I. Consequence of cellular cholesterol accumulation: Basic concepts and physiological implications. *J. Clin. Invest.* **2002**, *110*, 905–911. [CrossRef] [PubMed]

35. Monier, S.; Samadi, M.; Prunet, C.; Denance, M.; Laubriet, A.; Athias, A.; Berthier, A.; Steinmetz, E.; Jürgens, G.; Nègre-Salvayre, A.; et al. Impairment of the cytotoxic and oxidative activities of 7 beta-hydroxycholesterol and 7-ketocholesterol by esterification with oleate. *Biochem. Biophys. Res. Commun.* **2003**, *303*, 814–824. [CrossRef]

36. Vejux, A.; Guyot, S.; Montange, T.; Riedinger, J.M.; Kahn, E.; Lizard, G. Phospholipidosis and down-regulation of the PI3-K/PDK-1/Akt signalling pathway are vitamin E inhibitable events associated with 7-ketocholesterol-induced apoptosis. *J. Nutr Biochem.* **2009**, *20*, 45–61. [CrossRef]

37. Vejux, A.; Abed-Vieillard, D.; Hajji, K.; Zarrouk, A.; Mackrill, J.J.; Ghosh, S.; Nury, T.; Yammine, A.; Zaibi, M.; Mihoubi, W.; et al. 7-Ketocholesterol and 7β-hydroxycholesterol: In vitro and animal models used to characterize their activities and to identify molecules preventing their toxicity. *Biochem. Pharmacol.* **2020**, *173*, 113648. [CrossRef]
38. Ragot, K.; Delmas, D.; Athias, A.; Nury, T.; Baarine, M.; Lizard, G. α-Tocopherol impairs 7-ketocholesterol-induced caspase-3-dependent apoptosis involving GSK-3 activation and Mcl-1 degradation on 158N murine oligodendrocytes. *Chem. Phys. Lipids.* **2011**, *164*, 469–478. [CrossRef]
39. Bazan, N.G. Docosanoids and elovanoids from omega-3 fatty acids are pro-homeostatic modulators of inflammatory responses, cell damage and neuroprotection. *Mol. Asp. Med.* **2018**, *64*, 18–33. [CrossRef]
40. Olkkonen, V.M.; Hynynen, R. Interactions of oxysterols with membranes and proteins. *Mol. Asp. Med.* **2009**, *30*, 123–133. [CrossRef]
41. Hachem, M.; Belkouch, M.; Lo Van, A.; Picq, M.; Bernoud-Hubac, N.; Lagarde, M. Brain targeting with docosahexaenoic acid as a prospective therapy for neurodegenerative diseases and its passage across blood brain barrier. *Biochimie.* **2020**, *170*, 203–211. [CrossRef]
42. Miranda, A.R.; Albrecht, C.; Cortez, M.V.; Soria, E.A. Pharmacology and Toxicology of Polyphenols with Potential As Neurotropic Agents in Non-communicable Diseases. *Curr. Drug. Targets.* **2018**, *19*, 97–110. [CrossRef]
43. Savary, S.; Trompier, D.; Andréoletti, P.; Le Borgne, F.; Demarquoy, J.; Lizard, G. Fatty acids-induced lipotoxicity and inflammation. *Curr. Drug. Metab.* **2012**, *13*, 1358–1370. [CrossRef] [PubMed]
44. Samadi, A.; Sabuncuoglu, S.; Samadi, M.; Isikhan, S.Y.; Lay, I.; Yalcinkaya, A.; Chirumbolo, S.; Bjørklund, G.; Peana, M. A Comprehensive review on oxysterols and related diseases. *Curr. Med. Chem.* **2020**. [CrossRef] [PubMed]
45. Moore, K.; Hughes, C.F.; Ward, M.; Hoey, L.; McNulty, H. Diet, nutrition and the ageing brain: Current evidence and new directions. *Proc. Nutr. Soc.* **2018**, *77*, 152–163. [CrossRef] [PubMed]
46. Pedruzzi, E.; Guichard, C.; Ollivier, V.; Driss, F.; Fay, M.; Prunet, C.; Marie, J.C.; Pouzet, C.; Samadi, M.; Elbim, C.; et al. NAD(P)H oxidase Nox-4 mediates 7-ketocholesterol-induced endoplasmic reticulum stress and apoptosis in human aortic smooth muscle cells. *Mol. Cell Biol.* **2004**, *24*, 10703–10717. [CrossRef]
47. Attanzio, A.; Frazzitta, A.; Cilla, A.; Livrea, M.A.; Tesoriere, L.; Allegra, M. 7-Keto-Cholesterol and Cholestan-3beta, 5alpha, 6beta-Triol Induce Eryptosis through Distinct Pathways Leading to NADPH Oxidase and Nitric Oxide Synthase Activation. *Cell Physiol. Biochem.* **2019**, *53*, 933–947.
48. Nury, T.; Zarrouk, A.; Vejux, A.; Doria, M.; Riedinger, J.M.; Delage-Mourroux, R.; Lizard, G. Induction of oxiapoptophagy, a mixed mode of cell death associated with oxidative stress, apoptosis and autophagy, on 7-ketocholesterol-treated 158N murine oligodendrocytes: Impairment by α-tocopherol. *Biochem. Biophys. Res. Commun.* **2014**, *446*, 714–719. [CrossRef]
49. Klionsky, D.J.; Abdelmohsen, K.; Abe, A.; Abedin, M.J.; Abeliovich, H.; Acevedo Arozena, A. Guidelines for the use and interpretation of assays for monitoring autophagy (3rd edition). *Autophagy.* **2016**, *12*, 1–222.
50. Nury, T.; Zarrouk, A.; Ragot, K.; Debbabi, M.; Riedinger, J.M.; Vejux, A.; Aubourg, P.; Lizard, G. 7-Ketocholesterol is increased in the plasma of X-ALD patients and induces peroxisomal modifications in microglial cells: Potential roles of 7-ketocholesterol in the pathophysiology of X-ALD. *J. Steroid. Biochem. Mol. Biol.* **2017**, *169*, 123–136. [CrossRef]
51. Zarrouk, A.; Nury, T.; Karym, E.M.; Vejux, A.; Sghaier, R.; Gondcaille, C.; Andreoletti, P.; Trompier, D.; Savary, S.; Cherkaoui-Malki, M.; et al. Attenuation of 7-ketocholesterol-induced overproduction of reactive oxygen species, apoptosis, and autophagy by dimethyl fumarate on 158N murine oligodendrocytes. *J. Steroid. Biochem. Mol. Biol.* **2017**, *169*, 29–38. [CrossRef]
52. Bian, Y.; Wei, J.; Zhao, C.; Li, G. Natural polyphenols targeting senescence: a novel prevention and therapy strategy for cancer. *Int. J. Mol. Sci.* **2020**, *21*, 684. [CrossRef]
53. Fouache, A.; Zabaiou, N.; De Joussineau, C.; Morel, L.; Silvente-Poirot, S.; Namsi, A.; Lizard, G.; Poirot, M.; Makishima, M.; Baron, S.; et al. Flavonoids differentially modulate liver X receptors activity-Structure-function relationship analysis. *J. Steroid. Biochem. Mol. Biol.* **2019**, *190*, 173–182. [CrossRef] [PubMed]
54. Grygiel-Górniak, B. Peroxisome proliferator-activated receptors and their ligands: Nutritional and clinical implications–a review. *Nutr. J.* **2014**, *13*, 17. [CrossRef] [PubMed]
55. Cilla, A.; Alegría, A.; Attanzio, A.; Garcia-Llatas, G.; Tesoriere, L.; Livrea, M.A. Dietary phytochemicals in the protection against oxysterol-induced damage. *Chem. Phys. Lipids.* **2017**, *207*, 192–205. [CrossRef] [PubMed]

56. Azzi, J.; Jraij, A.; Auezova, L.; Fourmentin, S.; Greige-Gerges, H. Novel findings for quercetin encapsulation and preservation with cyclodextrins, liposomes, and drug-in-cyclodextrin-in-liposomes. *Food Hydrocoll.* **2018**, *81*, 328–340. [CrossRef]
57. Soukoulis, C.; Bohn, T. A comprehensive overview on the micro- and nano-technological encapsulation advances for enhancing the chemical stability and bioavailability of carotenoids. *Crit. Rev. Food Sci. Nutr.* **2018**, *58*, 1–36. [CrossRef]
58. Testa, G.; Gamba, P.; Badilli, U.; Gargiulo, S.; Maina, M.; Guina, T.; Calfapietra, S.; Biasi, F.; Cavalli, R.; Poli, G.; et al. Loading into nanoparticles improves quercetin's efficacy in preventing neuroinflammation induced by oxysterols. *PLoS One* **2014**, *9*, e96795. [CrossRef]
59. Varkuti, B.H.; Kepiro, M.; Liu, Z.; Vick, K.; Avchalumov, Y.; Pacifico, R.; MacMullen, C.M.; Kamenecka, T.M.; Puthanveettil, S.V.; Davis, R.L. Neuron-based high-content assay and screen for CNS active mitotherapeutics. *Sci. Adv.* **2020**, *6*, eaaw8702. [CrossRef]
60. Wen, R.; Banik, B.; Pathak, R.K.; Kumar, A.; Kolishetti, N.; Dhar, S. Nanotechnology inspired tools for mitochondrial dysfunction related diseases. *Adv. Drug. Deliv. Rev.* **2016**, *99*, 52–69. [CrossRef]
61. Zielonka, J.; Joseph, J.; Sikora, A.; Hardy, M.; Ouari, O.; Vasquez-Vivar, J.; Cheng, G.; Lopez, M.; Kalyanaraman, B. Mitochondria-Targeted Triphenylphosphonium-based compounds: Syntheses, mechanisms of action, and therapeutic and diagnostic Applications. *Chem. Rev.* **2017**, *117*, 10043–10120. [CrossRef]
62. Rothe, G.; Valet, G. Flow cytometric analysis of respiratory burst activity in phagocytes with hydroethidine and 2′,7′-dichlorofluorescin. *J. Leukoc. Biol.* **1990**, *47*, 440–448. [CrossRef]
63. Yeh, C.G.; His, B.; Faulk, W.P. Propidium iodide as a nuclear marker in immunofluorescence. II. Use with cellular identification and viahility studies. *J. Immunol. Method.* **1981**, *43*, 269–275. [CrossRef]
64. Lizard, G.; Fournel, S.; Genestier, L.; Dhedin, N.; Chaput, C.; Flacher, M.; Mutin, M.; Panaye, G.; Revillard, J.P. Kinetics of plasma membrane and mitochondrial alterations in cells undergoing apoptosis. *Cytometry* **1995**, *21*, 275–283. [CrossRef] [PubMed]

Sample Availability: Samples of the compounds are available from the authors

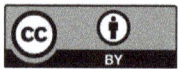

© 2020 by the authors. Licensee MDPI, Basel, Switzerland. This article is an open access article distributed under the terms and conditions of the Creative Commons Attribution (CC BY) license (http://creativecommons.org/licenses/by/4.0/).

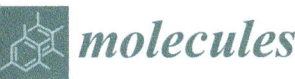

Review

The Neuroprotective Role of Polydatin: Neuropharmacological Mechanisms, Molecular Targets, Therapeutic Potentials, and Clinical Perspective

Sajad Fakhri [1], Mohammad Mehdi Gravandi [2], Sadaf Abdian [2], Esra Küpeli Akkol [3], Mohammad Hosein Farzaei [1,*] and Eduardo Sobarzo-Sánchez [4,5,*]

1. Pharmaceutical Sciences Research Center, Health Institute, Kermanshah University of Medical Sciences, Kermanshah 6734667149, Iran; sajad.fakhri@kums.ac.ir
2. Student Research Committee, Kermanshah University of Medical Sciences, Kermanshah 6714415153, Iran; mehdigravandi@yahoo.com (M.M.G.); abdian.ph@gmail.com (S.A.)
3. Department of Pharmacognosy, Faculty of Pharmacy, Gazi University, 06330 Ankara, Turkey; esrak@gazi.edu.tr
4. Department of Organic Chemistry, Faculty of Pharmacy, University of Santiago de Compostela, 15782 Santiago de Compostela, Spain
5. Instituto de Investigación y Postgrado, Facultad de Ciencias de la Salud, Universidad Central de Chile, Santiago 8330507, Chile
* Correspondence: mh.farzaei@gmail.com (M.H.F.); e.sobarzo@usc.es or eduardo.sobarzo@ucentral.cl (E.S.-S.)

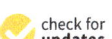

Abstract: Neurodegenerative diseases (NDDs) are one of the leading causes of death and disability in humans. From a mechanistic perspective, the complexity of pathophysiological mechanisms contributes to NDDs. Therefore, there is an urgency to provide novel multi-target agents towards the simultaneous modulation of dysregulated pathways against NDDs. Besides, their lack of effectiveness and associated side effects have contributed to the lack of conventional therapies as suitable therapeutic agents. Prevailing reports have introduced plant secondary metabolites as promising multi-target agents in combating NDDs. Polydatin is a natural phenolic compound, employing potential mechanisms in fighting NDDs. It is considered an auspicious phytochemical in modulating neuroinflammatory/apoptotic/autophagy/oxidative stress signaling mediators such as nuclear factor-κB (NF-κB), NF-E2–related factor 2 (Nrf2)/antioxidant response elements (ARE), matrix metalloproteinase (MMPs), interleukins (ILs), phosphoinositide 3-kinases (PI3K)/protein kinase B (Akt), and the extracellular regulated kinase (ERK)/mitogen-activated protein kinase (MAPK). Accordingly, polydatin potentially counteracts Alzheimer's disease, cognition/memory dysfunction, Parkinson's disease, brain/spinal cord injuries, ischemic stroke, and miscellaneous neuronal dysfunctionalities. The present study provides all of the neuroprotective mechanisms of polydatin in various NDDs. Additionally, the novel delivery systems of polydatin are provided regarding increasing its safety, solubility, bioavailability, and efficacy, as well as developing a long-lasting therapeutic concentration of polydatin in the central nervous system, possessing fewer side effects.

Keywords: polydatin; neurodegeneration; neuroprotection; therapeutic targets; pharmacology; novel delivery system

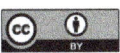

1. Introduction

Neurodegenerative diseases (NDDs) are amongst the most common factors of disability and death in humans, which refer to the gradual, symmetrical, and specific decreases in sensory, motor, and mental nerve activity resulting in the death of neurons [1,2]. Nerve death accounts for various signs of neurological dysregulations, both chronic and acute, consisting of Parkinson's disease (PD), Alzheimer's disease (AD), central nervous system (Brain/Spinal Cord) injuries, and stroke [3]. Additionally, autism, neuropathic pain, aging, and depression are other NDDs that result from nerve cell death [4,5]. From a mechanistic point of view, various factors cause neurological problems, such as oxidative stress [6], inflammation [7], and apoptosis [5,8]. The aforementioned pathological pathways play a harmful role in neuronal cell death mechanisms. The microglia activity, inflammatory cytokines, reactive oxygen species (ROS), and related mitochondrial disruption of oxidative pathways have shown negative results on the process of nerve regeneration that eventually leads to cell death [9,10].

Despite advances in clinical healthcare, neuroprotective agents are still clinically challenged in nerve destruction and NDDs. Thus, there is an emerging need to develop new multi-target therapies that further help to attenuate dysregulated signaling pathways in NDDs [11–13]. Several natural compounds isolated from edible and medicinal plants that exhibit anti-inflammatory properties have been investigated for potential application as pharmaceutical candidates [14]. Natural products are rich sources of polyphenolic compounds, consisting of stilbenoids, which are a big group of resveratrol substances such as monomers, dimers, and oligomers. Stilbenoids are naturally occurring compounds in a variety of plant families, such as Vitaceae, Gnetaceae, Cyperaceae, and Rocarpaceae. Consequently, the wine grape, *Vitis vinifera* L., is considered the primary nutritional source of these compounds [15].

Polydatin is a stilbenoid that passively penetrates cells. It also launches into the cells through an active mechanism by a glucose carrier. The glucose moiety of polydatin causes a higher resistance rate to enzymatic oxidation than resveratrol and has much better water solubility [16,17]. Polydatin has been shown to suppress oxidative stress, inflammation, and apoptosis as major pathways for nerve cell regeneration. The biological activity of polydatin and certain derivatives entails preventing or interfering with several neurodegenerative mechanisms [18].

In a previous study, the protective mechanisms of polydatin were evidenced in cerebral ischemia [19]. Recently, dementia-related disorders are also targeted by polydatin [20]. Besides, the general pharmacology and pharmacokinetic properties of polydatin were developed by Du et al. [21]. As of yet, no review article has discussed the entire set of neuroprotective mechanisms of polydatin. This review focuses on the pharmacological targets, molecular mechanisms, therapeutic potentials, and clinical perspectives of polydatin in NDDs. The pharmacological mechanisms of action of polydatin in the treatment or prevention of NDDs are provided.

2. Polydatin: Chemical Structure, Sources, and Pharmacokinetic Properties

Several studies concerning the chemical characterization of stilbenoids have been motivated by their numerous promising biological functions, especially those of polydatin. Polydatin (3,4′,5-trihydroxystilbene-3-β-D-glucoside) is a natural resveratrol glucoside known as resveratrol-3-β-mono-D-glucoside, an active product from the *Polygonum cuspidatum* Sieb. et Zucc roots (Figure 1). However, it is also found in grapes, red wines, hop cones, peanuts, cocoa/chocolate products, and several other meals [21].

Two isomeric types (*cis* and *trans*) of polydatin are found in nature. Cis-polydatin is often detected in lower levels. Moreover, they are less biologically active than the *trans* forms [22]. The most common sources of polydatin are grape juice and red/white wines. Cis-polydatin is the predominant isoform in carbonated wines and rosé, while the *trans* isomer is abundant in berries, peanuts, grapes, and pistachios [23]. The major sources of polydatin isomers are the rhizomes and roots of *Fallopia japonica* (Houtt.) Ronse Decraene (Polygonaceae), which have long been used in traditional Chinese and Japanese Medicine as an anticancer, diuretic, analgesic, anti-pyretic, and expectorant agent in the management of atherosclerosis [24]. However, this product is present in various other genera such as *Rumex, Picea, Rosa, Quercus,* and *Malus*. Polydatin has received similar consideration to resveratrol because glucoside concentrations are usually higher than aglycone ones in red wine and other grape products. The exact ratio of glycosylated forms to aglycones in wine relies on various aspects such as the fermentation method and ecological conditions in the vineyards [25].

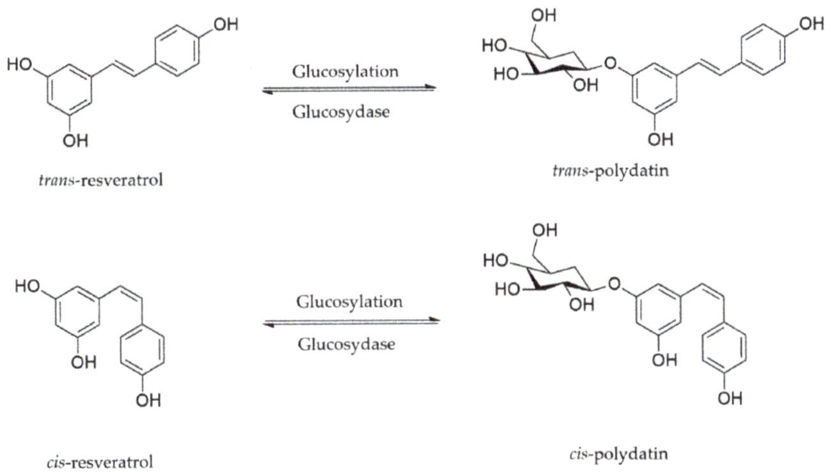

Figure 1. Polydatin, a glycosylated form of resveratrol.

Pharmacokinetic studies are often required for the effective and safe clinical use of drugs. The absorption, distribution, and metabolism of polydatin are connected to its bioactivity. Polydatin might have higher bioavailability and a better antioxidant function compared to resveratrol. In addition, intestinal absorption of polydatin is higher than resveratrol made by glucose groups [26]. Polydatin enters the cell through an active glucose carrier mechanism and passive diffusion, while resveratrol just passively penetrates cell membranes [27]. The active transport of polydatin mainly passes through a sodium-dependent glucose transporter 1 (SGLT1), chiefly present in the intestines and stomach [16]. Since the cell content of polydatin is not very low, it indicates an active transfer of polydatin by SGLT1 [21,27].

Polydatin employs two possible pathways to be deglycosylated from *trans*-resveratrol. The primary pathway is cleavage by cytosolic-β-glucosidase following the SGLT1 mediated by passing through the brush-border membrane. The second mechanism, which happens on the luminal side of the epithelium, is deglycosylation by the membrane-bound enzyme lactase-phlorizin hydrolase. This mechanism is followed by passive diffusion of the released aglycone and additional glucuronoconjugation [17]. Although resveratrol is more accumulated and leaves more residue in cells than polydatin, the half-life of polydatin is approximately four hours with a higher level of resveratrol Cmax at the same dose [27]. However, more analytical methods need to be investigated for the determination of *trans*-stilbene glycoside during pharmacokinetics studies [28].

Accordingly, polydatin as a glycosylated resveratrol could be a potential therapeutic agent with fewer pharmacokinetic limitations in comparison to resveratrol.

3. Polydatin against NDDs

Polydatin has demonstrated several biological/pharmacological effects, such as anti-inflammatory [29], anti-apoptotic [30], and antioxidant [31], against NDDs [32]. To combat oxidative stress, polydatin increased antioxidant capacity through associated antioxidant mediators, nuclear factor erythroid 2-related factor 2 (Nrf2) and sirtuin 1 (Sirt1), and antioxidant response elements (AREs) [18]. Polydatin suppresses oxidative stress through phosphoinositide 3-kinases (PI3K)/protein kinase B (Akt)-interconnected mediators [33]. It also blocks oxidative stress and reduces microglial apoptosis through the Nrf2/heme oxygenase (HO-1) pathway [34]. From the inflammatory point of view, by suppressing nuclear factor kappa B (NF-κB), polydatin can stop intercellular adhesion molecule-1 (ICAM-1) protein/mRNA production. Polydatin has also been shown to reduce pro-inflammatory cytokines (IL-1β, TNF-α, and IL-6) by down-regulating toll-like receptor-2 (TLR-2) and the

NF-κB p65 pathway [35]. As mitochondria are the major source of ROS in cells, when the intracellular mitochondria are damaged, electron transfer is abnormal, and ROS production is increased, which ultimately accelerates the onset of apoptosis [36]. Several studies have shown the beneficial influence of polydatin on mitochondria from a new perspective. Polydatin has been considered to suppress mitochondria-related cytochrome c release, moreover suppressing caspase-9 and caspase-3 [37]. Polydatin has been thought to decrease ROS release and improve mitochondrial activity by modulating the Sirt3/superoxide dismutase 2 (SOD2) pathway. SOD2 is a mitochondrial antioxidant enzyme whose activity is mediated by Sirt3 [38].

Overall, by modulating several mediators in inflammatory/apoptotic/autophagy/oxidative stress pathways, polydatin could be a hopeful candidate in combating NDDs.

3.1. Polydatin against AD, and Cognition/Memory Dysfunction

As the most common form of NDDs, AD is characterized by a gradual decline in memory and mental impairment in all aspects of a person's ability to perform daily activities, with unknown causes [39]. Studies have shown that the accumulation of old extracellular plaques, mainly consisting of the amyloid beta peptide (Aβ) and intracellular fiber nodules composed of hyperphosphorylated proteins, plays an essential role in the neuropathology of AD [40–42]. Besides, several inflammatory, apoptotic, and oxidative pathways are behind the pathogenesis of AD. Due to numerous pathophysiological mechanisms for AD, effective treatment has not yet been developed. Natural products have shown beneficial therapeutic effects on AD [43]. Amongst natural entities, oral administration of polydatin could dramatically reduce the production of malondialdehyde (MDA) and increase the activity of the antioxidants SOD and catalase (CAT) to protect learning and memory impairments in vivo. In addition, it lessened the damage caused by an oxygen-glucose deficiency in cultured neurons [44]. Tong et al. investigated the protective effect of polydatin in cancer patients undergoing chemotherapy, most of whom had cognitive impairments due to the use of chemotherapy drugs. In their study, polydatin, at a daily dose of 50 mg/kg, reduced doxorubicin-induced cognitive impairment and restored the hippocampal structure of the hippocampus. In addition, polydatin reduced doxorubicin-induced stress by regulating Nrf2, activating the NF-κB pathway, and reducing apoptosis [45,46]. In another study, polydatin was reported to defend against learning and memory failure in neonatal rats with hypoxic-ischemic brain injury (HIBI) caused by unilateral carotid artery ligation. In addition, polydatin decreased memory deficiency and increased the expression of the hippocampal brain-derived neurotrophic factor (BDNF) in rats with HIBI [47]. Moreover, in a study on rat's cognitive function exposed to chronic ethanol, polydatin increased cell survival while decreasing the expression level of cyclin-dependent kinase 5 (cdk5), and reversed functional defects in ethanol-treated mice evaluated by the Morris water test [48]. In another recent study, polydatin has shown protective roles against dementia-related disorders by attenuating several dysregulated pathways, including suppressing neuroapoptosis, oxidative stress, N-methyl D-aspartate receptor subtype 2B (NR2B), senile plaques, neurofibrillary tangles, and cholinergic dysfunctions [20]. Polydatin-mediated in vitro inhibition of Aβ25–35 polymerization and associated fibrils/oligomers was also reported by Rivière et al. [49,50]. As another anti-AD mechanism of polydatin, an in vitro increase in α3 and α7 nicotinic acetylcholine receptors (nAChRs) could help combat NDDs [51]. During an in vivo study, the modulation of NR2B by polydatin in rats' prefrontal cortex reduced learning and memory impairments [52].

Therefore, polydatin could be a helpful candidate in preventing AD and cognitive/memory impairment in various cases. Such an effect is exerted through the modulation of several dysregulated mechanisms, including neurological deficit scores, oxidative stress (e.g., Nrf2, SOD, CAT), inflammation (e.g., NF-κB), as well as Aβ, BDNF, and nAChRs.

3.2. Polydatin against PD

PD is an aging-associated condition and the second-most significant reason for NDDs [53]. PD is known for midbrain dopaminergic neuronal loss and the accumulation of α-synucleins called Lewy bodies. Furthermore, damages to non-dopaminergic pathways cause non-motor and motor malfunctions [54]. Owing to their poor effectiveness and adverse side effects, traditional therapies for PD are challenging to implement, and the development of novel innovative and safe agents is now needed. Oxidative stress and neuroinflammation play a significant role in PD pathogenesis [55]. Therefore, preventing the dysregulated mediators of these pathways has a considerable role in prohibiting the dissemination of PD. From a pathophysiological perspective, the degradation of substantia nigra dopaminergic neurons is caused by the hereditary sensitivity and response to harmful environmental stimuli [56]. Bai et al. reported that polydatin could play a critical role in combating PD. Besides, polydatin meaningfully decreased apoptosis and mitochondrial dysfunction during rotenone/Parkin deficiency induced in a human dopaminergic neuronal cell line, SH-SY5Y. In their study, polydatin suppressed the rotenone-induced cell death, mitochondrial membrane potential (MMP), Sirt 1, DJ1, and ROS production. Their study found that when autophagy-related gene 5 (Atg5) is biologically inhibited, the beneficial effects of polydatin are partly inhibited, implying Atg5-mediated neuroprotection [57]. Parkin knockdown-induced oxidative stress, mitochondrial malfunction autophagy deficiency, and mitochondrial fusion expansion were all alleviated by polydatin [58]. Polydatin therapy may also reverse abnormalities in mitochondrial morphology and motor malfunction in a Drosophila model of PD caused by Parkin insufficiency [57].

In the pathogenicity of PD, neuroinflammation hyperactivates microglia and results in the destruction of dopaminergic neurons. As a result, reducing microglial activity could help in the management of PD [59]. Polydatin crosses the blood–brain barrier to protect motor deterioration of substantia nigra and preserves dopaminergic neurons and motor function by suppressing pro-inflammatory mediators and microglia [60,61]. Huang et al. indicated that polydatin caused an increase in Nrf2, p-Akt, and p-glycogen synthase kinase-3β (GSK-3β) Ser9, activated microglial BV-2 cells, and suppressed NF-κB and pro-inflammatory mediators in the substantia nigra of PD rat-induced by lipopolysaccharide (LPS). Polydatin also inhibited dopaminergic neurodegeneration caused by microglial activation through modulating the Akt/GSK-3β/Nrf2/NF-κB signaling pathway [62]. It is worth noting the discrepancies on the anti/pro-inflammatory cytokines following microglia activation. It reveals the complexity of the brain microglial regulation, including the critical M1 (inflammatory microglia) and M2 (anti-inflammatory microglia). Microglia activations, especially the M1 type, have been considered a critical orchestrator in triggering inflammatory responses during NDDs. However, the production/release of inflammatory cytokines has been highlighted as a common feature associated with the microglial response, which is closely related to imbalanced protein homeostasis in NDDs [63]. So, modulating microglia activation could be a promising strategy for polydatin in combating NDDs.

The disturbance of glycolysis and the decrease in ATP production are other factors involved in the dysfunction of dopaminergic neurons and developing PD [64]. Zhang et al. showed that polydatin might improve glycolysis, glucose metabolism, ATP production, and motor dysfunction in mice with 1-methyl-4-phenyl-1,2,3,6-tetrahydropyridine (MPTP)-induced early dopaminergic neuronal degeneration. In their study, polydatin prevented the loss of dopaminergic neurons in the striatum and substantia nigra, thereby suppressing neural apoptosis (Bax and cleaved caspase-3) and improving motor function in mice [65]. Suppressing complex I of the electron transport chain and heightened oxidative stress are among the first triggers in the pathogenesis of PD [66]. In an in vitro study, reducing lipid peroxidation, inhibiting apoptosis, and activating the mitogen-activated protein kinase (MAPK) are introduced as the primary neuroprotective mechanisms of polydatin on dopaminergic neurons [67]. A study by Ahmed et al. showed that polydatin (3 mg/kg, intraperitoneally) possessed a neuroprotective effect in attenuating the degeneration of dopaminergic neurons in nigro-striatal regions of the brain. They also indicated that polydatin improved neuromotor behavior in a rat model of rotenone-induced PD. Thus, the protective effect of polydatin against striatal degeneration is presented in their report [68]. In a similar report, polydatin meaningfully prevented the rotenone-induced dysregulations of MDA, manganese SOD, glutathione, and thioredoxin in the striatum. Besides, polydatin inhibited the rotenone-induced neurodegeneration of dopaminergic neurons in the substantia nigra [61].

Polydatin, as a balancer, may thus be a treatment strategy in PD by reducing oxidative stress, as well as controlling autophagic mechanisms and mitochondrial fusion.

3.3. Polydatin against Central Nervous System (Brain/Spinal Cord) Injuries

Traumatic brain injury (TBI) is the leading cause of corporality, and permanent dysfunction has become a global public health problem [69]. People with severe TBI sometimes necessitate lengthy therapy. Treatments are missing due to the complexity and obscurity of the pathophysiological pathways in TBI [70]. TBI induced mitochondrial neuronal damage, as evidenced by an increase in ROS mitochondria and a reduction in MMP, causing the previous mitochondrial transition pore to open [69]. Polydatin has shown various pharmacological benefits, including antioxidation, anti-inflammation, anti-apoptosis, and brain-associated injuries [71,72].

Sprague–Dawley rats receiving 30 mg/kg polydatin intraperitoneally after TBI decreased in ROS and blocked TBI-induced MDA expression while increasing SOD levels in damaged cortices. In their study, polydatin prevented MMP collapse and the previous mitochondrial transition pore from opening TBI and reduced the endoplasmic reticulum stress response following TBI [69]. Consistently, polydatin significantly lowered endoplasmic reticulum stress-related unfolded protein activation, containing blocked p-extracellular regulated kinase (ERK) phosphorylation, declined spliced XBP-1, and cleaved activating transcription factor 6 (ATF6) production, as well as increasing the expression of glucose-regulated proteins (GRP78). Besides, polydatin regulated the p38MAPK signaling pathway and the mitochondrial apoptotic pathway (e.g., caspase-3/9) and improved neurological scores and the length of survival in TBI rats [69]. In another report, polydatin protected against SCI by suppressing oxidative stress and apoptosis passing through Nrf2/HO-1 signaling in vitro and in vivo [34]. Polydatin also increased neuronal viability and protected against oxygen-glucose deprivation/re-oxygenation-induced mitochondrial injury and apoptosis in a dose-dependent manner. Besides, polydatin modulated the activity of neuronal mitochondria, including MMP, intracellular calcium levels, the opening of the mitochondrial permeability transition pore (mPTP), ROS generation, and adenosine triphosphate levels. From a mechanistic perspective, polydatin suppressed Keap1 and upregulated Nrf2/HO-1 and NAD(P)H Quinone Dehydrogenase 1 (NQO-1) in oxygen-glucose deprivation/re-oxygenation-treated spinal cord motor neurons. Additionally, polydatin reversed the mitochondrial and neuronal damage induced by spinal cord ischemia/reperfusion in a mouse model, partially suppressed by the Nrf2 inhibitor. This represents that the neuroprotective effects of polydatin pass through the Nrf2/ARE pathway [73]. The engagement of Nrf2 on neuronal differentiation in both in vivo and in vitro studies are also provided by Zhan et al. [74]. The involvement of Nrf2/ARE in the protective effects of polydatin is also presented in other reports [75]. In this line, the inhibitory effect of polydatin on ferroptosis was shown both in vitro and in TBI mice. Those responses were applied by preventing the accumulation of free Fe^{2+}, increasing MDA, and decreasing glutathione peroxidase (GPx) [76].

The most common causes of traumatic spinal cord injury (SCI) are motor/car collisions, abuse, and falls [77]. Not unexpectedly, epidemiological trials discovered that SCI mainly existed in young males and resulted in lifelong cognitive defects that significantly reduce their life quality [78]. SCI is characterized by various symptoms, including limb paralysis, a loss of feeling in the lower extremities, and uracratia or uroschesis. A growing body of research suggests the aggregation of inflammatory cytokines across the compromised spinal cord and is amongst the main risk aspects for SCI pathological symptoms [10,11].

Findings indicated that several pro-inflammatory cytokines, including the macrophage migration inhibitory factor (MIF), interleukin-1 (IL-1), IL-6, and tumor necrosis factor-α, are intensified steadily after compression-induced SCI [9]. To modulate these mechanisms, polydatin was injected into adult male Sprague–Dawley rats in a single intraperitoneal dose. In this line, polydatin significantly reduced spinal cord edema and morphological changes in vivo. It also decreased nitric oxide (NO) in spinal cord tissues of SCI rats, which was consistent with the pattern of inducible nitric oxide synthase (iNOS) production. Accordingly, LPS increased protein and mRNA levels of iNOS in BV2 cells, and polydatin reversed these changes [78]. Consequently, polydatin decreased the LPS-induced rise in NO and response to inflammatory microglia. Polydatin also significantly reduced IL-6, IL-1, and TNF-α after a single injection and inhibited the development of inflammatory cytokines in spinal cord tissues following SCI. Besides, polydatin blocked LPS-induced NF-κB activation in BV2 microglia and inhibited the activity of NLRP3 inflammasomes [78]. This stilbene attenuated TBI-induced acute lung injury by suppressing the S100B-mediated formation of neutrophil extracellular traps [79]. Polydatin also meaningfully decreased MDA while increasing SOD, GPx, CAT, and the level of total antioxidant capacity in the brain and liver. Besides, polydatin reduced inflammatory mediators of serum, such as IL-6, IL-1β, and TNF-α. It also modulated the D-galactose-induced caspase-3 and Bcl-2/Bax ratio elevation in the liver and brain [30].

Altogether, the critical role of polydatin in the modulation of Nrf2/ARE, ERK/MAPK, and interconnected apoptotic/inflammatory pathways could pave the road in the modulation of brain/SCI injuries.

3.4. Polydatin against Stroke: As a Coupled Complication to NDDs

Stroke is one of the most severe cerebrovascular disorders, affecting patients' quality of life [80]. Further pieces of evidence and mechanisms of polydatin protect against cerebral ischemia. Two different shreds of evidence have been mentioned, namely the inhibition of the neurological deficit score and limiting the brain infarction volume in rats with middle cerebral artery occlusion after being treated with polydatin. Several mechanisms have been provided for these two effects of polydatin [81].

Ischemic stroke increases neuroinflammation and ROS. Shah et al. investigated the neuroprotective activity of polydatin against ischemic brain damage in a rat model of chronic middle cerebral artery occlusion (MCAO). Their results indicated that polydatin minimized infarction volume and mitigated neurobehavioral defects by limiting the activation of p38MAPK and c-Jun N-terminal kinase, thereby suppressing neuroinflammation and ROS. They also demonstrated that polydatin upregulated the endogenous antioxidants Nrf2, HO-1, and the thioredoxin pathway, and reduced inflammation and ROS in cortical tissue [82]. As previously mentioned, inflammation and oxidative stress are two major factors in cerebral ischemic pathogenesis. In this line, NF-κB activation plays a critical role in inflammation. Besides, low levels of glioma-associated oncogene Patched-1 (Ptch1), homolog1 (Gli1), and SOD1 will lead to oxidative stress. Ji et al. demonstrated that polydatin could protect the brain of rats with permanent MCAO. Such effects were exerted by modulating inflammation via lowering NF-κB and the attenuation of oxidative stress through increasing Ptch1, Gli1, SOD1 expression, as well as ameliorating blood–brain barrier permeability [83]. Besides, the neuroprotective effects of polydatin on neurological function and the Nrf2 pathway of rats with cerebral hemorrhage were identified. Their study showed that polydatin enhanced neurological function and decreased oxidative stress in rats by controlling the Nrf2/ARE pathway and downstream gene production [84]. Mitochondrial dysfunction and apoptosis are involved in the process of ischemic stroke. In the study of Gao et al., the neuroprotective effect of polydatin was evaluated. Their results demonstrated the anti-apoptotic effect of polydatin and improved mitochondrial dysfunction due to ischemic/reperfusion injury in a rat MCAO model. Increasing Bcl-2 and decreasing cytochrome c, Bax, and caspases-3/9 are centrally associated protective mechanisms [37].

Considering the role of cell adhesion molecules (CAMs) in developing ischemia/reperfusion-induced cerebrovascular diseases in a rat MCAO model, Cheng et al. found that polydatin can reduce the volume of brain infarction by decreasing the levels of CAMs in comparison to the control group, as well as the involvement of E-selectin, L-selectin, integrins, ICAM-1, and vascular cell adhesion molecule-1 (VCAM-1) [85]. Metastasis-associated lung adenocarcinoma transcript 1 (MALAT1) is a non-coding RNA that has a role in protecting the blood–brain barrier after an ischemic event. In the study of Ruan et al., it has been demonstrated that polydatin could upregulate the expression of MALAT1. Polydatin initiated a MALAT1/CREB/PGC-1α/PPARγ cascade that eventually led to protecting cerebrovascular endothelium and blood–brain barrier integrity from ischemia [81]. Moreover, Chen et al. discovered that high doses of polydatin could reduce edema, inflammation, and apoptosis after an ischemic event in the brain tissue of rat models with MCAO by regulating the expression of p53 and Notch1. The scores for the neurological function and behavioral scores were also improved in such models [86]. During an in vitro study, the protective effects of polydatin have also been shown in influencing the regulation of neuroglobin (Ngb) promotor activity and mRNA expression [87]. Polydatin might also regulate gene expression of Ngb through the attenuation of CREB, HIF-1α, p56, and early growth response protein 1 (Egr1). Besides, a polydatin-associated reduction in NO was also related to Ngb up-regulation [88,89]. From another point of view, polydatin meaningfully inhibited cerebral edema in cerebral hemorrhage rats by suppressing excitatory amino acids [90].

Beyond the stroke, polydatin has shown several other neuroprotective effects. For instance, in the study of Guan et al., polydatin potentially showed anxiolytic effects and suppressed neuroinflammation in a chronic pain mouse model by reducing pro-inflammatory cytokines, including TNF-α and IL-1β in the amygdala [91].

Different mechanisms are employed by polydatin to combat stroke and anxiety, including Nrf2/HO-1/ARE, Bax/caspases, Egr1/Ngb, CREB, and PGC-1. Additionally, antioxidant activity, an improvement in mitochondrial health, free-radical scavenging, anti-apoptotic/anti-inflammatory activities, up-regulation of BDNF/Shh/Ngb pathway, and down-regulation of CAMs are other protective mechanisms of polydatin [19,92].

The entire set of neuropharmacological characteristics of polydatin against AD, PD, TBI/SCI, and stroke are presented in Table 1. Overall, by employing several mechanisms and the modulation of various dysregulated pathways, polydatin could be a promising neuroprotective phytochemical against PD, AD, TBI/SCI, and stroke (Figure 2).

Table 1. Neuropharmacological mechanisms of polydatin against different NDDs.

NDDs	Methods	Models	Neuropharmacological Mechanisms	References
AD	Chronic cerebral hypoperfusion	in vivo: Sprague–Dawley rats	↓MDA, ↑CAT, ↑SOD	[44]
	Doxorubicin-induced cognitive impairment	in vivo: Sprague–Dawley rats	↓Nrf2, ↑NF-κB, ↓caspase-3, ↓caspase-9	[45,46]
	HIBI	in vivo: Sprague–Dawley rats	↓Memory deficient, ↑BDNF	[47]
	Chronic ethanol exposure	in vivo: Sprague–Dawley rats	↑Cell survival, ↓cdk5, ↓functional defects	[48]
	Polymerization of Aβ	in vitro: Aβ$_{25-35}$	↓Aβ25–35 polymerization	[49,50]
	D-galactose-induced	in vitro: DPPH in vivo: Male Kunming mice	↑Body weight, ↓MDA, ↑CAT, ↑SOD, ↑GSH, ↓IL-1β, ↓TNF-α, ↓IL-6, ↓ Bax/Bcl-2, ↓caspase-3	[30]

Table 1. Cont.

NDDs	Methods	Models	Neuropharmacological Mechanisms	References
PD	Rotenone-induced	in vitro: Human neuroblastoma SH-SY5Y	↓Mitochondrial dysfunction, Atg5-mediated autophagy, modulating MMP, ↑Sirt 1, ↓ROS	[57]
	LPS-induced	in vitro: Microglial BV-2 cells in vivo: Wistar rats	↑p-GSK-3β, ↑p-Akt, ↑Ser9, ↑Nrf2, ↓NF-κB	[62]
	MPTP-induced	in vivo: Adult male BALB/c mice	↑Glycolysis, ↑ATP production, ↓motor dysfunction	[65]
	Rotenone-induced	in vivo: Sprague–Dawley rats	↑ATP, ↑SOD, ↑thioredoxin,	[61]
		in vitro: Dopaminergic SH-SY5Y cells	↑MAPK, ↓caspase-3, caspase-7, ↓LPO, ↑ERK1/2/5	[67]
TBI/SCI	Brain injury	in vivo: Wistar albino male rats	↓MDA, ↑antioxidant potential	[93]
	SCI	in vitro: murine microglia BV2 cells in vivo: Sprague-Dawley rats	↑Nrf2, ↑HO-1, ↓caspase-3, ↓Bax/Bcl-2 ratio	[34]
	Oxygen glucose deprivation/re-oxygenation-induced mitochondrial injury	in vivo: C57BL/6J mice in vitro: SMNs	↑Intracellular calcium levels, ↑mPTP, ↓ROS, ↓apoptosis, ↑ATP, ↓Keap1, ↑Nrf2, ↑HO-1, ↑NQO-1	[73]
	Neuronal differentiation of BMSCs	in vivo: C57BL/6 mice in vitro: Bone marrow mesenchymal stem cell (BMSC)	↑Nrf2	[74,75]
	Secondary damage of TBI	in vivo: TBI mouse model in vitro: Neuro2A cells	↓GPx, ↑MDA, ↓accumulation of free Fe^{2+}	[76]
	SCI	in vivo: Sprague-Dawley rats in vitro: Murine microglia BV2 cells	↓TNF-α, ↓IL-1β, ↓NO, ↓iNOS, ↓IL-6, ↓NF-κB	[94]
	D-galactose-induced	in vivo: Male Kunming mice in vitro: DPPH	↓TNF-α, ↓IL-1β, ↓IL-6, ↓caspase-3, ↓Bax/Bcl-2	[30]
Stroke	MCAO	in vivo: Sprague–Dawley rats	↑Nrf2, ↑HO-1, ↓ROS, ↓p38, ↑Gli1, ↑Ptch1, ↑SOD1	[82,83]
	Intracerebral hemorrhage	in vivo: Wistar rat	↑Neurological function, ↑NO, ↑SOD, ↑MDA, ↑GSSG, ↑GSH, ↑Nrf2	[95]
	MCAO	in vivo: Sprague–Dawley rats	↑Bcl-2, ↓IL-1β, ↓TNF-α, ↓IL-6, ↓Bax, ↓caspases-3/9	[37]
	Ischemia–reperfusion injury	in vivo: Sprague–Dawley rats	↓CAMs, ↓E-selectin, ↓L-selectin, ↓ICAM-1	[85]
	OGD	in vitro: Human embryonic kidney cells (HEK-293T) in vivo: Sprague–Dawley rats	↑MALAT1, ↑CREB, ↑PGC-1α	[81]
	MCAO	in vivo: Sprague–Dawley rats	↓Edema, ↓apoptosis, p53/Notch1 modulation	[86]
	OGD	in vitro: PC12 cell	↓CREB, ↓HIF-1α, ↓p56, ↓Egr1, ↑Ngb, ↓NO	[87–89]
	Hypoxia/ischemia and oxidative stress-induced injury	in vitro: N2a cells	↓CREB, ↑BDNF, ↑Shh, ↑Ngb, ↓apoptosis	[19,92]

AD: Alzheimer's disease, Akt: Protein kinase B, Atg5: Autophagy Related 5, ATP: Adenosine triphosphate, Aβ: Amyloid beta, Bcl-2: B-cell lymphoma 2, BDNF: Brain-derived neurotrophic factor, BMSCs: Bone marrow mesenchymal stem cell, CAT: Catalase, Cdk5: Cyclin dependent kinase 5, DPPH: 2,2-diphenyl-1-picrylhydrazyl, Egr1: Early growth response 1, ERK: Extracellular-signal-regulated kinase, GRP78: Glucose-regulated protein, GPx: Glutathione peroxidase, GSH: Glutathione, GSK-3β: Glycogen synthase kinase-3β, GSSG: Glutathione disulfide, HEK-293T: Human embryonic kidney cells, HIBI: Hypoxic-ischemic brain injury, HIF-1α: Hypoxia-inducible factor 1-alpha, HO-1: Heme oxygenase-1, ICAM-1: Intercellular adhesion molecule-1, IL: Interleukin, iNOS: Inducible nitric oxide synthase, LPO: Lipid peroxidation, LPS: Lipopolysaccharides, MALAT1: Metastasis associated lung adenocarcinoma transcript 1, MAPK: Mitogen-activated protein kinase, MCAO: Middle cerebral artery occlusion, MDA: Malondialdehyde, MMP: Matrix metalloproteinase, MPTP: 1-methyl-4-phenyl-1,2,3,6-tetrahydropyridine, NF-κB: Nuclear factor kappa-light-chain-enhancer of activated B cells, Ngb: Neuroglobin, NO: Nitric oxide, Nrf2: Nuclear factor E2-related factor 2, OGD: Oxygen-glucose deprivation, PD: Parkinson's disease, PTCH1: Protein patched homolog 1, ROS: Reactive oxygen species, SCI: Spinal cord injury, SMNs: spinal motor neurons, SOD: Superoxide dismutase, TBI: Traumatic brain injury, TNF-α: Tumor necrosis factor α.

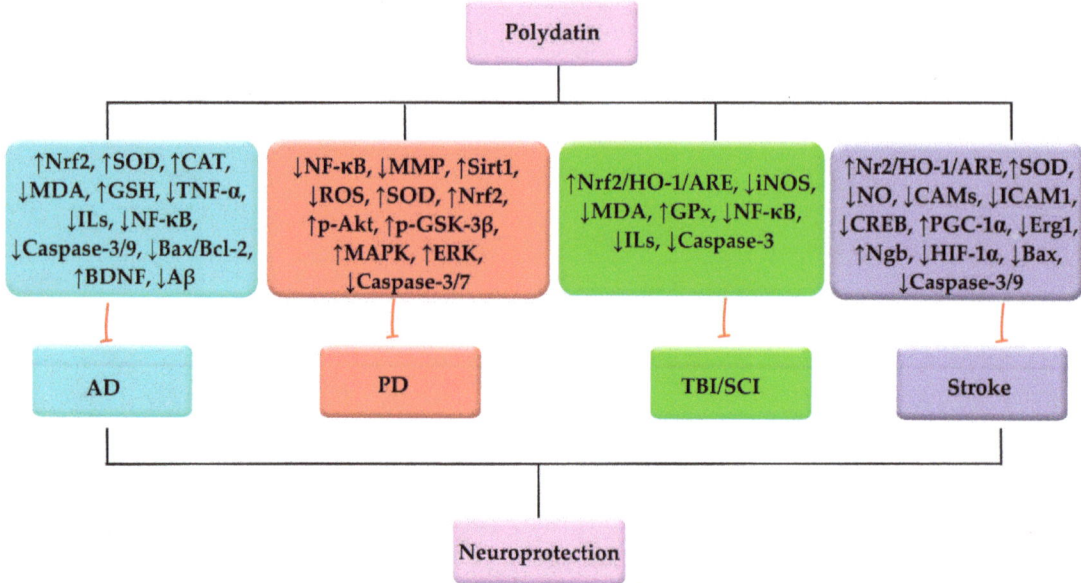

Figure 2. Polydatin employs several mediators to combat PD, AD, TBI/SCI, and stroke.

4. Polydatin Novel Delivery Systems: Nanoformulations, and Targeted Therapy

Nanomedicine is the medicinal use of nanotechnology that employs biocompatible, low-toxicity nanomaterials and nanoparticles to control drug pharmacokinetics, administration rate, and bioavailability [96]. In addition, polydatin may guard against brain injury, kidney problems, heart failure, and improve glucose and lipid metabolism [97,98]. However, therapeutic activities of polydatin are constrained due to weak water solubility, the chemical imbalance in aqueous alkaline medium, and substantial first-pass metabolism. To address these limitations, recyclable nanostructures have sparked wide attention because of their potential in drug delivery and successful removal from the body [11]. In this way, chitosan-loaded nanoparticles administrated daily by gastric intubation for about one month improved the effect of polydatin in male Wistar albino rats [99].

In diabetes mellitus (DM), polydatin was used because of its various therapeutic mechanisms consisting of controlling free-radical production and mitochondrial activity, as well as regulation of inflammation and oxidative stress [97,98]. The anti-hyperglycemic and antioxidant effects of polydatin resulted in a substantial reduction in hemoglobin A1C in treated diabetic rats, and treatment resulted in a significant increase in hepatic glycogen levels, which may be secondary to improved insulin levels and intervention [98].

Apart from its low water solubility, the reduced effectiveness and safety risk of polydatin must be addressed before being used in clinical trials. In this way, microenvironment-sensitive nanoparticles have shown considerable promise in increasing the bioavailability of lipophilic substances [100]. The depletion of liver fibrosis in mice given a polydatin-loaded micelle (PD-MC) was verified by measuring hydroxyproline and fibrotic parameters, including collagen type 1 (Col1), tissue inhibitor of metalloproteinases 1 (TIMP-1), transforming growth factor-beta (TGF-β), and PD-MC, which not only inhibited hepatocyte apoptotic cell death but also showed anti-inflammatory properties. The anti-inflammatory activity of PD-MC was linked to its ability to suppress the ROS and TLR4/NF-B p65 signaling pathway. The mice treated with PD-MC had significantly less hepatic oxidative stress due to the lower levels of 4-Hydroxynonenal (4-HNE) [101].

Polydatin has a clear impact on the cardiac system, acting as an anticoagulant, anti-inflammatory, anti-atherosclerotic, anti-hypercholesterolemic, and anti-ischemic agent. It reduces platelet accumulation, increases microcirculation, strengthens the endothelium and nervous system, and relieves coughing and asthma, which can be found to manage shock [21]. However, the limited oral bioavailability (half-life 8–14 min) and low solubility (the highest solubility is estimated to be 30 g/mL in water at 25 °C) of polydatin has restricted its administration [21,102]. Accordingly, liposomes have shown increased solubilization and stabilization while also providing good drug concentrations for water-soluble and lipid-soluble medicines. The polydatin-loaded liposomes (10 mg/kg) system was balanced in Sprague–Dawley rats. The long-lasting characteristics of the polydatin-loaded liposomal system can improve the absorbance of polydatin in the digestive system, but there are no organ histopathologic modifications after treatment with the polydatin-loaded liposome [102].

In cancer, the traditional treatment options, such as surgery, chemotherapy, radioactivity, immunotherapy, and hormonal treatments, are inadequate for controlling cancer progression [103]. In this way, polydatin possesses various properties such as anti-proliferative, antioxidant, anti-inflammation, and immunomodulatory. For improving the anticancer effectiveness of polydatin and other novel therapies, the production of nanoparticles has received much attention [104]. So, oral administration of polydatin-loaded poly (lactic-co-glycolic acid) [PLGA] nanoparticles (polydatin-PLGA-NPs) in Syrian hamsters resulted in lower amounts of lipid peroxidative byproducts. Polydatin-PLGA-NP therapy decreased tumor histological symptoms from extreme to mild and blocked the development of squamous cell carcinoma. Besides, the administration of polydatin-PLGA-NPs led to a substantial reduction in tumor volume and occurrence. Polydatin-PLGA-NPs significantly increased enzymatic antioxidant rates such as SOD, CAT, and GPx, while decreasing the rate of cytochrome (Cyt) p450, Cyt b5, glutathione S-transferase, gammaglutamil transferase, and glutathione reductase activities, which are among the metabolizing enzymes of phases I and II. Polydatin-PLGA-NPs treatment caused apoptosis via sheared caspase-3 overexpression and the prevention of dimethyl benzyl anthracene-induced mutant p53 and cyclin-D1 production in a dose-dependent manner [105]. As another disorder, irritable bowel syndrome is currently thought to result from dysfunction in the brain—gut axis, including both central and peripheral pathways concerned, and in particular, involving cannabinoid receptors and affecting the activity of most cells. To modulate these dysregulated mechanisms, the effect of a co-micronized form of palmitoylethanolamide/polydatin was examined in 157 patients with irritable bowel syndrome [106].

Altogether, in addition to its high effectiveness and the more appropriate pharmacokinetic characteristics of polydatin, using novel delivery systems for this secondary metabolite could increase the associated efficacy and reduce some of the remaining limitations of phytochemicals, by increasing solubility/bioavailability and decreasing safety risks. Figure 3 shows the novel delivery systems of polydatin.

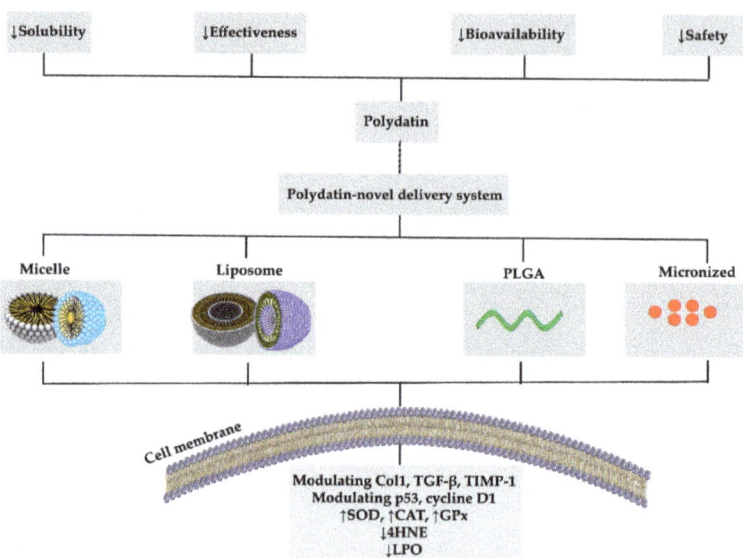

Figure 3. Novel delivery systems of polydatin: Reduction in the pharmacokinetic limitations.

5. Conclusions

Polydatin is a multi-target stilbenoid secondary metabolite extracted from herbal sources. As polydatin is a glycosylated form of resveratrol, several biological activities and health benefits are connected to the administration of polydatin, including cardioprotective, hepatoprotective, and neuroprotective factors. Prevailing studies focus on the neuroprotective potential of polydatin by employing several mechanisms, including Nrf2/Keap1/ARE, PI3K/Akt, ERK/MAPK, TLR/NF-κB/TNF-α/ILs, and Bax/Bcl-2/caspases (Figure 4). In this line, polydatin critically modulates inflammatory, apoptotic, and oxidative mediators towards combating AD, PD, stroke, CNS injuries, and miscellaneous neuroprotective responses. On the other hand, the pharmacokinetic drawbacks of polydatin, including their poor bioavailability, low solubility/selectivity, low plasma concentration, rapid metabolism, and chemical degradation, limit the associated therapeutic uses. It reveals the importance of novel drug delivery systems to reduce the restrictions in modulating tumor cell senescence. It is also worth noting that providing a novel delivery system could potentially help the polydatin to pass through the blood–brain barrier and develop a long-lasting therapeutic concentration of drugs in the CNS, while possessing fewer side effects [107–109].

In the present study, the pharmacological targets, molecular mechanisms, and therapeutic potentials of polydatin are highlighted through the attenuation of inflammatory/apoptotic/oxidative pathways to tackle multiple dysregulated pathways in NDDs. The need to provide novel delivery systems of polydatin, including nanoformulations, and targeted therapy is also considered. Further pre-clinical studies are needed to elucidate the precise neuroprotective mechanisms of polydatin followed by well-controlled clinical trials.

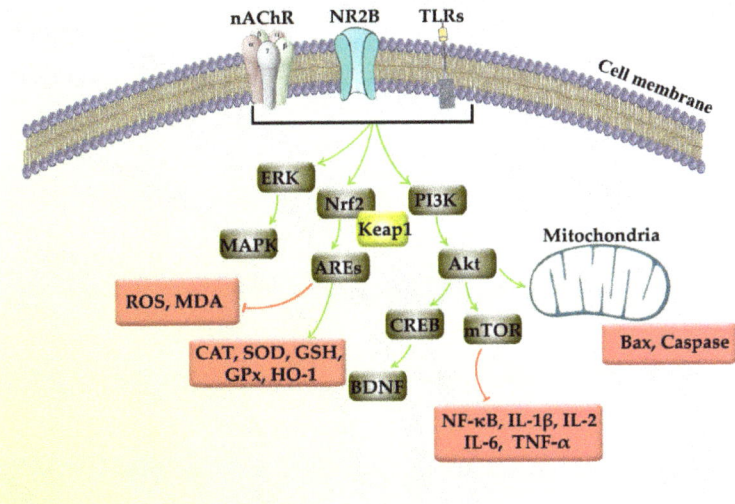

Figure 4. Neuroprotective mechanisms of polydatin.

Author Contributions: Conceptualization, S.F., M.H.F. and E.S.-S.; drafting of the manuscript, S.F., M.M.G. and S.A.; software, S.F., reviewing and editing of the paper: S.F., E.K.A., M.H.F. and E.S.-S.; All authors have read and agreed to the published version of the manuscript.

Funding: This research received no external funding.

Institutional Review Board Statement: Not applicable.

Informed Consent Statement: Not applicable.

Acknowledgments: E.S.-S. thanks Proyecto Interno I+D+I UCEN (CIP2020036) for financial support.

Conflicts of Interest: The authors declare that the research was conducted in the absence of any commercial or financial relationships that could be construed as a potential conflict of interest.

Abbreviations

AD	Alzheimer's disease
Akt	Protein kinase B
Atg5	Autophagy Related 5
ATF6	Activating transcription factor 6 (ATF6)
ATP	Adenosine triphosphate
Aβ	Amyloid beta
Bcl-2	B-cell lymphoma 2
ARE	Antioxidant response element
BDNF	Brain-derived neurotrophic factor
BMSCs	Bone marrow mesenchymal stem cell
CAMs	Cell adhesion molecules
CAT	Catalase
Cdk5	Cyclin dependent kinase 5
Col1	Collagen type 1
Cyt	Cytochrome
DM	Diabetes mellitus

DPPH	2,2-diphenyl-1-picrylhydrazyl
Egr1	Early growth response 1
ERK	Extracellular-signal-regulated kinase
Gli1	Homolog1
GRP78	Glucose-regulated protein
GPx	Glutathione peroxidase
GSH	Glutathione
GSK-3β	Glycogen synthase kinase-3β
GSSG	Glutathione disulfide
HEK-293T	Human embryonic kidney cells
HIBI	Hypoxic-ischemic brain injury
HIF-1α	Hypoxia-inducible factor 1-alpha
HO-1	Heme oxygenase-1
ICAM-1	Intercellular adhesion molecule-1
IL	Interleukin
iNOS	Inducible nitric oxide synthase
LPO	Lipid peroxidation
LPS	Lipopolysaccharides
MALAT1	Metastasis associated lung adenocarcinoma transcript 1
MAPK	Mitogen-activated protein kinase
MCAO	Middle cerebral artery occlusion
MDA	Malondialdehyde
MIF	Macrophage migration inhibitory factor
MMP	Mitochondrial membrane potential
MPTP	1-methyl-4-phenyl-1,2,3,6-tetrahydropyridine
nAChRs	Nicotinic acetylcholine receptors
NDDs	Neurodegenerative diseases
mPTP	Mitochondrial permeability transition pore
NF-κB	Nuclear factor kappa-light-chain-enhancer of activated B cells
Ngb	Neuroglobin
NO	Nitric oxide
Nrf2	Nuclear factor E2-related factor 2
NQO-1	NAD(P)H Quinone Dehydrogenase 1
OGD	Oxygen-glucose deprivation
Ptch1	Patched-1
PD	Parkinson's disease
PD-MC	Polydatin-loaded micelle
PI3K	Phosphoinositide 3-kinases
PLGA	Poly (lactic-co-glycolic acid)
ROS	Reactive oxygen species
SCI	Spinal cord injury
SD	Sprague–Dawley
SGLT1	Sodium-dependent glucose transporter
Sirt1	Sirtuin 1
SMNs	Spinal motor neurons
SOD	Superoxide dismutase
TBI	Traumatic brain injury
TGF-β	Transforming growth factor-beta
TIMP-1	Tissue inhibitor of metalloproteinases 1
TLR	Toll-like receptor
TNF-α	Tumor necrosis factor α
VCAM-1	Vascular cell adhesion molecule-1
4-HNE	4-Hydroxynonenal
6-OHDA	6-hydroxydopamine

References

1. Trapp, B.D.; Nave, K.-A. Multiple sclerosis: An immune or neurodegenerative disorder? *Annu. Rev. Neurosci.* **2008**, *31*, 247–269. [CrossRef]
2. Heneka, M.T.; McManus, R.M.; Latz, E. Inflammasome signalling in brain function and neurodegenerative disease. *Nat. Rev. Neurosci.* **2018**, *19*, 610–621. [CrossRef]
3. LaFerla, F.M.; Oddo, S. Alzheimer's disease: Aβ, tau and synaptic dysfunction. *Trends Mol. Med.* **2005**, *11*, 170–176. [CrossRef]
4. Mamik, M.K.; Power, C. Inflammasomes in neurological diseases: Emerging pathogenic and therapeutic concepts. *Brain* **2017**, *140*, 2273–2285. [CrossRef] [PubMed]
5. Abbaszadeh, F.; Fakhri, S.; Khan, H. Targeting apoptosis and autophagy following spinal cord injury: Therapeutic ap-proaches to polyphenols and candidate phytochemicals. *Pharmacol. Res.* **2020**, *160*, 105069. [CrossRef] [PubMed]
6. Floyd, R.A. Antioxidants, Oxidative Stress, and Degenerative Neurological Disorders. *Proc. Soc. Exp. Boil. Med.* **1999**, *222*, 236–245. [CrossRef]
7. Degan, D.; Ornello, R.; Tiseo, C.; Carolei, A.; Sacco, S.; Pistoia, F. The Role of Inflammation in Neurological Disorders. *Curr. Pharm. Des.* **2018**, *24*, 1485–1501. [CrossRef] [PubMed]
8. Wu, Y.; Chen, M.; Jiang, J. Mitochondrial dysfunction in neurodegenerative diseases and drug targets via apoptotic signaling. *Mitochondrion* **2019**, *49*, 35–45. [CrossRef] [PubMed]
9. Fakhri, S.; Abbaszadeh, F.; Dargahi, L.; Jorjani, M. Astaxanthin: A mechanistic review on its biological activities and health benefits. *Pharmacol. Res.* **2018**, *136*, 1–20. [CrossRef] [PubMed]
10. Fakhri, S.; Abbaszadeh, F.; Jorjani, M. On the therapeutic targets and pharmacological treatments for pain relief following spinal cord injury: A mechanistic review. *Biomed. Pharmacother.* **2021**, *139*, 111563. [CrossRef] [PubMed]
11. Zarneshan, S.N.; Fakhri, S.; Farzaei, M.H.; Khan, H.; Saso, L. Astaxanthin targets PI3K/Akt signaling pathway toward potential therapeutic applications. *Food. Chem. Toxicol.* **2020**, *145*, 111714. [CrossRef]
12. Gravandi, M.M.; Fakhri, S.; Zarneshan, S.N.; Yarmohammadi, A.; Khan, H. Flavonoids modulate AMPK/PGC-1α and inter-connected pathways toward potential neuroprotective activities. *Metab. Brain Dis.* **2021**, *36*, 1501–1521. [CrossRef] [PubMed]
13. Fakhri, S.; Iranpanah, A.; Gravandi, M.M.; Moradi, S.Z.; Ranjbari, M.; Majnooni, M.B.; Echeverría, J.; Qi, Y.; Wang, M.; Liao, P.; et al. Natural products attenuate PI3K/Akt/mTOR signaling pathway: A promising strategy in regulating neurodegeneration. *Phytomedicine* **2021**, *91*, 153664. [CrossRef] [PubMed]
14. Dvorakova, M.; Landa, P. Anti-inflammatory activity of natural stilbenoids: A review. *Pharmacol. Res.* **2017**, *124*, 126–145. [CrossRef] [PubMed]
15. Xiao, K.; Zhang, H.-J.; Xuan, L.-J.; Zhang, J.; Xu, Y.-M.; Bai, D.-L. Stilbenoids: Chemistry and bioactivities. In *Bioactive Natural Products (Part L)*; Attaur, R., Ed.; Elsevier: Amsterdam, The Netherlands, 2008; Volume 34, pp. 453–646.
16. Henry, C.; Vitrac, X.; Decendit, A.; Ennamany, R.; Krisa, S.; Mérillon, J.-M. Cellular uptake and efflux of trans-piceid and its aglycone trans-resveratrol on the apical membrane of human intestinal Caco-2 cells. *J. Agric. Food Chem.* **2005**, *53*, 798–803. [CrossRef] [PubMed]
17. Henry-Vitrac, C.; Desmoulière, A.; Girard, D.; Mérillon, J.-M.; Krisa, S. Transport, deglycosylation, and metabolism of trans-piceid by small intestinal epithelial cells. *Eur. J. Nutr.* **2006**, *45*, 376–382. [CrossRef] [PubMed]
18. Zhao, X.-J.; Yu, H.-W.; Yang, Y.-Z.; Wu, W.-Y.; Chen, T.-Y.; Jia, K.-K.; Kang, L.-L.; Jiao, R.-Q.; Kong, L.-D. Polydatin prevents fructose-induced liver inflammation and lipid deposition through increasing miR-200a to regulate Keap1/Nrf2 pathway. *Redox Biol.* **2018**, *18*, 124–137. [CrossRef] [PubMed]
19. Tang, K.S.; Tan, J.S. The protective mechanisms of polydatin in cerebral ischemia. *Eur. J. Pharmacol.* **2019**, *842*, 133–138. [CrossRef]
20. Tang, K.S. Protective Effects of Polydatin Against Dementia-Related Disorders. *Curr. Neuropharmacol.* **2020**, *19*, 127–135. [CrossRef]
21. Du, Q.-H.; Peng, C.; Zhang, H. Polydatin: A review of pharmacology and pharmacokinetics. *Pharm. Biol.* **2013**, *51*, 1347–1354. [CrossRef]
22. Ribeiro de Lima, M.T.; Waffo-Téguo, P.; Teissedre, P.L.; Pujolas, A.; Vercauteren, J.; Cabanis, J.C.; Mérillon, J.M. Determination of stilbenes (trans-astringin, cis- and trans- piceid, and cis- and trans- resveratrol) in Portuguese wines. *J. Agric. Food Chem.* **1999**, *47*, 2666–2670. [CrossRef]
23. Zamora-Ros, R.; Andres-Lacueva, C.; Lamuela-Raventós, R.M.; Berenguer, T.; Jakszyn, P.; Martínez, C.; Sánchez, M.J.; Navarro, C.; Chirlaque, M.D.; Tormo, M.-J.; et al. Concentrations of resveratrol and derivatives in foods and estimation of dietary intake in a Spanish population: European Prospective Investigation into Cancer and Nutrition (EPIC)-Spain cohort. *Br. J. Nutr.* **2008**, *100*, 188–196. [CrossRef]
24. Jensen, J.S.; Wertz, C.F.; O'Neill, V.A. Preformulation Stability of trans-Resveratrol and trans-Resveratrol Glucoside (Piceid). *J. Agric. Food Chem.* **2010**, *58*, 1685–1690. [CrossRef]
25. Galeano-Díaz, T.; Durán-Merás, I.; Airado-Rodríguez, D. Isocratic chromatography of resveratrol and piceid after previous generation of fluorescent photoproducts: Wine analysis without sample preparation. *J. Sep. Sci.* **2007**, *30*, 3110–3119. [CrossRef]
26. Wang, H.-L.; Gao, J.-P.; Han, Y.-L.; Xu, X.; Wu, R.; Gao, Y.; Cui, X.-H. Comparative studies of polydatin and resveratrol on mutual transformation and antioxidative effect in vivo. *Phytomedicine* **2015**, *22*, 553–559. [CrossRef] [PubMed]
27. He, H.; Zhao, Y.; Chen, X.; Zheng, Y.; Wu, X.; Wang, R.; Li, T.; Yu, Q.; Jing, J.; Ma, L.; et al. Quantitative determination of trans-polydatin, a natural strong anti-oxidative compound, in rat plasma and cellular environment of a human colon ade-nocarcinoma cell line for pharmacokinetic studies. *J. Chromatogr. B* **2007**, *855*, 145–151. [CrossRef]

28. Lv, G.; Lou, Z.; Chen, S.; Gu, H.; Shan, L. Pharmacokinetics and tissue distribution of 2,3,5,4′-tetrahydroxystilbene-2-O-β-d-glucoside from traditional Chinese medicine Polygonum multiflorum following oral ad-ministration to rats. *J. Ethnopharmacol.* **2011**, *137*, 449–456. [CrossRef] [PubMed]
29. Lanzilli, G.; Cottarelli, A.; Nicotera, G.; Guida, S.; Ravagnan, G.; Fuggetta, M.P. Anti-inflammatory Effect of Resveratrol and Polydatin by In Vitro IL-17 Modulation. *Inflammation* **2011**, *35*, 240–248. [CrossRef] [PubMed]
30. Xu, L.-Q.; Xie, Y.-L.; Gui, S.-H.; Zhang, X.; Mo, Z.-Z.; Sun, C.-Y.; Li, C.-L.; Luo, D.-D.; Zhang, Z.-B.; Su, Z.-R.; et al. Polydatin attenuates D-galactose-induced liver and brain damage through its anti-oxidative, anti-inflammatory and anti-apoptotic effects in mice. *Food Funct.* **2016**, *7*, 4545–4555. [CrossRef] [PubMed]
31. Jayalakshmi, P.; Devika, P. Assessment of in vitro antioxidant activity study of polydatin. *J. Pharm. Phytochem.* **2019**, *8*, 55–58.
32. Zeng, Z.; Chen, Z.; Li, T.; Zhang, J.; Gao, Y.; Xu, S.; Cai, S.; Zhao, K.-S. Polydatin: A new therapeutic agent against multiorgan dysfunction. *J. Surg. Res.* **2015**, *198*, 192–199. [CrossRef]
33. Liu, H.-B.; Meng, Q.-H.; Huang, C.; Wang, J.-B.; Liu, X.-W. Nephroprotective effects of polydatin against ischemia/reperfusion injury: A role for the PI3K/Akt signal pathway. *Oxidative Med. Cell. Longev.* **2015**, *2015*, 362158. [CrossRef]
34. Lv, R.; Du, L.; Zhang, L.; Zhang, Z. Polydatin attenuates spinal cord injury in rats by inhibiting oxidative stress and microglia apoptosis via Nrf2/HO-1 pathway. *Life Sci.* **2019**, *217*, 119–127. [CrossRef]
35. Jiang, K.-F.; Zhao, G.; Deng, G.-Z.; Wu, H.-C.; Yin, N.-N.; Chen, X.-Y.; Qiu, C.-W.; Peng, X.-L. Polydatin ameliorates Staphylococcus aureus-induced mastitis in mice via inhibiting TLR2-mediated activation of the p38 MAPK/NF-κB pathway. *Acta Pharmacol. Sin.* **2017**, *38*, 211–222. [CrossRef] [PubMed]
36. Starkov, A.A. The Role of Mitochondria in Reactive Oxygen Species Metabolism and Signaling. *Ann. N. Y. Acad. Sci.* **2008**, *1147*, 37–52. [CrossRef] [PubMed]
37. Gao, Y.; Chen, T.; Lei, X.; Li, Y.; Dai, X.; Cao, Y.; Ding, Q.; Lei, X.; Li, T.; Lin, X. Neuroprotective effects of polydatin against mitochondrial-dependent apoptosis in the rat cerebral cortex following ischemia/reperfusion injury. *Mol. Med. Rep.* **2016**, *14*, 5481–5488. [CrossRef]
38. Zeng, Z.; Yang, Y.; Dai, X.; Xu, S.; Li, T.; Zhang, Q.; Zhao, K.-S.; Chen, Z. Polydatin ameliorates injury to the small intestine induced by hemorrhagic shock via SIRT3 activation-mediated mitochondrial protection. *Expert Opin. Ther. Targets* **2016**, *20*, 645–652. [CrossRef]
39. Mathys, H.; Davila-Velderrain, J.; Peng, Z.; Gao, F.; Mohammadi, S.; Young, J.Z.; Menon, M.; He, L.; Abdurrob, F.; Jiang, X.; et al. Single-cell transcriptomic analysis of Alzheimer's disease. *Nature* **2019**, *570*, 332–337. [CrossRef] [PubMed]
40. Cheignon, C.; Tomas, M.; Bonnefont-Rousselot, D.; Faller, P.; Hureau, C.; Collin, F. Oxidative stress and the amyloid beta peptide in Alzheimer's disease. *Redox Boil.* **2018**, *14*, 450–464. [CrossRef]
41. Milanini, B.; Valcour, V. Differentiating HIV-Associated Neurocognitive Disorders From Alzheimer's Disease: An Emerging Issue in Geriatric NeuroHIV. *Curr. HIV/AIDS Rep.* **2017**, *14*, 123–132. [CrossRef]
42. Schneider, J.A.; Arvanitakis, Z.; Leurgans, S.E.; Bennett, D.A. The neuropathology of probable Alzheimer disease and mild cognitive impairment. *Ann. Neurol. Off. J. Am. Neurol. Assoc. Child Neurol. Soc.* **2009**, *66*, 200–208. [CrossRef]
43. Fakhri, S.; Pesce, M.; Patruno, A.; Moradi, S.Z.; Iranpanah, A.; Farzaei, M.H.; Sobarzo-Sánchez, E. Attenuation of Nrf2/Keap1/ARE in Alzheimer's disease by plant secondary metabolites: A mechanistic review. *Molecules* **2020**, *25*, 4926. [CrossRef] [PubMed]
44. Li, R.-P.; Wang, Z.-Z.; Sun, M.-X.; Hou, X.-L.; Sun, Y.; Deng, Z.-F.; Xiao, K. Polydatin protects learning and memory impair-ments in a rat model of vascular dementia. *Phytomedicine* **2012**, *19*, 677–681. [CrossRef] [PubMed]
45. Tong, Y.; Wang, K.; Sheng, S.; Cui, J. Polydatin ameliorates chemotherapy-induced cognitive impairment (chemobrain) by inhibiting oxidative stress, inflammatory response, and apoptosis in rats. *Biosci. Biotechnol. Biochem.* **2020**, *84*, 1201–1210. [CrossRef] [PubMed]
46. Cauli, O. Oxidative Stress and Cognitive Alterations Induced by Cancer Chemotherapy Drugs: A Scoping Review. *Antioxidants* **2021**, *10*, 1116. [CrossRef] [PubMed]
47. Sun, J.; Qu, Y.; He, H.; Fan, X.; Qin, Y.; Mao, W.; Xu, L. Protective effect of polydatin on learning and memory impairments in neonatal rats with hypoxic-ischemic brain injury by up-regulating brain-derived neurotrophic factor. *Mol. Med. Rep.* **2014**, *10*, 3047–3051. [CrossRef]
48. Zhang, Y.; Li, S.; Wang, W.; Xu, C.; Liang, S.; Liu, M.; Hao, W.; Zhang, R. Beneficial effects of polydatin on learning and memory in rats with chronic ethanol exposure. *Int. J. Clin. Exp. Pathol.* **2015**, *8*, 11116–11123.
49. Rivière, C.; Richard, T.; Quentin, L.; Krisa, S.; Mérillon, J.-M.; Monti, J.-P. Inhibitory activity of stilbenes on Alzheimer's β-amyloid fibrils in vitro. *Bioorg. Med. Chem.* **2007**, *15*, 1160–1167. [CrossRef]
50. Rivière, C.; Delaunay, J.-C.; Immel, F.; Cullin, C.; Monti, J.-P. The Polyphenol Piceid Destabilizes Preformed Amyloid Fibrils and Oligomers In Vitro: Hypothesis on Possible Molecular Mechanisms. *Neurochem. Res.* **2008**, *34*, 1120–1128. [CrossRef]
51. Xiao, H.-T.; Qi, X.-L.; Liang, Y.; Lin, C.-Y.; Wang, X.; Guan, Z.-Z.; Hao, X.-Y. Membrane permeability-guided identification of neuroprotective components from Polygonum cuspidatun. *Pharm. Biol.* **2013**, *52*, 356–361. [CrossRef]
52. Xu, C.-Y.; Li, S.; Chen, L.; Hou, F.-J.; Zhng, R.-L. [Effect of polydatin on learning and memory and expression of NR2B in the prefrontal cortex of rats with chronic alcoholism]. *Chin. J. Appl. Physiol.* **2011**, *27*, 213–235.
53. de Lau, L.M.L.; Breteler, M.M.B. Epidemiology of Parkinson's disease. *Lancet Neurol.* **2006**, *5*, 525–535. [CrossRef]
54. Shtilbans, A.; Henchcliffe, C. Biomarkers in Parkinson's disease. *Curr. Opin. Neurol.* **2012**, *25*, 460–465. [CrossRef]

55. Jiang, T.; Sun, Q.; Chen, S. Oxidative stress: A major pathogenesis and potential therapeutic target of antioxidative agents in Parkinson's disease and Alzheimer's disease. *Prog. Neurobiol.* **2016**, *147*, 1–19. [CrossRef]
56. Roy, S. Synuclein and dopamine: The Bonnie and Clyde of Parkinson's disease. *Nat. Neurosci.* **2017**, *20*, 1514–1515. [CrossRef]
57. Bai, H.; Ding, Y.; Li, X.; Kong, D.; Xin, C.; Yang, X.; Zhang, C.; Rong, Z.; Yao, C.; Lu, S.; et al. Polydatin protects SH-SY5Y in models of Parkinson's disease by promoting Atg5-mediated but parkin-independent autophagy. *Neurochem. Int.* **2020**, *134*, 104671. [CrossRef] [PubMed]
58. Kang, L.; Liu, S.; Li, J.; Tian, Y.; Xue, Y.; Liu, X. Parkin and Nrf2 prevent oxidative stress-induced apoptosis in intervertebral endplate chondrocytes via inducing mitophagy and anti-oxidant defenses. *Life Sci.* **2020**, *243*, 117244. [CrossRef]
59. Yun, S.P.; Kam, T.-I.; Panicker, N.; Kim, S.; Oh, Y.; Park, J.-S.; Kwon, S.-H.; Park, Y.J.; Karuppagounder, S.S.; Park, H.; et al. Block of A1 astrocyte conversion by microglia is neuroprotective in models of Parkinson's disease. *Nat. Med.* **2018**, *24*, 931–938. [CrossRef] [PubMed]
60. Kujawska, M.; Jodynis-Liebert, J. Polyphenols in Parkinson's Disease: A Systematic Review of In Vivo Studies. *Nutrients* **2018**, *10*, 642. [CrossRef] [PubMed]
61. Chen, Y.; Zhang, D.-Q.; Liao, Z.; Wang, B.; Gong, S.; Wang, C.; Zhang, M.-Z.; Wang, G.-H.; Cai, H.; Liao, F.-F.; et al. Anti-oxidant polydatin (piceid) protects against substantia nigral motor degeneration in multiple rodent models of Parkinson's disease. *Mol. Neurodegener.* **2015**, *10*, 1–14. [CrossRef] [PubMed]
62. Huang, B.; Liu, J.; Meng, T.; Li, Y.; He, D.; Ran, X.; Chen, G.; Guo, W.; Kan, X.; Fu, S.; et al. Polydatin prevents lipopolysaccharide (LPS)-induced Parkinson's disease via regulation of the AKT/GSK3β-Nrf2/NF-κB signaling axis. *Front. Immunol.* **2018**, *9*, 2527. [CrossRef]
63. Bachiller, S.; Jiménez-Ferrer, I.; Paulus, A.; Yang, Y.; Swanberg, M.; Deierborg, T.; Boza-Serrano, A. Microglia in neurological diseases: A road map to brain-disease dependent-inflammatory response. *Front. Cell. Neurosci.* **2018**, *12*, 488. [CrossRef]
64. Hong, C.T.; Chau, K.-Y.; Schapira, A.H.V. Meclizine-induced enhanced glycolysis is neuroprotective in Parkinson disease cell models. *Sci. Rep.* **2016**, *6*, 25344. [CrossRef] [PubMed]
65. Zhang, S.; Wang, S.; Shi, X.; Feng, X. Polydatin alleviates parkinsonism in MPTP-model mice by enhancing glycolysis in dopaminergic neurons. *Neurochem. Int.* **2020**, *139*, 104815. [CrossRef] [PubMed]
66. Guo, C.; Sun, L.; Chen, X.; Zhang, D. Oxidative stress, mitochondrial damage and neurodegenerative diseases. *Neural Regen. Res.* **2013**, *8*, 2003–2014. [CrossRef] [PubMed]
67. Potdar, S.; Parmar, M.S.; Ray, S.D.; Cavanaugh, J.E. Protective effects of the resveratrol analog piceid in dopaminergic SH-SY5Y cells. *Arch. Toxicol.* **2018**, *92*, 669–677. [CrossRef] [PubMed]
68. Ahmed, M.R.; Shaikh, M.A.; Baloch, N.A.; Nazir, S.; Abrar, H.; Ulhaq, H.S.I. Neuroprotective Potential of Polydatin Against Motor Abnormalities and Dopaminergic Neuronal Loss in Rotenone Induced Parkinson Model. *Int. J. Morphol.* **2018**, *36*, 584–591. [CrossRef]
69. Fakhri, S.; Tomas, M.; Capanoglu, E.; Hussain, Y.; Abbaszadeh, F.; Lu, B.; Hu, X.; Wu, J.; Zou, L.; Smeriglio, A. Antioxidant and anticancer potentials of edible flowers: Where do we stand? *Crit. Rev. Food Sci. Nutr.* **2021**, 1–57. [CrossRef]
70. Shi, K.; Zhang, J.; Dong, J.-F.; Shi, F.-D. Dissemination of brain inflammation in traumatic brain injury. *Cell. Mol. Immunol.* **2019**, *16*, 523–530. [CrossRef]
71. Fakhri, S.; Piri, S.; Majnooni, M.B.; Farzaei, M.H.; Echeverría, J. Targeting neurological manifestations of coronaviruses by candidate phytochemicals: A mechanistic approach. *Front. Pharmacol.* **2020**, *11*, 621099. [CrossRef] [PubMed]
72. Nouri, Z.; Fakhri, S.; Nouri, K.; Wallace, C.E.; Farzaei, M.H.; Bishayee, A. Targeting multiple signaling pathways in cancer: The rutin therapeutic approach. *Cancers* **2020**, *12*, 2276. [CrossRef]
73. Zhan, J.; Li, X.; Luo, D.; Yan, W.; Hou, Y.; Hou, Y.; Chen, S.; Luan, J.; Zhang, Q.; Lin, D. Polydatin Attenuates OGD/R-Induced Neuronal Injury and Spinal Cord Ischemia/Reperfusion Injury by Protecting Mitochondrial Function via Nrf2/ARE Signaling Pathway. *Oxidative Med. Cell. Longev.* **2021**, *2021*, 6687212. [CrossRef] [PubMed]
74. Zhan, J.; Li, X.; Luo, D.; Hou, Y.; Hou, Y.; Chen, S.; Xiao, Z.; Luan, J.; Lin, D. Polydatin promotes the neuronal differentiation of bone marrow mesenchymal stem cells in vitro and in vivo: Involvement of Nrf2 signalling pathway. *J. Cell. Mol. Med.* **2020**, *24*, 5317–5329. [CrossRef]
75. Chen, M.; Hou, Y.; Lin, D. Polydatin Protects Bone Marrow Stem Cells against Oxidative Injury: Involvement of Nrf 2/ARE Pathways. *Stem Cells Int.* **2016**, *2016*, 9394150. [CrossRef] [PubMed]
76. Huang, L.; He, S.; Cai, Q.; Li, F.; Wang, S.; Tao, K.; Xi, Y.; Qin, H.; Gao, G.; Feng, D. Polydatin alleviates traumatic brain injury: Role of inhibiting ferroptosis. *Biochem. Biophys. Res. Commun.* **2021**, *556*, 149–155. [CrossRef] [PubMed]
77. Prochazka, A. Targeted stimulation of the spinal cord to restore locomotor activity. *Nat. Med.* **2016**, *22*, 125–126. [CrossRef] [PubMed]
78. Fakhri, S.; Kiani, A.; Jalili, C.; Abbaszadeh, F.; Piri, S.; Farzaei, M.H.; Rastegari-Pouyani, M.; Mohammadi-Noori, E.; Khan, H. Intrathecal Administration of Melatonin Ameliorates the Neuroinflammation-mediated Sensory and Motor Dysfunction in a rat Model of Compression Spinal Cord Injury. *Curr. Mol. Pharmacol.* **2020**. [CrossRef]
79. Gu, Z.; Li, L.; Li, Q.; Tan, H.; Zou, Z.; Chen, X.; Zhang, Z.; Zhou, Y.; Wei, D.; Liu, C.; et al. Polydatin alleviates severe traumatic brain injury induced acute lung injury by inhibiting S100B mediated NETs formation. *Int. Immunopharmacol.* **2021**, *98*, 107699. [CrossRef]
80. Wolfe, C.D.A. The impact of stroke. *Br. Med. Bull.* **2000**, *56*, 275–286. [CrossRef]

81. Ruan, W.; Li, J.; Xu, Y.; Wang, Y.; Zhao, F.; Yang, X.; Jiang, H.; Zhang, L.; Saavedra, J.M.; Shi, L.; et al. MALAT1 up-regulator poly-datin protects brain microvascular integrity and ameliorates stroke through C/EBPβ/MALAT1/CREB/PGC-1α/PPARγ path-way. *Cell. Mol. Neurobiol.* **2019**, *39*, 265–286. [CrossRef] [PubMed]
82. Shah, F.A.; Kury, L.A.; Li, T.; Zeb, A.; Koh, P.O.; Liu, F.; Zhou, Q.; Hussain, I.; Khan, A.U.; Jiang, Y.; et al. Polydatin attenuates neu-ronal loss via reducing neuroinflammation and oxidative stress in rat MCAO models. *Front. Pharmacol.* **2019**, *10*, 663. [CrossRef]
83. Ji, H.; Zhang, X.; Du, Y.; Liu, H.; Li, S.; Li, L. Polydatin modulates inflammation by decreasing NF-κB activation and oxidative stress by increasing Gli1, Ptch1, SOD1 expression and ameliorates blood–brain barrier permeability for its neuroprotective effect in pMCAO rat brain. *Brain Res. Bull.* **2012**, *87*, 50–59. [CrossRef] [PubMed]
84. Bheereddy, P.; Yerra, V.G.; Kalvala, A.K.; Sherkhane, B.; Kumar, A. SIRT1 activation by polydatin alleviates oxidative damage and elevates mitochondrial biogenesis in experimental diabetic neuropathy. *Cell Mol. Neurobiol.* **2020**, 1–15. [CrossRef]
85. Cheng, Y.; Zhang, H.-T.; Sun, L.; Guo, S.; Ouyang, S.; Zhang, Y.; Xu, J. Involvement of cell adhesion molecules in polydatin protection of brain tissues from ischemia–reperfusion injury. *Brain Res.* **2006**, *1110*, 193–200. [CrossRef] [PubMed]
86. Chen, F.Y.; Fang, X.Y.; Zhang, H. Effect of polydatin on expression of p53 and Notch1 in brain tissue of ischemic cerebrovascular disease. *J. Biol. Regul. Homeost. Agents* **2018**, *32*, 133–138. [PubMed]
87. Liu, N.; Yu, Z.; Gao, X.; Yun, S.S.; Yuan, J.; Xun, Y.; Wang, T.; Yan, F.; Yuan, S.; Zhang, J.; et al. Establishment of cell-based neu-roglobin promoter reporter assay for neuroprotective compounds screening. *CNS Neurol. Disord.-Drug Targets (Former. Curr. Drug Targets-CNS Neurol. Disord.)* **2016**, *15*, 629–639.
88. Xu, B.; Lin, H.-B.; Zhou, H.; Xu, J.-P. [Protective effect of polydatin on a PC12 cell model of oxygen-glucose deprivation]. *Nan fang yi ke da xue xue bao J. South. Med Univ.* **2010**, *30*, 1041–1043.
89. Liu, N.; Yu, Z.; Xiang, S.; Zhao, S.; Tjärnlund-Wolf, A.; Xing, C.; Zhang, J.; Wang, X. Transcriptional regulation mechanisms of hypoxia-induced neuroglobin gene expression. *Biochem. J.* **2012**, *443*, 153–164. [CrossRef] [PubMed]
90. Liu, H.; Zhang, G.; Bie, X.; Liu, M.; Yang, Y.; Wan, H.; Zhang, Y. Effect of polydatin on dynamic changes of excitatory amino acids in cerebrospinal fluid of cerebral hemorrhage rats. *China J. Chin. Mater. Med.* **2010**, *35*, 3038–3042.
91. Guan, S.-Y.; Zhang, K.; Wang, X.-S.; Yang, L.; Feng, B.; Tian, D.-D.; Gao, M.-R.; Liu, S.-B.; Liu, A.; Zhao, M.-G. Anxiolytic effects of polydatin through the blockade of neuroinflammation in a chronic pain mouse model. *Mol. Pain* **2020**, *16*, 1744806919900717. [CrossRef] [PubMed]
92. Liu, N.; Yu, Z.; Li, Y.; Yuan, J.; Zhang, J.; Xiang, S.; Wang, X. Transcriptional regulation of mouse neuroglobin gene by cyclic AMP responsive element binding protein (CREB) in N2a cells. *Neurosci. Lett.* **2013**, *534*, 333–337. [CrossRef] [PubMed]
93. Li, L.; Tan, H.-P.; Liu, C.-Y.; Yu, L.-T.; Wei, D.-N.; Zhang, Z.-C.; Lu, K.; Zhao, K.-S.; Maegele, M.; Cai, D.-Z.; et al. Polydatin prevents the induction of secondary brain injury after traumatic brain injury by protecting neuronal mitochondria. *Neural Regen. Res.* **2019**, *14*, 1573–1582. [CrossRef]
94. Lv, R.; Du, L.; Liu, X.; Zhou, F.; Zhang, Z.; Zhang, L. Polydatin alleviates traumatic spinal cord injury by reducing microglial inflammation via regulation of iNOS and NLRP3 inflammasome pathway. *Int. Immunopharmacol.* **2019**, *70*, 28–36. [CrossRef] [PubMed]
95. Zhao, X.; Qin, J.; Li, H.; Feng, X.; Lv, Y.; Yang, J. Effect of Polydatin on Neurological Function and the Nrf2 Pathway during Intracerebral Hemorrhage. *J. Mol. Neurosci.* **2020**, *70*, 1332–1337. [CrossRef] [PubMed]
96. Pelaz, B.; Alexiou, C.; Alvarez-Puebla, R.A.; Alves, F.; Andrews, A.M.; Ashraf, S.; Balogh, L.P.; Ballerini, L.; Bestetti, A.; Brendel, C.; et al. Diverse Applications of Nanomedicine. *ACS Nano* **2017**, *11*, 2313–2381. [CrossRef] [PubMed]
97. Yousef, A.I.; Shawki, H.H.; El-Shahawy, A.A.; El-Twab, S.M.A.; Abdel-Moneim, A.; Oishi, H. Polydatin mitigates pancreatic β-cell damage through its antioxidant activity. *Biomed. Pharmacother.* **2021**, *133*, 111027. [CrossRef] [PubMed]
98. Abdel-Moneim, A.; El-Shahawy, A.; Yousef, A.I.; El-Twab, S.M.A.; Elden, Z.E.; Taha, M. Novel polydatin-loaded chitosan nanoparticles for safe and efficient type 2 diabetes therapy: In silico, in vitro and in vivo approaches. *Int. J. Biol. Macromol.* **2020**, *154*, 1496–1504. [CrossRef] [PubMed]
99. Mostafa, F.; Galaly, S.R.; Mohamed, H.M.; Abdel-Moneim, A.; Abdul-Hamid, M. Ameliorative effect of polydatin and poly-datin-loaded chitosan nanoparticles against diabetes-induced pulmonary disorders in rats. *J. Taibah Univ. Sci.* **2021**, *15*, 37–49. [CrossRef]
100. Fabris, S.; Momo, F.; Ravagnan, G.; Stevanato, R. Antioxidant properties of resveratrol and piceid on lipid peroxidation in micelles and monolamellar liposomes. *Biophys. Chem.* **2008**, *135*, 76–83. [CrossRef] [PubMed]
101. Lin, L.; Gong, H.; Li, R.; Huang, J.; Cai, M.; Lan, T.; Huang, W.; Guo, Y.; Zhou, Z.; An, Y.; et al. Nanodrug with ROS and pH Dual-Sensitivity Ameliorates Liver Fibrosis via Multicellular Regulation. *Adv. Sci.* **2020**, *7*, 1903138. [CrossRef] [PubMed]
102. Guan, Q.; Chen, W.; Hu, X.; Wang, X.; Li, L. Novel nanoliposomal delivery system for polydatin: Preparation, characterization, and in vivo evaluation. *Drug Des. Dev. Ther.* **2015**, *9*, 1805–1813. [CrossRef] [PubMed]
103. Fakhri, S.; Abbaszadeh, F.; Jorjani, M.; Pourgholami, M.H. The effects of anticancer medicinal herbs on vascular endothelial growth factor based on pharmacological aspects: A review study. *Nutr. Cancer* **2021**, *73*, 1–15. [CrossRef]
104. Xiao, J. Dietary Flavonoid Aglycones and Their Glycosides: Which Show Better Biological Significance? *Crit. Rev. Food Sci. Nutr.* **2017**, *57*, 1874–1905. [CrossRef] [PubMed]

105. Vijayalakshmi, S.; Mariadoss, A.V.A.; Ramachandran, V.; Shalini, V.; Agilan, B.; Sangeetha, C.C.; Balupillai, A.; Kotakadi, V.S.; Karthikkumar, V.; Ernest, D. Polydatin Encapsulated Poly [Lactic-co-glycolic acid] Nanoformulation Counteract the 7,12-Dimethylbenz[a] Anthracene Mediated Experimental Carcinogenesis through the Inhibition of Cell Proliferation. *Antioxidants* **2019**, *8*, 375. [CrossRef] [PubMed]
106. Cremon, C.; Stanghellini, V.; Barbaro, M.R.; Cogliandro, R.F.; Bellacosa, L.; Santos, J.; Vicario, M.; Pigrau, M.; Cotoner, C.A.; Lobo, B.; et al. Randomised clinical trial: The analgesic properties of dietary supplementation with palmitoylethanolamide and polydatin in irritable bowel syndrome. *Aliment. Pharmacol. Ther.* **2017**, *45*, 909–922. [CrossRef] [PubMed]
107. Lagoa, R.; Silva, J.; Rodrigues, J.R.; Bishayee, A. Advances in phytochemical delivery systems for improved anticancer activity. *Biotechnol. Adv.* **2020**, *38*, 107382. [CrossRef]
108. Kashyap, D.; Tuli, H.S.; Yerer, M.B.; Sharma, A.; Sak, K.; Srivastava, S.; Pandey, A.; Garg, V.K.; Sethi, G.; Bishayee, A. Natural product-based nanoformulations for cancer therapy: Opportunities and challenges. *Semin. Cancer Biol.* **2021**, *69*, 5–23. [CrossRef]
109. Fakhri, S.; Moradi, S.Z.; Farzaei, M.H.; Bishayee, A. Modulation of dysregulated cancer metabolism by plant secondary metabolites: A mechanistic review. *Semin. Cancer Biol.* **2020**, *74*, 1–156. [CrossRef]

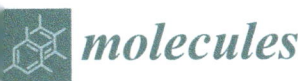

Review
Effects of Wine Components in Inflammatory Bowel Diseases

Josip Vrdoljak [1,2], Marko Kumric [1], Tina Ticinovic Kurir [1,2], Ivan Males [3], Dinko Martinovic [1], Marino Vilovic [1] and Josko Bozic [1,*]

[1] Department of Pathophysiology, University of Split School of Medicine, 21000 Split, Croatia; josip.vrdoljak@mefst.hr (J.V.); marko.kumric@mefst.hr (M.K.); tticinov@mefst.hr (T.T.K.); dinko.martinovic@mefst.hr (D.M.); marino.vilovic@mefst.hr (M.V.)
[2] Department of Endocrinology, Diabetes and Metabolic Diseases, University Hospital of Split, 21000 Split, Croatia
[3] Department of Surgery, University Hospital of Split, 21000 Split, Croatia; ivmales@kbsplit.hr
* Correspondence: josko.bozic@mefst.hr

Abstract: With the rising prevalence of Inflammatory bowel disease (IBD) worldwide, and the rising cost of treatment with novel biological drugs, there is an increasing interest in various diets and natural foods as a potential way to control/modulate IBD. As recent data indicates that diet can modify the metabolic responses essential for the resolution of inflammation, and as wine compounds have been shown to provide substantial anti-inflammatory effect, in this review we aimed to discuss the current evidence concerning the impact of biological compounds present in wine on IBD. A number of preclinical studies brought forth strong evidence on the mechanisms by which molecules in wine, such as resveratrol or piceatannol, provide their anti-inflammatory, anti-oxidative, anti-tumor, and microbiota-modulation effects. However, concerning the effects of alcohol, it is still unclear how the amount of ethanol ingested within the framework of moderate wine consumption (1–2 glasses a day) affects patients with IBD, as human studies regarding the effects of wine on patients with IBD are scarce. Nevertheless, available evidence justifies the conductance of large-scale RCT trials on human subjects that will finally elucidate whether wine can offer real benefits to the IBD population.

Keywords: wine; inflammatory bowel disease; resveratrol; polyphenols; Crohn's disease; ulcerative colitis; diet; inflammation

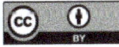

1. Introduction

Inflammatory bowel disease (IBD) consists of a spectrum of chronic, non-communicable, multifactorial diseases of the gastrointestinal tract. Two main types of IBD are Crohn´s disease (CD) and ulcerative colitis (CD) [1]. The global prevalence of IBD is rising, increasing the load on the working population and the healthcare system [2–4]. There are a lot of unknowns in the etiology and pathophysiology of IBD. It is considered that IBD occurs in a complex interplay of susceptible genes, an ill-fitted diet, changed intestinal microbiota, and a pathologic immune response to dietary elements and intestinal microbes [5–7]. The current treatment modalities for IBD consist of anti-inflammatory drugs (salicylates etc.), immunosuppressants (azathioprine, corticosteroids, etc.), biological medications (anti-TNF-α, anti-integrin, cytokine-targeted therapy), and surgical treatment [8–10]. Besides these therapeutic modalities, there are also dietary therapies such as Exclusive Enteral Nutrition [11,12]. In addition, there is an increasing interest in various diets and natural foods as a potential way to control/modulate IBD [13]. The usual suspects being the Paleolithic diet, low-FODMAP diet, gluten-free diet, specific carbohydrate-based diet, and the Mediterranean diet (MedDiet) [12–14]. Interestingly, recent data indicates that diet can modify the metabolic responses essential for the optimal healing of injury-induced inflammation, as nutrients can act as signaling agents [14]. Lately, the MedDiet, primarily through the usage of red wine and olive oil, is coming to the forefront of prevention and management of chronic diseases, including cardiovascular disease (CVD), diabetes mellitus type 2, cancer, and IBD [15–17].

The Mediterranean diet is a dietary pattern commonly found in the olive oil tree-growing parts of the Mediterranean basin [15,18]. Red wine and olive oil have been a central part of the Mediterranean diet since the days of the ancient Greeks and Romans. Even since those days, people have talked about the health benefits of olive oil and wine, but only now, in modern times, can we dissect these foods and look at the molecules that give them the desired effects on health.

This review will discuss the current evidence concerning the impact of biological compounds found in wine on IBD. We will describe the composition of wine and the impacts of wine as a whole or its isolated compounds on IBD pathophysiology by reviewing in vitro, animal, and human studies, whilst respecting that a limited amount of these compounds are found in wine.

1.1. Wine Composition

Wine, one of the oldest alcoholic beverages, is created during a process of grape must fermentation. The main constituents of wine are water, ethanol (usually between 9–15%), carbohydrates, organic acids (malic acid, citric acid, tartaric acid, etc.), as well as polyphenols, and volatile compounds [19,20]. The technological process of winemaking and the different types of grapes used offer a plethora of different wines with varying levels of alcohol and polyphenols [19,21]. Specifically, the concentration of phenolic compounds within grapes is dependent on grape variety, growing season, soil type, maturity of wine, as well as environmental and climatic conditions [22]. The phenolic composition (both concentration and composition) changes mainly in the first steps of vinification and continues during storage. In line with this, it is important to address that phenolic composition of the final wine differs from the composition of the corresponding grapes as a consequence of production of new derivatives, such as tyrosol, flavenes, and free phenolic acids [23]. The total content of phenolic compounds in grapes is affected by several factors: cultivar, the geographic origin, year of production, soil chemistry, degree of maturation, as well as solar radiation and temperature [23]. For all these reasons, estimation of polyphenol content in wine is rather challenging, and consequently, it represents a major obstacle in creation of "standardized moderate consumption" of wine.

Polyphenols are considered the main bioactive components in wine that positively affect health (prevention and management of non-communicable diseases) [19,24]. Because all grape parts are used during the winemaking process of red wine, the polyphenolic content is much higher in red wine when compared to white wine (1–5 g/L vs. 0.2–0.5 g/L) [18]. Polyphenols consist of a wide variety of chemical compounds that are generally classified into two main branches: flavonoids, and non-flavonoids [25]. Flavonoids are represented by flavonols (quercetin and myricetin), chalcones, flavononols, flavanols (catechin and epicatechin), flavones, anthocyanidins and isoflavonoids. Non-flavonoids are represented by phenolic acids, stilbenes (resveratrol), coumarins, lignans, and tannins [25,26]. Most of these compounds have demonstrated some or all of these desired effects: antioxidant, anti-inflammatory, anti-cancer, and anti-microbial (Figure 1) [27,28].

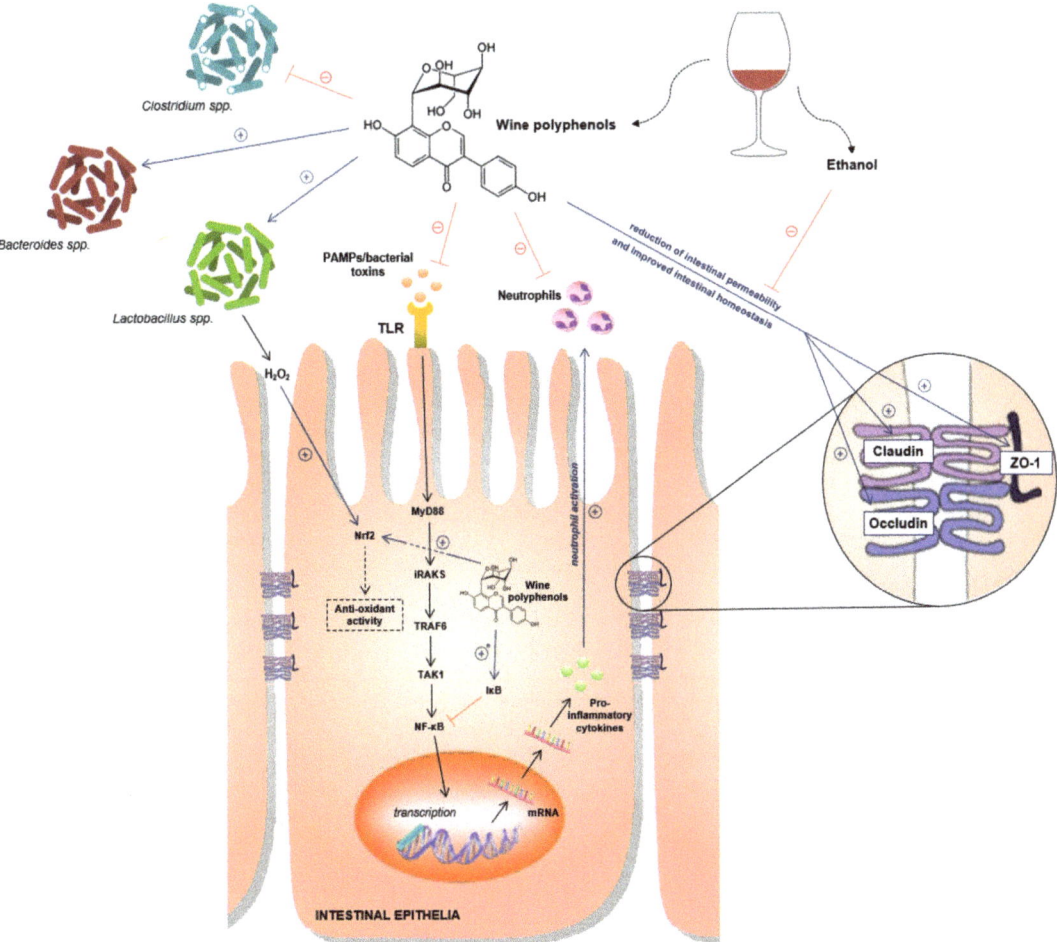

Figure 1. Multiple molecular targets of wine polyphenols contributing to its anti-inflammatory and anti-oxidant effects, changes in intestinal permeability and gut microbiota. Abbreviations: PAMPs: Pathogen-associated molecular patterns; ZO-1: Zonula occludens-1; TLR: Toll-like receptor; Nrf2: nuclear factor erythroid-derived 2; MyD88: Myeloid differentiation primary response 88; iRAKS: Interleukin-1 receptor associated kinase; TRAF6: Tumor necrosis factor receptor (TNFR)-associated factor 6; TAK1: transforming growth factor-β-activated kinase 1; NF-κB: nuclear factor kappa-light-chain-enhancer of activated B cells; IκB: inhibitor of nuclear factor kappa B.

1.2. Wine Composition

Since IBD is a chronic, non-communicable, inflammatory disease, a rising number of research papers are trying to ascertain the potential positive effects of wine or its components on IBD. Many of the phenolic compounds in wine have low bioavailability, and hence, reach low concentrations in the bloodstream, while their high content present in the gut can produce a more significant effect on enterocytes and the bacterial flora [29,30].

1.2.1. The Evidence In Vitro

The pathophysiology of IBD consists of an aberrant immune response of the gut, with an increased expression of pro-inflammatory cytokines and an increased creation of reactive oxygen species (ROS). This cascade's main factors are COX-2, iNOS, IL-8, TNF-α, and NF-κB. Furthermore, a critical mechanistic determinant of IBD is a dysfunctional intestinal barrier, as seen through altered expression and subcellular distribution of tight junction (TJ) proteins [31]. Nunes et al. have demonstrated how a polyphenolic extract from Portuguese red wine decreased the paracellular permeability in cytokine-stimulated HT-29 colon epithelial cells. The red wine extract induced a significant increase in the mRNA of the barrier-forming TJ proteins occludin, claudin-5, and *zonula occludens* (ZO)-1 compared to control cells. It also led to less formation of claudin-2 mRNA, which is a channel-forming protein usually induced by pro-inflammatory conditions [31]. One other paper that focused on the impact of wine-digested fluids on gut microbiota has shown an increase in *Akkermansia*, *Selenomonadaceae*, and *Megasphaera* genus levels, as well as a positive change in short-chain fatty acid (SCFA) levels which could lead to decreased paracellular permeability [32].

On the other hand, a study by Asai et al. exhibited how a low and acute dose of ethanol leads to apoptotic cell death in confluent Caco-2 cells and, therefore, impairs intestinal barrier function [33]. Interestingly, these positive impacts of wine polyphenols on intestinal permeability in vitro are in contrast to in vivo findings by Swanson et al., where moderate wine consumption led to increased intestinal permeability [34].

Considering intestinal permeability, in vitro evidence on the impact of red wine extract and wine digested fluids suggests a protective effect on the cellular barrier [31,32]. This is in stark contrast to the in vitro evidence using an acute dose of ethanol and the in vivo evidence provided by Swanson et al. [33,34]. Hence, it is probable that the polyphenolic content per se has a positive effect on intestinal permeability, while the alcoholic content potentially negates that effect.

Moreover, another study with Portuguese red-wine extract enriched in anthocyanins exhibited an anti-inflammatory effect in HT-29 colon epithelial cells stimulated with pro-inflammatory factors (TNF-α, IFN-γ, and IL-1). It was shown how the wine extract decreases COX-2 activity, the synthesis of iNOS and IL-8, as well as decreases the degradation of inhibitor of NF-κB [35]. Nevertheless, the polyphenol-enriched red wine extract contains a higher concentration of polyphenols than the concentration ingested in the usually recommended one glass of wine a day.

Considering the role of oxidative stress in IBD pathophysiology, many researchers have investigated the potential benefits of antioxidants. A study by Deiana et al. has shown how extracts from three different Sardinian grape varieties applied to Caco-2 cell monolayers counteracted the oxidative activity in a tert-butyl hydroperoxide (TBH)-induced oxidative damage model [36]. Furthermore, Tannin procyanidin B2 has also exhibited protective activity against oxidative stress in the human colonic Caco-2 cell model by up-regulating glutathione S-transferase P1 (GSTP1) via s ERK and p38 MAPK activation and Nrf2 translocation [37]. A study on the potential anti-oxidative effect of resveratrol on porcine intestinal-epithelial cell line (IPEC-J2) treated with deoxynivalenol (DON), has shown a reduction in ROS levels via Nrf2 signaling pathway activation [38]. Moreover, numerous studies have exhibited the anti-inflammatory effects of resveratrol in intestinal cells. In one study on Caco-2 cells exposed to bacterial lipopolysaccharide, resveratrol reduced the rate of degradation of an endogenous NF-κB inhibitor (IκB), and therefore led to a reduction of NF-κB activity with a decrease in COX-2 expression [39]. Another beneficial effect of resveratrol is on alleviating mitochondrial dysfunction [40]. When resveratrol was applied in extremely high concentrations it prevented indomethacin-induced mitochondrial dysfunction in Caco-2 cells [40,41]. In another study on Caco-2 cells stimulated with LPS, where researchers studied the effects of polyphenols from red wine, cocoa and green tea they found how a dietary dose moderately modulates intestinal inflammation, but does not increase HDL production [42].

A number of in vitro experiments using batch culture fermentation have shown beneficial effects of wine components on fecal microbiota. The common impact seen is a growth enhancement of *Bifidobacterium* spp. and *Lactobacillus* spp., with growth inhibition of the *Clostridium* group [43–47]. These experiments show how wine and its components have a prebiotic effect on the "good" gut bacteria while also showing anti-microbial results on those bacteria that could lead to intestinal pathology.

Overall, the above-mentioned in vitro experiments provide evidence that wine and wine polyphenols have the following benefits: (i) they decrease the activity of NF-κB and therefore decrease the production of pro-inflammatory cytokines, (ii) activate Nrf2 signalling pathway and therefore reduce ROS levels, (iii) polyphenols (quercetin) bind to the ubiquinone site of complex I protecting it from inhibitors like indomethacin and decreasing mitochondrial dysfunction, (iv) wine polyphenols support the growth of healthy microbiota and inhibit the growth of pathologic microbiota (Table 1).

Table 1. In vitro studies on wine polyphenols and intestinal inflammation.

Study	Cell Type	Intervention	Results
Nunes et al. [31]	Cytokine-stimulated HT-29 colon epithelial cells	Polyphenolic extract from Portuguese red wine	↑ mRNA of TJ-proteins ↓ mRNA of channel forming proteins
Zorraquín-Peña et al. [32]	Caco-2 cell monolayers grown in Transwell® inserts	Intestinal-digested wine (IDW) and colonic-digested wine (CDW)	Reduction in *Bacteroides* and an increase in *Veillonella*, *Escherichia/Shigella* and *Akkermansia*. ↑ SCFA levels
Nunes et al. [35]	HT-29 colon epithelial cells stimulated with pro-inflammatory factors	Portuguese red-wine extract enriched in anthocyanins	↓ degradation of IκB ↓ COX2 ↓ iNOS ↓ Interleukin 8
Deiana et al. [36]	Caco-2 cell monolayers stimulated with tert-butyl hydroperoxide	Wine extracts from three different Sardinian grape varieties	Scavenging of reactive oxygen species and/or prevention of their formation
Rodriguez-Ramiro et al. [37]	Human colonic Caco-2 cell model	Tannin procyanidin B2	Up-regulation of glutathione S-transferase P1 (GSTP1)
Yang et al. [38]	porcine intestinal-epithelial cell line (IPEC-J2) treated with deoxynivalenol	Resveratrol	Reduction in ROS levels via Nrf2 signaling pathway activation
Cianciulli et al. [39]	Caco-2 cells exposed to bacterial lipopolysaccharide	Resveratrol	↓ degradation of IκB
Carrasco-Pozo et al. [41]	Caco-2 cells exposed to indomethacin	Quercetin, resveratrol, rutin and epigallocatechin gallate	Reduction of mitochondrial dysfunction
Nicod et al. [42]	Caco-2 cells stimulated with LPS	Polyphenols from red wine, cocoa and green tea	Moderate reduction in intestinal inflammation markers
Hidalgo et al. [43]	pH-controlled, stirred, batch-culture fermentation system	Anthocyanins and gallic acid	↑ *Bifidobacterium* spp. ↑ *Lactobacillus*–*Enterococcus* spp.
Cueva et al. [44]	Faecal batch-culture fermentation	Two purified fractions from grape seed extract (GSE): GSE-M (70% monomers and 28% procyanidins) and GSE-O (21% monomers and 78% procyanidins)	↑ *Lactobacillus/Enterococcus* ↓ *Clostridium histolyticum*

1.2.2. The Evidence on Animal Models

As reviewed by Nunes et al., the benefits of resveratrol, a key active molecule present in red wine, have also been confirmed in animal models of IBD and intestinal cancer [38]. For example, Martin et al. have shown that, in an early colonic inflammation model caused by trinitrobenzenesulphonic acid (TNBS) instillation in rats, resveratrol (5–10 mg/kg/day) administration has significantly decreased the index of neutrophil infiltration and levels of proinflammatory cytokine IL-1β, whilst reducing the degree of colonic injury [48]. Furthermore, the same researches later showed how resveratrol extended its benefits to a rat model of chronic gut inflammation caused by TNBS. Resveratrol treatment led to decreased neutrophil infiltration, reduced TNF-α levels, reduced COX-2 and the NF-κB p65 protein expression, and also led to a significant increase of TNBS-induced apoptosis in colonic cells [49]. Moreover, another study on the DSS-induced colitis mouse model, but with a diet enriched with resveratrol, showed attenuation of colitis signs and symptoms. The mice that ate a resveratrol enriched diet (at 20 mg/kg of diet) maintained their body weight and had less diarrhoea and rectal bleeding. All the mice in the treatment group survived compared to the 40% mortality rate in the non-resveratrol group. The same study also showed a significant reduction in proinflammatory cytokines, TNF-alpha and IL-1beta, and an increase of the anti-inflammatory cytokine IL-10 [50].

Moreover, Larrosa and associates demonstrated on rats with DSS-induced colitis how low doses of resveratrol, similar to the dosage contained in a hypothetical daily diet of a person weighing 70 kg, lead to a reduction in mucosal levels of inflammatory markers [51]. Similar to the previously mentioned studies, prostaglandin E (PGE)-2, COX-2, and PGE synthase-1 were affected. In addition, this study showed an increase in *Bifidobacterium* and *Lactobacillus* spp. with a reduction in *E. coli* growth [51]. This is in line with other studies that have shown that resveratrol enhances the growth of *Lactococcus lactis*, whilst inhibiting the growth of *Enterococcus faecalis* [52]. Importantly, the relation between resveratrol and gut microbiota is a two-way street [53]. On one hand, resveratrol modulates gut microbiota, yet on the other, resveratrol can be transformed by gut microbiota into various bioactive metabolites.

In a DSS-induced colitis mouse model, Li et al. have exhibited that mice fed with muscadine grape phytochemicals (MGP) or muscadine wine phytochemicals (MWP) for 14 days had decreased levels of proinflammatory cytokines (IL-6, TNF-α), reduced myeloperoxidase activity, while also preventing weight loss and preserving colonic length [54]. A study researching the effects of grape seed extract (GSE) in a rat model of DSS-induced ulcerative colitis yielded promising results. Male Sprague-Dawley rats were fed daily (days 0–10) with GSE (400 mg/kg), and compared with no-GSE controls, GSE-fed rats had significantly decreased ileal villus height (14%; $p < 0.01$) and mucosal thickness (13%; $p < 0.01$), approaching the values of healthy controls. GSE also reduced the qualitative histological severity score ($p < 0.05$) in the proximal colon, but there was no significant effect in the distal colon [55]. In a study investigating the effects of proanthocyanidins from grape seed (GSPE) in a TNBS-induced recurrent ulcerative colitis rat model, Wang et al. demonstrated how GSPE treatment led to a recovery of pathologic changes in the colon, reduced the colonic weight/length ratio, and improved the macroscopic and microscopic damage scores. Furthermore, iNOS and myeloperoxidase activities were significantly reduced in the GSPE group, while the superoxide dismutase and gluthatione peroxidase activities were significantly increased [56].

These data indicate that proanthocyandins and wine/grape phytochemicals have similar and probably synergistic effects on the colonic mucosa. The main characteristics exhibited were modulation of the inflammatory response, inhibition of inflammatory cell infiltration, a reduction in ROS-damage, and a promotion of colonic tissue repair and regeneration [53–56].

Correspondingly, and as reviewed previously, a number of animal studies have exhibited the benefits of resveratrol in decreasing the risk of colon cancer in animal models with chronic intestinal inflammation [40]. In one study on a DSS colitis mouse model, they found how resveratrol inhibited the formation of polyps, and also reduced cell damage and subsequent proliferation of epithelial cells in the intestinal mucosa [57]. By these effects, resveratrol inhibited the tumour initiation process, and we can argue that by these mechanisms it can potentially lead to a decrease in colon cancer incidence in chronic intestinal inflammation, such as IBD-. Moreover, in a study by Cui et al., the authors demonstrated that resveratrol reduces tumour incidence and tumour multiplicity. In mice treated with azoxymethane (AOM) + DSS, tumour incidence was 80%, while the mice treated with AOM + DSS + resveratrol (300 ppm) had a 20% tumour incidence. Moreover,

AOM + DSS-treated mice had 2.4 +/−0.7 tumours per animal, while the resveratrol treated group had 0.2 +/− 0.13 tumours per animal [58]. In another study, rats were fed with processed meat, and red wine and pomegranate extracts were added to their diet. The rats that were fed polyphenols had significantly less precancerous lesions, with a full suppression of faecal excretion of nitrosyl iron, therefore suggesting that nitrozation could be a promoter of carcinogenesis [59].

Additionally, Dolara et al. have showed how red wine polyphenols can influence carcinogenesis, intestinal microflora, oxidative damage and gene expression profiles in rats [60]. The rats were treated with Azoxymethane (AOM) and 1,2-dimethylhydrazine dihydrochloride (DMH) for colon cancer/adenoma induction, and statistically significant reduction in adenoma number was seen in DMH group, while a significant reduction in total tumor number (cancer + adenoma) was seen in AOM group. What's more, the main bacterial strains in the polyphenol treated group were *Bacteroides*, *Lactobacillus* and *Bifidobacterium* spp., whereas in the control group the predominant strains were *Bacteroides*, *Clostridium* and *Propionibacterium* spp. [60]. The authors used wine polyphenols which contained 4.4% anthocyanins, 0.8% flavonols, 2.0% phenolic acids, 1.4% catechin, 1.0% epicatechin and 28.0% proanthocyanidin units, consisting of 18.0% epigallocatechin, 13.2% catechin, 65.0% epicatechin and 3.8% epicatechin gallate [59]. In addition, in a study by Femia et al., the authors researched the effects of red wine polyphenols on AOM-induced colon carcinogenesis in rats [61]. The results showed that rats treated with total polyphenolic extracts from red wine (WE) had significantly less colorectal adenomas, while there was no noticeable difference in rats treated with high molecular weight polyphenols (HMWP) or low molecular weight polyphenols (LMWP), respectively, suggesting that a synergistic effect of polyphenols is needed to exert a beneficial outcome [61].

Interestingly, a recent study investigated piceatannol, an analogue of resveratrol found in grapes and wine as well, different just by an additional hydroxyl group located at the 3′-carbon and metabolically more stable than resveratrol [61–63]. They showed how piceatannol significantly inhibited VEGF-mediated signalling and cell proliferation in VEGF-treated colon cancer cells (HT-29), as well as suppressed VEGF-mediated angiogenesis in zebrafish embryos [64]. Piceatannol is abundant in wine, with an average concentration of 13.1 ng/mL in French red wine (3× that of resveratrol) [65]. Furthermore, as it was shown that piceatannol has a higher oral bioavailability than resveratrol, added that it is also more metabolically stable than resveratrol, whilst having similar anti-inflammatory, anti-cancer, and cardioprotective properties, piceatannol positioned itself as a molecule on which additional future research should be focused [61,64,65].

Overall, the presented studies on animal models confirm the findings from in vitro studies (Table 2). These studies show how bioactive compounds found in wine (resveratrol, piceatannol, proanthocyanidins, total phenolic extracts) exert an anti-inflammatory, anti-oxidative, and anti-tumor effect, as well as positive effect on intestinal flora [39,50,51,58,59,61].

Table 2. Animal studies on wine polyphenols and IBD.

Study	Animal Model	Intervention	Results
Martin et al. [48]	TNBS instillation in rats	resveratrol (5–10 mg/kg/day)	↓ neutrophil infiltration ↓ Interleukin-1β
Martin et al. [49]	rat model of chronic gut inflammation caused by TNBS	resveratrol 10 mg/kg/day	↓ TNF-α ↓ COX-2 ↓ NF-κBp65 protein expression
Sánchez-Fidalgo et al. [50]	DSS-induced colitis mouse model	Diet enriched with resveratrol (20 mg/kg of diet)	↓ rectal bleeding ↓ diarrhoea ↓ mortality
Larrosa et al. [51]	DSS-induced colitis rat model	diet with resveratrol, similar to dosage contained in a hypothetical daily diet of a person weighing 70 kg	↓ PGE-2 ↓ COX-2 ↓ PGE synthase-1 ↑ *Bifidobacterium* and *Lactobacillus* spp. ↓ *E. coli*
Qiao et al. [52]	mice fed with high fat diet	diet with resveratrol (200 mg/kg)	↑ *Lactococcus lactis* ↓ *Enterococcus faecalis*

Table 2. Cont.

Study	Animal Model	Intervention	Results
Li et al. [54]	DSS-induced colitis mouse model	diet with MGP or MWP	↓ Interleukin-6, TNF-α ↓ myeloperoxidase activity ↓ weight loss
Cheah et al. [55]	DSS-induced rat model of ulcerative colitis	grape seed extract (400 mg/kg) gavage	↓ ileal villus height ↓ mucosal thickness ↓ proximal colon qualitative histological severity score
Wang et al. [56]	TNBS-induced recurrent ulcerative colitis rat model	proanthocyanidins from grape seed (GSPE)	↓ colonic weight/length ratio ↓ iNOS and myeloperoxidase activity
Altamemi et al. [57]	DSS colitis mouse model	resveratrol treatment via oral gavage	↓ formation of polyps ↓ cell damage and subsequent proliferation of epithelial cells
Cui et al. [58]	mice treated with AOM + DSS,	resveratrol (300 ppm)	↓ reduces tumour incidence and tumour multiplicity
Bastide et al. [59]	rats were fed with processed meat	diet with red wine and pomegranate extracts	↓ less precancerous lesions ↓ faecal excretion of nitrosyl iron
Dolara et al. [60]	rats were treated with AOM and DMH for colon cancer/adenoma induction	diet enriched with red wine polyphenols	↓ adenoma number in DMH group ↓ total tumor number in AOM group
Femia et al. [61]	AOM-induced colon carcinogenesis in rats	rats treated with WE, HMWP or LMWP	↓ less colorectal adenomas in WE group ↔ No noticeable difference in HMWP and LMWP groups
Kwon et al. [64]	VEGF-treated colon cancer cells (HT-29), and VEGF-mediated angiogenesis in zebrafish embryos	treatment with piceatannol	↓ cell proliferation ↓ VEGF induced angiogenesis

1.2.3. The Evidence on Humans

While the evidence of the beneficial effects of wine and/or wine polyphenols on intestinal inflammation are plentiful in in vitro and animal models, the human in vivo studies are still lacking large randomized control trials (RCTs) and meta-analyses. Nevertheless, the current evidence is also promising and mandates further research on the matter.

An RCT study investigating the effects of resveratrol on patients with ulcerative colitis, in which the patients were given 500 mg resveratrol or placebo capsule for 6 weeks, showed that resveratrol supplementation led to a significant decrease in plasma levels of TNF-a, hs-CRP, as well as decrease in activity of NF-kB in PBMCs [66]. Moreover, the score of inflammatory bowel disease questionnaire-9 (IBDQ-9) increased, while the clinical colitis activity index score has significantly decreased in the treatment group [66]. In a small sample study by Sabzevary-Ghahfarokhi et al., it was demonstrated on patients with UC that resveratrol can reverse the inflammatory effects of TNF-α by reducing IL-1β and increasing IL-11 production, thereby providing protective effects on UC patients [67]. Additionally, a study by Gonzalez et al. analyzed intestinal immune markers in healthy volunteers before and after red wine consumption. They demonstrated that in a subgroup of participants with a high basal cytokine level, red wine ingestion led to a significant reduction in pro-inflammatory markers (TNF-α, IL-6, and IFN-γ) that usually promote initial inflammation [68]. However, poor water solubility and low bioavailability of resveratrol limit its clinical applications [69]. Hence, Intagliata et al. recently reported multiple modalities that could reverse these issues using different delivery systems such as liposomes, polymeric and lipid nanoparticles, but also by chemical modifications thus improving its physicochemical properties [70].

Furthermore, the aforementioned study by Swanson et al. investigated the effects of moderate red wine consumption on intestinal permeability and stool calprotectin, which are associated with recurrent IBD disease activity [34]. Interestingly, the study had mixed results, as 1–3 glasses of daily red wine consumption led to decreased stool calprotectin levels in inactive IBD patients, while it also led to increased intestinal permeability measured by urinary lactulose/mannitol excretion (small bowel permeability) and urinary sucralose secretion (large bowel permeability). Nevertheless, the study had several notable limitations: small sample size (21 subjects), short follow-up duration (1 week), and a lack of assessment of mucosal activity. We can argue that these effects result from harmful effects of alcohol on those areas of the gut that are sensitive because of previous inflammatory damage and match the location of the disease. Given all the evidence from in vitro and animal studies regarding the anti-inflammatory effects from compounds found in wine, we hypothesize how these biologically active compounds are causing the decrease in stool calprotectin levels. In a previous study, the same author found how patients with inactive IBD drink alcohol in quantities similar to the general population, and how 75% of IBD patients reported a worsening of GI symptoms after drinking alcohol [71]. Another prospective cohort study also indicated how alcohol consumption increases the risk of exacerbation in patients with UC [72].

Moreover, in a crossover study, Hey et al. investigated the effects of five different alcoholic drinks on patients with CD [73]. Twenty patients with CD in remission and twelve healthy controls were randomly given red wine, white wine, Smirnoff Ice, Elephant Beer and pure ethanol. No differences in alcohol absorption were found between the groups, but CD patients reported a higher abdominal pain symptom score after ingesting Smirnoff Ice and Elephant beer. Authors argue how high sugar content present in these drinks leads to more intestinal fermentation that could present itself with symptoms of abdominal pain and bloating [73].

In our previous observational study investigating MedDiet adherence in patients with IBD, only 4.5% of patients in the UC group and 8% of patients in the CD group reported daily red wine intake in the MedDiet framework. Notably, when the participants were asked about the suspected foods that aggravate IBD-related symptoms, 50% in the UC group and 36% in the CD group reported alcohol as a suspect [74]. Interestingly, in a Swedish prospective cohort study that showed how the MedDiet lowers the risk of late-onset Crohn's disease, moderate alcohol intake increased with the MedDiet adherence score. In the highest MedDiet score bracket [6–8], 61% of participants moderately consumed alcohol, while the number of moderate alcohol consumers in the lowest bracket [0–2] was only 14% [75]. While some of the IBD patients associate wine intake with symptom aggravation, it seems that moderate wine consumption in the framework of the MedDiet could lead to IBD prevention [74,75].

2. Precautions and Future Directions

In general, alcohol was shown to increase gut permeability by causing transepithelial and paracellular permeability [76]. Chronic alcohol ingestion also leads to gut dysbiosis (less *Lactobacillus* and *Bifidobacterium* spp.), bacterial overgrowth, and a disruption of intestinal immune response [76–78]. The research shows that chronic and uncontrolled ethanol ingestion disrupts intestinal homeostasis and increases intestinal and, later on, systemic inflammation [76,79]. The other well-established deleterious effects of wine on liver function, metabolism, brain, and alcohol addiction, must not be neglected as well [80]. On the other hand, as we have discussed in this review, other studies show how biologically active compounds found in alcoholic beverages such as wine (polyphenols, tannins, organic acids) have a completely different effect on intestinal homeostasis, and exert anti-inflammatory, anti-oxidative, and positive microbiota effects, making wine capable of assisting in disease control and affecting disease monitoring [29,40]. Nevertheless, most of the alcohol-mediated effects seem to aggravate intestinal inflammation and consequently impact disease onset, recurrence, and control of symptoms. Furthermore, British Society of Gastroenterology consensus guidelines address the importance of alcohol reduction because alcohol further reduces bone mineral density, which is already substantially struck by corticosteroids [81]. Finally, alcohol use interferes with the metabolism of most IBD medications, leading to either increase in side effect occurrence rate or loss of drug's effect [82]. Specifically, mesalamine, azathioprine, methotrexate, and biologic medications can all be affected by concomitant alcohol intake via a variety of mechanisms. Nevertheless, a large number of authors advocates moderate wine consumption based on inferences drawn from large-scale populational studies. Although questioned by certain authors, the

J-shaped curve explaining the relationship between alcohol use and total mortality has been well established [83,84]. Namely, the lowest mortality risk was observed at 6 g/day of alcohol (half of a drink/day), but with lower mortality with up to 4 drinks/day in men and 2 drinks/day in women when compared with no alcohol consumption, even after adjustment for a myriad of confounding variables. Furthermore, as presented by Xi et al., light alcohol consumption appears to be protective against cancer mortality, unlike heavy alcohol use which is associated with increased cancer risk [85–87]. Unlike the cardiovascular effects of wine, which have been extensively studied, the role of wine in IBD, or any other gastrointestinal pathology for that matter, has been poorly elucidated. Although certain inferences from studies exploiting the effects of wine on vascular function can be drawn to IBD because of the overlapping mechanisms, such as anti-inflammatory properties and protection from oxidative stress, the evidence on the effect of wine and alcohol on IBD course is still inconclusive.

Hence, as detrimental effects seem to prevail, at least for now, future research should focus on finding the optimal dose of red wine for these patients. We are casting about for dosage (if it exists) in which the beneficial effects of polyphenols, tannins, and organic acids will outweigh the detrimental effects of ethanol. It should also be noted that even if we found optimal dosage, adherence to the exact dosage of wine will be very challenging, markedly owing to the addictive nature of alcohol consumption. In summary, before we have firm evidence from more extensive prospective studies, caution should be advised in recommending red wine consumption to patients with IBD.

3. Conclusions

This review summarized the current evidence concerning the effects of wine compounds on IBD. A number of in vitro and animal model studies provide strong evidence on the mechanisms by which molecules found in wine, such as resveratrol or piceatannol provide their anti-inflammatory, anti-oxidative, anti-tumor, and microbiota-modulation effects. However, concerning the effects of alcohol, it is still unclear how the amount of ethanol ingested within the framework of moderate wine consumption (1–2 glasses a day) affects patients with IBD, as human studies on the effects of wine and its molecules on IBD/intestinal inflammation are scarce. In addition, it is doubtful whether the above-noted effects can be obtained by drinking wine exclusively, as this beverage contains only scarce amount of these compounds. Since more and more patients are turning to dietary options, such as the Mediterranean diet, as a means to control their diseases, there is an increasing need for high-quality, evidence-based information. Therefore, we have a strong foundation for translation into clinical studies and human research. With the rising prevalence of IBD worldwide and the rising cost of treatment with novel biological drugs, wine polyphenols could serve as a cheaper therapeutic modality accessible to more patients. We conclude that the evidence provided can serve as a basis for large-scale RCT trials on human subjects that will finally elucidate whether wine can offer real benefits to the IBD population.

Author Contributions: Conceptualization, J.V., T.T.K. and I.M.; writing—original draft preparation, M.K., D.M., M.V. and J.V.; writing—review and editing, I.M., T.T.K. and J.B.; visualization, J.V.; supervision, D.M., M.V. and J.B.; project administration, M.K. and J.B. All authors have read and agreed to the published version of the manuscript.

Funding: This research received no external funding.

Institutional Review Board Statement: Not applicable.

Informed Consent Statement: Not applicable.

Data Availability Statement: Not applicable.

Acknowledgments: The paper has been proofread by language professional Dalibora Behmen, M.A. The figure was kindly provided by Zrinka Miocic M. Arch.

Conflicts of Interest: The authors declare no conflict of interest.

Abbreviations

TJ-protein	Tight Junction protein
SCFA	Short-chain fatty acid
COX2	Cyclooxygenase-2
I-κB	inhibitor of nuclear factor kappa B
iNOS	Inducible nitric oxide synthase
LPS	Lipopolysaccharides
TNBS	trinitrobenzenesulphonic acid
WE	total polyphenolic extracts from red wine
HMWP	high molecular weight polyphenols
LMWP	low molecular weight polyphenols
MGP	muscadine grape phytochemicals
MWP	muscadine wine phytochemicals
VEGF	Vascular endothelial growth factor
DSS	dextran sulfate sodium
AOM	azoxymethane
DMH	1,2-dimethylhydrazine dihydrochloride
PGE2	Prostaglandin E_2
TNF-α	tumor necrosis factor alpha

References

1. Guan, Q. A Comprehensive Review and Update on the Pathogenesis of Inflammatory Bowel Disease. *J. Immunol. Res.* **2019**, *2019*, 7247238. [CrossRef] [PubMed]
2. Kaplan, G.G. The global burden of IBD: From 2015 to 2025. *Nat. Rev. Gastroenterol. Hepatol.* **2015**, *12*, 720–727. [CrossRef] [PubMed]
3. Longobardi, T.; Jacobs, P.; Bernstein, C.N. Work losses related to inflammatory bowel disease in the United States: Results from the National Health Interview Survey. *Am. J. Gastroenterol.* **2003**, *98*, 1064–1072. [CrossRef] [PubMed]
4. Park, K.T.; Ehrlich, O.G.; Allen, J.I.; Meadows, P.; Szigethy, E.M.; Henrichsen, K.; Kim, S.C.; Lawton, R.C.; Murphy, S.M.; Regueiro, M.; et al. The Cost of Inflammatory Bowel Disease: An Initiative From the Crohn's & Colitis Foundation. *Inflamm. Bowel Dis.* **2020**, *26*, 1–10. [CrossRef] [PubMed]
5. Zivkovic, P.M.; Matetic, A.; Tadin Hadjina, I.; Rusic, D.; Vilovic, M.; Supe-Domic, D.; Borovac, J.A.; Mudnic, I.; Tonkic, A.; Bozic, J. Serum Catestatin Levels and Arterial Stiffness Parameters Are Increased in Patients with Inflammatory Bowel Disease. *J. Clin. Med.* **2020**, *9*, 628. [CrossRef]
6. Brnić, D.; Martinovic, D.; Zivkovic, P.M.; Tokic, D.; Hadjina, I.T.; Rusic, D.; Vilovic, M.; Supe-Domic, D.; Tonkic, A.; Bozic, J. Serum adropin levels are reduced in patients with inflammatory bowel diseases. *Sci. Rep.* **2020**, *10*, 9264. [CrossRef]
7. Ananthakrishnan, A.N.; Bernstein, C.N.; Iliopoulos, D.; Macpherson, A.; Neurath, M.F.; Ali, R.A.R.; Vavricka, S.R.; Fiocchi, C. Environmental triggers in IBD: A review of progress and evidence. *Nat. Rev. Gastroenterol. Hepatol.* **2018**, *15*, 39–49. [CrossRef] [PubMed]
8. Yeshi, K.; Ruscher, R.; Hunter, L.; Daly, N.L.; Loukas, A.; Wangchuk, P. Revisiting Inflammatory Bowel Disease: Pathology, Treatments, Challenges and Emerging Therapeutics Including Drug Leads from Natural Products. *J. Clin. Med.* **2020**, *9*, 1273. [CrossRef]
9. Knutson, D.; Greenberg, G.; Cronau, H. Management of Crohn's disease—A practical approach. *Am. Fam. Phys.* **2003**, *68*, 707–714.
10. Ungaro, R.; Mehandru, S.; Allen, P.B.; Peyrin-Biroulet, L.; Colombel, J.F. Ulcerative colitis. *Lancet* **2017**, *389*, 1756–1770. [CrossRef]
11. Wark, G.; Samocha-Bonet, D.; Ghaly, S.; Danta, M. The Role of Diet in the Pathogenesis and Management of Inflammatory Bowel Disease: A Review. *Nutrients* **2020**, *13*, 135. [CrossRef]
12. Kakodkar, S.; Mutlu, E.A. Diet as a Therapeutic Option for Adult Inflammatory Bowel Disease. *Gastroenterol. Clin. N. Am.* **2017**, *46*, 745–767. [CrossRef]
13. Jiang, Y.; Jarr, K.; Layton, C.; Gardner, C.D.; Ashouri, J.F.; Abreu, M.T.; Sinha, S.R. Therapeutic Implications of Diet in Inflammatory Bowel Disease and Related Immune-Mediated Inflammatory Diseases. *Nutrients* **2021**, *13*, 890. [CrossRef]
14. Sears, B.; Saha, A.K. Dietary Control of Inflammation and Resolution. *Front. Nutr.* **2021**, *8*, 709435. [CrossRef]
15. Trichopoulou, A.; Martinez-Gonzalez, M.A.; Tong, T.Y.; Forouhi, N.G.; Khandelwal, S.; Prabhakaran, D.; Mozaffarian, D.; de Lorgeril, M. Definitions and potential health benefits of the Mediterranean diet: Views from experts around the world. *BMC Med.* **2014**, *12*, 112. [CrossRef] [PubMed]
16. Stromsnes, K.; Correas, A.G.; Lehmann, J.; Gambini, J.; Olaso-Gonzalez, G. Anti-Inflammatory Properties of Diet: Role in Healthy Aging. *Biomedicines* **2021**, *9*, 922. [CrossRef] [PubMed]
17. Babio, N.; Toledo, E.; Estruch, R.; Ros, E.; Martinez-Gonzalez, M.A.; Castaner, O.; Bullo, M.; Corella, D.; Aros, F.; Gomez-Gracia, E.; et al. Mediterranean diets and metabolic syndrome status in the PREDIMED randomized trial. *CMAJ* **2014**, *186*, E649–E657. [CrossRef] [PubMed]

18. Davis, C.; Bryan, J.; Hodgson, J.; Murphy, K. Definition of the Mediterranean Diet; a Literature Review. *Nutrients* **2015**, *7*, 9139–9153. [CrossRef]
19. Gutierrez-Escobar, R.; Aliano-Gonzalez, M.J.; Cantos-Villar, E. Wine Polyphenol Content and Its Influence on Wine Quality and Properties: A Review. *Molecules* **2021**, *26*, 718. [CrossRef]
20. Castaldo, L.; Narváez, A.; Izzo, L.; Graziani, G.; Gaspari, A.; Minno, G.D.; Ritieni, A. Red Wine Consumption and Cardiovascular Health. *Molecules* **2019**, *24*, 3626. [CrossRef]
21. Mendoza, L.; Matsuhiro, B.; Aguirre, M.; Isaacs, M.; SotÉS, G.; Milena, C.; Melo, R. Characterization of phenolic acids profile from chilean red wines by high-performance liquid chromatography. *J. Chil. Chem. Soc.* **2010**, *56*, 688–691. [CrossRef]
22. Lorrain, B.; Ky, I.; Pechamat, L.; Teissedre, P.L. Evolution of analysis of polyphenols from grapes, wines, and extracts. *Molecules* **2013**, *18*, 1076–1100. [CrossRef]
23. Kennedy, J.A.; Mathews, M.A.; Waterhouse, A.L. Effect of maturity and vine water status on grape skin and wine flavonoids. *Am. J. Enol. Vitic.* **2002**, *53*, 268–274.
24. Arranz, S.; Chiva-Blanch, G.; Valderas-Martinez, P.; Medina-Remon, A.; Lamuela-Raventos, R.M.; Estruch, R. Wine, beer, alcohol and polyphenols on cardiovascular disease and cancer. *Nutrients* **2012**, *4*, 759–781. [CrossRef] [PubMed]
25. Radonjic, S.; Maras, V.; Raicevic, J.; Kosmerl, T. Wine or Beer? Comparison, Changes and Improvement of Polyphenolic Compounds during Technological Phases. *Molecules* **2020**, *25*, 4960. [CrossRef] [PubMed]
26. Minzer, S.; Estruch, R.; Casas, R. Wine Intake in the Framework of a Mediterranean Diet and Chronic Non-Communicable Diseases: A Short Literature Review of the Last 5 Years. *Molecules* **2020**, *25*, 5045. [CrossRef]
27. Banc, R.; Socaciu, C.; Doina, M.; Lorena, F.; Cozma, A.; Oana, S.; Loghin, F. Benefits of Wine Polyphenols on Human Health: A Review. *Bull. UASVM Food Sci. Technol.* **2014**, *71*, 79–87. [CrossRef]
28. Latruffe, N.; Rifler, J.-P. Special Issue: Wine and Vine Components and Health. *Diseases* **2019**, *7*, 30. [CrossRef]
29. Biasi, F.; Deiana, M.; Guina, T.; Gamba, P.; Leonarduzzi, G.; Poli, G. Wine consumption and intestinal redox homeostasis. *Redox Biol.* **2014**, *2*, 795–802. [CrossRef]
30. Giovinazzo, G.; Grieco, F. Functional Properties of Grape and Wine Polyphenols. *Plant. Foods Hum. Nutr.* **2015**, *70*, 454–462. [CrossRef]
31. Nunes, C.; Freitas, V.; Almeida, L.; Laranjinha, J. Red wine extract preserves tight junctions in intestinal epithelial cells under inflammatory conditions: Implications for intestinal inflammation. *Food Funct.* **2019**, *10*, 1364–1374. [CrossRef]
32. Zorraquín-Peña, I.; Taladrid, D.; Tamargo, A.; Silva, M.; Molinero, N.; de Llano, D.G.; Bartolomé, B.; Moreno-Arribas, M.V. Effects of Wine and Its Microbial-Derived Metabolites on Intestinal Permeability Using Simulated Gastrointestinal Digestion/Colonic Fermentation and Caco-2 Intestinal Cell Models. *Microorganisms* **2021**, *9*, 1378. [CrossRef] [PubMed]
33. Asai, K.; Buurman, W.A.; Reutelingsperger, C.P.; Schutte, B.; Kaminishi, M. Low concentrations of ethanol induce apoptosis in human intestinal cells. *Scand. J. Gastroenterol.* **2003**, *38*, 1154–1161. [CrossRef] [PubMed]
34. Swanson, G.R.; Tieu, V.; Shaikh, M.; Forsyth, C.; Keshavarzian, A. Is moderate red wine consumption safe in inactive inflammatory bowel disease? *Digestion* **2011**, *84*, 238–244. [CrossRef] [PubMed]
35. Nunes, C.; Ferreira, E.; Freitas, V.; Almeida, L.; Barbosa, R.M.; Laranjinha, J. Intestinal anti-inflammatory activity of red wine extract: Unveiling the mechanisms in colonic epithelial cells. *Food Funct.* **2013**, *4*, 373–383. [CrossRef]
36. Deiana, M.; Loru, D.; Incani, A.; Rosa, A.; Atzeri, A.; Melis, M.P.; Cabboi, B.; Hollecker, L.; Pinna, M.B.; Argiolas, F.; et al. Wine extracts from Sardinian grape varieties attenuate membrane oxidative damage in Caco-2 cell monolayers. *Food Chem.* **2012**, *134*, 2105–2113. [CrossRef]
37. Rodriguez-Ramiro, I.; Ramos, S.; Bravo, L.; Goya, L.; Martin, M.A. Procyanidin B2 induces Nrf2 translocation and glutathione S-transferase P1 expression via ERKs and p38-MAPK pathways and protect human colonic cells against oxidative stress. *Eur. J. Nutr.* **2012**, *51*, 881–892. [CrossRef]
38. Yang, J.; Zhu, C.; Ye, J.; Lv, Y.; Wang, L.; Chen, Z.; Jiang, Z. Protection of Porcine Intestinal-Epithelial Cells from Deoxynivalenol-Induced Damage by Resveratrol via the Nrf2 Signaling Pathway. *J. Agric. Food Chem* **2019**, *67*, 1726–1735. [CrossRef]
39. Cianciulli, A.; Calvello, R.; Cavallo, P.; Dragone, T.; Carofiglio, V.; Panaro, M.A. Modulation of NF-kappaB activation by resveratrol in LPS treated human intestinal cells results in downregulation of PGE2 production and COX-2 expression. *Toxicol. Vitr.* **2012**, *26*, 1122–1128. [CrossRef]
40. Nunes, S.; Danesi, F.; Del Rio, D.; Silva, P. Resveratrol and inflammatory bowel disease: The evidence so far. *Nutr. Res. Rev.* **2018**, *31*, 85–97. [CrossRef]
41. Carrasco-Pozo, C.; Mizgier, M.L.; Speisky, H.; Gotteland, M. Differential protective effects of quercetin, resveratrol, rutin and epigallocatechin gallate against mitochondrial dysfunction induced by indomethacin in Caco-2 cells. *Chem Biol. Interact.* **2012**, *195*, 199–205. [CrossRef]
42. Nicod, N.; Chiva-Blanch, G.; Giordano, E.; Dávalos, A.; Parker, R.S.; Visioli, F. Green tea, cocoa, and red wine polyphenols moderately modulate intestinal inflammation and do not increase high-density lipoprotein (HDL) production. *J. Agric. Food Chem.* **2014**, *62*, 2228–2232. [CrossRef]
43. Hidalgo, M.; Oruna-Concha, M.J.; Kolida, S.; Walton, G.E.; Kallithraka, S.; Spencer, J.P.; de Pascual-Teresa, S. Metabolism of anthocyanins by human gut microflora and their influence on gut bacterial growth. *J. Agric. Food Chem.* **2012**, *60*, 3882–3890. [CrossRef]

44. Cueva, C.; Sanchez-Patan, F.; Monagas, M.; Walton, G.E.; Gibson, G.R.; Martin-Alvarez, P.J.; Bartolome, B.; Moreno-Arribas, M.V. In vitro fermentation of grape seed flavan-3-ol fractions by human faecal microbiota: Changes in microbial groups and phenolic metabolites. *FEMS Microbiol. Ecol.* **2013**, *83*, 792–805. [CrossRef] [PubMed]
45. Barroso, E.; Sánchez-Patán, F.; Martín-Alvarez, P.J.; Bartolomé, B.; Moreno-Arribas, M.V.; Peláez, C.; Requena, T.; van de Wiele, T.; Martínez-Cuesta, M.C. *Lactobacillus* plantarum IFPL935 favors the initial metabolism of red wine polyphenols when added to a colonic microbiota. *J. Agric. Food Chem.* **2013**, *61*, 10163–10172. [CrossRef]
46. Dueñas, M.; Cueva, C.; Muñoz-González, I.; Jiménez-Girón, A.; Sánchez-Patán, F.; Santos-Buelga, C.; Moreno-Arribas, M.V.; Bartolomé, B. Studies on Modulation of Gut Microbiota by Wine Polyphenols: From Isolated Cultures to Omic Approaches. *Antioxidants* **2015**, *4*, 1–21. [CrossRef] [PubMed]
47. Nash, V.; Ranadheera, C.S.; Georgousopoulou, E.N.; Mellor, D.D.; Panagiotakos, D.B.; McKune, A.J.; Kellett, J.; Naumovski, N. The effects of grape and red wine polyphenols on gut microbiot—A systematic review. *Food Res. Int.* **2018**, *113*, 277–287. [CrossRef] [PubMed]
48. Martín, A.R.; Villegas, I.; La Casa, C.; de la Lastra, C.A. Resveratrol, a polyphenol found in grapes, suppresses oxidative damage and stimulates apoptosis during early colonic inflammation in rats. *Biochem. Pharm.* **2004**, *67*, 1399–1410. [CrossRef] [PubMed]
49. Martín, A.R.; Villegas, I.; Sánchez-Hidalgo, M.; de la Lastra, C.A. The effects of resveratrol, a phytoalexin derived from red wines, on chronic inflammation induced in an experimentally induced colitis model. *Br. J. Pharm.* **2006**, *147*, 873–885. [CrossRef]
50. Sánchez-Fidalgo, S.; Cárdeno, A.; Villegas, I.; Talero, E.; de la Lastra, C.A. Dietary supplementation of resveratrol attenuates chronic colonic inflammation in mice. *Eur. J. Pharm.* **2010**, *633*, 78–84. [CrossRef]
51. Larrosa, M.; Yañéz-Gascón, M.J.; Selma, M.V.; González-Sarrías, A.; Toti, S.; Cerón, J.J.; Tomás-Barberán, F.; Dolara, P.; Espín, J.C. Effect of a low dose of dietary resveratrol on colon microbiota, inflammation and tissue damage in a DSS-induced colitis rat model. *J. Agric. Food Chem.* **2009**, *57*, 2211–2220. [CrossRef] [PubMed]
52. Qiao, Y.; Sun, J.; Xia, S.; Tang, X.; Shi, Y.; Le, G. Effects of resveratrol on gut microbiota and fat storage in a mouse model with high-fat-induced obesity. *Food Funct.* **2014**, *5*, 1241–1249. [CrossRef] [PubMed]
53. Hu, Y.; Chen, D.; Zheng, P.; Yu, J.; He, J.; Mao, X.; Yu, B. The Bidirectional Interactions between Resveratrol and Gut Microbiota: An Insight into Oxidative Stress and Inflammatory Bowel Disease Therapy. *BioMed. Res. Int.* **2019**, *2019*, 5403761. [CrossRef]
54. Li, R.; Kim, M.-H.; Sandhu, A.K.; Gao, C.; Gu, L. Muscadine Grape (*Vitis rotundifolia*) or Wine Phytochemicals Reduce Intestinal Inflammation in Mice with Dextran Sulfate Sodium-Induced Colitis. *J. Agric. Food Chem.* **2017**, *65*, 769–776. [CrossRef]
55. Cheah, K.Y.; Bastian, S.E.; Acott, T.M.; Abimosleh, S.M.; Lymn, K.A.; Howarth, G.S. Grape seed extract reduces the severity of selected disease markers in the proximal colon of dextran sulphate sodium-induced colitis in rats. *Dig. Dis Sci.* **2013**, *58*, 970–977. [CrossRef]
56. Wang, Y.H.; Yang, X.L.; Wang, L.; Cui, M.X.; Cai, Y.Q.; Li, X.L.; Wu, Y.J. Effects of proanthocyanidins from grape seed on treatment of recurrent ulcerative colitis in rats. *Can. J. Physiol. Pharm.* **2010**, *88*, 888–898. [CrossRef]
57. Altamemi, I.; Murphy, E.A.; Catroppo, J.F.; Zumbrun, E.E.; Zhang, J.; McClellan, J.L.; Singh, U.P.; Nagarkatti, P.S.; Nagarkatti, M. Role of microRNAs in resveratrol-mediated mitigation of colitis-associated tumorigenesis in Apc(Min/+) mice. *J. Pharm. Exp.* **2014**, *350*, 99–109. [CrossRef]
58. Cui, X.; Jin, Y.; Hofseth, A.B.; Pena, E.; Habiger, J.; Chumanevich, A.; Poudyal, D.; Nagarkatti, M.; Nagarkatti, P.S.; Singh, U.P.; et al. Resveratrol suppresses colitis and colon cancer associated with colitis. *Cancer Prev. Res.* **2010**, *3*, 549–559. [CrossRef]
59. Bastide, N.M.; Naud, N.; Nassy, G.; Vendeuvre, J.L.; Taché, S.; Guéraud, F.; Hobbs, D.A.; Kuhnle, G.G.; Corpet, D.E.; Pierre, F.H. Red Wine and Pomegranate Extracts Suppress Cured Meat Promotion of Colonic Mucin-Depleted Foci in Carcinogen-Induced Rats. *Nutr. Cancer* **2017**, *69*, 289–298. [CrossRef] [PubMed]
60. Dolara, P.; Luceri, C.; De Filippo, C.; Femia, A.P.; Giovannelli, L.; Caderni, G.; Cecchini, C.; Silvi, S.; Orpianesi, C.; Cresci, A. Red wine polyphenols influence carcinogenesis, intestinal microflora, oxidative damage and gene expression profiles of colonic mucosa in F344 rats. *Mutat. Res.* **2005**, *591*, 237–246. [CrossRef] [PubMed]
61. Femia, A.P.; Caderni, G.; Vignali, F.; Salvadori, M.; Giannini, A.; Biggeri, A.; Gee, J.; Przybylska, K.; Cheynier, V.; Dolara, P. Effect of polyphenolic extracts from red wine and 4-OH-coumaric acid on 1,2-dimethylhydrazine-induced colon carcinogenesis in rats. *Eur. J. Nutr.* **2005**, *44*, 79–84. [CrossRef]
62. Setoguchi, Y.; Oritani, Y.; Ito, R.; Inagaki, H.; Maruki-Uchida, H.; Ichiyanagi, T.; Ito, T. Absorption and metabolism of piceatannol in rats. *J. Agric. Food Chem.* **2014**, *62*, 2541–2548. [CrossRef]
63. Hu, W.-H.; Dai, D.K.; Zheng, B.Z.-Y.; Duan, R.; Dong, T.T.-X.; Qin, Q.-W.; Tsim, K.W.-K. Piceatannol, a Natural Analog of Resveratrol, Exerts Anti angiogenic Efficiencies by Blockage of Vascular Endothelial Growth Factor Binding to Its Receptor. *Molecules* **2020**, *25*, 3769. [CrossRef]
64. Kwon, G.T.; Jung, J.I.; Song, H.R.; Woo, E.Y.; Jun, J.G.; Kim, J.K.; Her, S.; Park, J.H. Piceatannol inhibits migration and invasion of prostate cancer cells: Possible mediation by decreased interleukin-6 signaling. *J. Nutr. Biochem.* **2012**, *23*, 228–238. [CrossRef]
65. Roupe, K.A.; Remsberg, C.M.; Yáñez, J.A.; Davies, N.M. Pharmacometrics of stilbenes: Seguing towards the clinic. *Curr. Clin. Pharm.* **2006**, *1*, 81–101. [CrossRef]
66. Samsami-Kor, M.; Daryani, N.E.; Asl, P.R.; Hekmatdoost, A. Anti-Inflammatory Effects of Resveratrol in Patients with Ulcerative Colitis: A Randomized, Double-Blind, Placebo-controlled Pilot Study. *Arch. Med. Res.* **2015**, *46*, 280–285. [CrossRef] [PubMed]

67. Sabzevary-Ghahfarokhi, M.; Soltani, A.; Luzza, F.; Larussa, T.; Rahimian, G.; Shirzad, H.; Bagheri, N. The protective effects of resveratrol on ulcerative colitis via changing the profile of Nrf2 and IL-1β protein. *Mol. Biol. Rep.* **2020**, *47*, 6941–6947. [CrossRef] [PubMed]
68. Muñoz-González, I.; Espinosa-Martos, I.; Rodríguez, J.M.; Jiménez-Girón, A.; Martín-Álvarez, P.J.; Bartolomé, B.; Moreno-Arribas, M.V. Moderate Consumption of Red Wine Can Modulate Human Intestinal Inflammatory Response. *J. Agric. Food Chem.* **2014**, *62*, 10567–10575. [CrossRef] [PubMed]
69. Shi, Y.; Zhou, J.; Jiang, B.; Miao, M. Resveratrol and inflammatory bowel disease. *Ann. N. Y. Acad. Sci.* **2017**, *1403*, 38–47. [CrossRef] [PubMed]
70. Intagliata, S.; Modica, M.N.; Santagati, L.M.; Montenegro, L. Strategies to Improve Resveratrol Systemic and Topical Bioavailability: An Update. *Antioxidants* **2019**, *8*, 244. [CrossRef] [PubMed]
71. Swanson, G.R.; Sedghi, S.; Farhadi, A.; Keshavarzian, A. Pattern of alcohol consumption and its effect on gastrointestinal symptoms in inflammatory bowel disease. *Alcohol* **2010**, *44*, 223–228. [CrossRef]
72. Jowett, S.L.; Seal, C.J.; Pearce, M.S.; Phillips, E.; Gregory, W.; Barton, J.R.; Welfare, M.R. Influence of dietary factors on the clinical course of ulcerative colitis: A prospective cohort study. *Gut* **2004**, *53*, 1479–1484. [CrossRef]
73. Hey, H.; Schmedes, A.; Nielsen, A.A.; Winding, P.; Grønbaek, H. Effects of five different alcoholic drinks on patients with Crohn's disease. *Scand. J. Gastroenterol.* **2007**, *42*, 968–972. [CrossRef]
74. Vrdoljak, J.; Vilovic, M.; Zivkovic, P.M.; Tadin Hadjina, I.; Rusic, D.; Bukic, J.; Borovac, J.A.; Bozic, J. Mediterranean Diet Adherence and Dietary Attitudes in Patients with Inflammatory Bowel Disease. *Nutrients* **2020**, *12*, 3429. [CrossRef]
75. Khalili, H.; Håkansson, N.; Chan, S.S.; Chen, Y.; Lochhead, P.; Ludvigsson, J.F.; Chan, A.T.; Hart, A.R.; Olén, O.; Wolk, A. Adherence to a Mediterranean diet is associated with a lower risk of later-onset Crohn's disease: Results from two large prospective cohort studies. *Gut* **2020**, *69*, 1637–1644. [CrossRef] [PubMed]
76. Bishehsari, F.; Magno, E.; Swanson, G.; Desai, V.; Voigt, R.M.; Forsyth, C.B.; Keshavarzian, A. Alcohol and Gut-Derived Inflammation. *Alcohol Res.* **2017**, *38*, 163–171. [PubMed]
77. Bajaj, J.S. Alcohol, liver disease and the gut microbiota. *Nat. Rev. Gastroenterol. Hepatol.* **2019**, *16*, 235–246. [CrossRef]
78. Dubinkina, V.B.; Tyakht, A.V.; Odintsova, V.Y.; Yarygin, K.S.; Kovarsky, B.A.; Pavlenko, A.V.; Ischenko, D.S.; Popenko, A.S.; Alexeev, D.G.; Taraskina, A.Y.; et al. Links of gut microbiota composition with alcohol dependence syndrome and alcoholic liver disease. *Microbiome* **2017**, *5*, 141. [CrossRef] [PubMed]
79. Patel, S.; Behara, R.; Swanson, G.R.; Forsyth, C.B.; Voigt, R.M.; Keshavarzian, A. Alcohol and the Intestine. *Biomolecules* **2015**, *5*, 2573–2588. [CrossRef] [PubMed]
80. Rehm, J. The risks associated with alcohol use and alcoholism. *Alcohol Res. Health* **2011**, *34*, 135–143.
81. Lamb, C.A.; Kennedy, N.A.; Raine, T.; Hendy, P.A.; Smith, P.J.; Limdi, J.K.; Hayee, B.; Lomer, M.C.E.; Parkes, G.C.; Selinger, C.; et al. British Society of Gastroenterology consensus guidelines on the management of inflammatory bowel disease in adults. *Gut* **2019**, *68*, s1–s106. [CrossRef] [PubMed]
82. White, B.A.; Ramos, G.P.; Kane, S. The Impact of Alcohol in Inflammatory Bowel Diseases. *Inflamm. Bowel Dis.* **2021**, izab089. [CrossRef] [PubMed]
83. Stockwell, T.; Zhao, J.; Panwar, S.; Roemer, A.; Naimi, T.; Chikritzhs, T. Do "Moderate" Drinkers Have Reduced Mortality Risk? A Systematic Review and Meta-Analysis of Alcohol Consumption and All-Cause Mortality. *J. Stud. Alcohol Drugs.* **2016**, *77*, 185–198. [CrossRef] [PubMed]
84. De Gaetano, G.; Costanzo, S. Alcohol and Health: Praise of the J Curves. *J. Am. Coll Cardiol.* **2017**, *70*, 923–925. [CrossRef] [PubMed]
85. Xi, B.; Veeranki, S.P.; Zhao, M.; Ma, C.; Yan, Y.; Mi, J. Relationship of Alcohol Consumption to All-Cause, Cardiovascular, and Cancer-Related Mortality in U.S. Adults. *J. Am. Coll. Cardiol.* **2017**, *70*, 913–922. [CrossRef]
86. Poli, A.; Marangoni, F.; Avogaro, A.; Barba, G.; Bellentani, S.; Bucci, M.; Cambieri, R.; Catapano, A.L.; Costanzo, S.; Cricelli, C. Moderate alcohol use and health: A consensus document. *Nutr. Metab. Cardiovasc. Dis.* **2013**, *23*, 487–504. [CrossRef]
87. Jin, M.; Cai, S.; Guo, J.; Zhu, Y.; Li, M.; Yu, Y.; Zhang, S.; Chen, K. Alcohol drinking and all cancer mortality: A meta-analysis. *Ann. Oncol.* **2013**, *24*, 807–816. [CrossRef]

Wine, Polyphenols, and Mediterranean Diets. What Else Is There to Say?

Celestino Santos-Buelga *, Susana González-Manzano and Ana M. González-Paramás

Grupo de Investigación en Polifenoles (GIP-USAL), Universidad de Salamanca, E-37007 Salamanca, Spain; susanagm@usal.es (S.G.-M.); paramas@usal.es (A.M.G.-P.)
* Correspondence: csb@usal.es; Tel.: +34-923-294-500

Abstract: A considerable amount of literature has been published claiming the cardiovascular benefits of moderate (red) wine drinking, which has been considered a distinguishing trait of the Mediterranean diet. Indeed, red wine contains relevant amounts of polyphenols, for which evidence of their biological activity and positive health effects are abundant; however, it is also well-known that alcohol, even at a low level of intake, may have severe consequences for health. Among others, it is directly related to a number of non-communicable diseases, like liver cirrhosis or diverse types of cancer. The IARC classifies alcohol as a Group 1 carcinogen, causally associated with the development of cancers of the upper digestive tract and liver, and, with sufficient evidence, can be positively associated with colorectum and female breast cancer. In these circumstances, it is tricky, if not irresponsible, to spread any message on the benefits of moderate wine drinking, about which no actual consensus exists. It should be further considered that other hallmarks of the Mediterranean diet are the richness in virgin olive oil, fruits, grains, and vegetables, which are also good sources of polyphenols and other phytochemicals, and lack the risks of wine. All of these aspects are reviewed in this article.

Keywords: olive oil; resveratrol; alcohol; phytochemicals; tyrosol

1. Introduction

In November 2010, following a transnational nomination submitted by Spain, Greece, Italy, and Morocco, the UNESCO decided to inscribe the Mediterranean Diet as an Intangible Cultural Heritage of Humanity (https://ich.unesco.org/en/Decisions/5.COM/6.41, accessed on 1 September 2021), further enlarged in December 2013 with the incorporation of three other countries: Croatia, Cyprus, and Portugal (https://ich.unesco.org/en/Decisions/8.COM/8.10, accessed on 1 September 2021). In its decision, the UNESCO recognized the Mediterranean diet (MedDiet) as "a set of skills, knowledge, practices and traditions ranging from the landscape to the table, including the crops, harvesting, fishing, conservation, processing, preparation and, particularly, consumption of food (. . .) characterized by a nutritional model that has remained constant over time and space, (. . .) always respecting beliefs of each community."

Consistent associations of this Mediterranean dietary pattern with cardiovascular benefits were first reported in the 1960's from the earlier results of the Seven Countries Study (https://www.sevencountriesstudy.com/, accessed on 1 September 2021), describing significantly lower mortality rates and incidences of cardiovascular diseases in the Italian, Greek, and Croatian cohorts than in the rest of the included (non-Mediterranean) countries [1]. Further confirmation of these outcomes was obtained from the HALE project (Healthy Ageing—a Longitudinal study in Europe), analysing data on lifestyle, dietary, and biological determinants of healthy ageing from individuals of 13 European countries, collected from the Seven Countries, as well as the FINE (Finland, Italy, Netherlands Elderly study) and SENECA (Survey in Europe on Nutrition in the Elderly—a Concerted Action) prospections. It was found that adherence to a MedDiet, together with a healthful lifestyle (i.e., being physically active, non-smoking for more than 15 years, and moderate alcohol intake) was associated with a more than 50% lower rate of all-causes and cause-specific mortality, including coronary heart disease (CHD), cardiovascular disease (CVD), and cancer [2].

Similar observations were made from many other epidemiological and intervention studies. A comprehensive analysis of the results from observational studies and randomised clinical trials—comprising a total population of over 12,800,000 individuals—was made by Dinu et al. [3], concluding that there was robust evidence to suggest that greater adherence to a Mediterranean diet style is associated with a reduced risk of overall mortality, CVD, overall cancer incidence, neurodegenerative diseases, and type-2 diabetes. In a previous screening across intervention trials, Serra-Majem et al. [4] also concluded that there was good evidence to suggest that a MedDiet improves the lipid profile, endothelial function, and blood pressure, despite the fact that the authors also highlighted that there were discrepancies on how the different studies defined and formulated the Mediterranean diet.

Indeed, the Mediterranean diet does not constitute a close and unique nutritional model, but it is rather a compendium of diverse dietary habits traditionally followed by countries around the Mediterranean basin. In spite of their heterogeneity, some common patterns are observed across these countries, namely a high consumption of plant products such as fruits, vegetables, legumes, and nuts, as well as cereals (bread, pasta, rice, and whole grains); a moderate intake of dairy products, fish, poultry, and eggs as main protein sources, with small amounts of red and processed meat; the use of olive oil as a main fat source and water as a beverage of choice. Additionally, the diet is characterized by infusions and optional moderate amounts of wine taken with meals, and a preference for seasonal, fresh, and locally low-processed products. This was summarized in the Pyramid of the Mediterranean diet proposed by the "Fundación Dieta Mediterránea" (https://dietamediterranea.com/en/fundacion, accessed on 1 September 2021) (Figure 1).

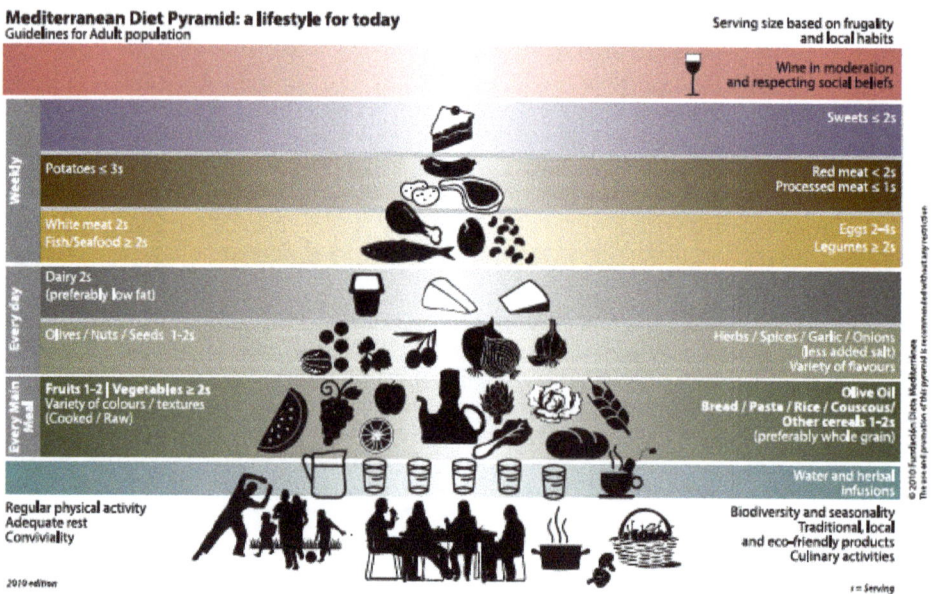

Figure 1. Pyramid of the Mediterranean diet (https://dietamediterranea.com/en/fundacion, accessed on 1 September 2021).

Relevant nutrients and bioactive compounds contributed by the main food items in the Mediterranean diet are summarized in Table 1.

Table 1. Main bioactive compounds provided by representative foodstuffs of the Mediterranean diets.

Food Item	Main Bioactive Compounds
Fresh fruit	Vitamin C, polyphenols, dietary fiber
Citrus fruits	Vitamin C, flavonoids
Nuts	Polyunsaturated fatty acids, phytosterols, vitamin E
Whole grains	Complex carbohydrates, dietary fiber
Legumes	Proteins, dietary fiber, saponins
Raw vegetables (tomatoes, carrots)	Hydrosoluble vitamins, carotenoids
Leafy green vegetables	Folic acid, dietary fiber
Cruciferous	Glucosinolates
Fish	n-3 Long-chain polyunsaturated fatty acids, high-quality proteins
Dairy products	Calcium, bioactive peptides, high-quality proteins
Eggs and poultry	High-quality proteins
Extra virgin olive oil	Monounsaturated fatty acids, polyphenols, phytosterols
Red wine	Polyphenols
Allium compounds	Sulphur compounds

The dietary patterns of the MedDiet have been suggested to likely overlap with those for optimal prevention of both cardiovascular diseases and cancer. Thus, it is considered that, whatever the particular food choices, Mediterranean diets provide adequate intakes of total fat and long-chain polyunsaturated fatty acids, dietary fiber, antioxidant vitamins, carotenoids, and polyphenols, as well as a balanced n-6/n-3 ratio of essential fatty acids and low amounts of saturated fatty acids (SFA) [5–7]. All of these characteristics are related to beneficial effects on endothelial and cardiovascular function. Furthermore, monounsaturated fatty acids (MUFA) present in olive oil (i.e., oleic acid) are acknowledged to improve the blood lipid profiles [8]. Actually, a common and consistent feature of the MedDiet seems to be the existence of a high MUFA/SFA ratio (estimated to be around 2.0 on average) [5], which has been significantly associated with low CVD mortality and overall mortality [9]. Complex carbohydrates and dietary fiber contributed by whole grain products, legumes, and vegetables have also been related with gut health and protection against different cancers, especially colorectal cancer [10,11]. There are also glucosinolates and other organosulphur compounds present in cruciferous vegetables and allium condiments, which have acknowledged anti-inflammatory properties [12]. Another feature of the MedDiet which is usually associated with its health-promoting properties is the supply of significant amounts of different classes of antioxidant polyphenols, which are even higher than those of other dietary antioxidants, such as vitamin C, vitamin E, or carotenoids [13]. Regular intake of these compounds has been related to beneficial effects on the lipids profile, blood pressure, glucose metabolism, adiposity, or inflammatory processes, and are also associated with a reduction in the incidence of several chronic diseases, like cardiovascular diseases, type-2 diabetes, metabolic syndrome, neurodegenerative disorders, or different cancers [14–16].

The purpose of the present review is to discuss the role of wine and wine polyphenols in the health benefits of the Mediterranean diet. A particular mention is made to resveratrol, owing to the special attention that has been paid to its possible contribution to the beneficial effects of moderate wine intake, as associated with the MetDiet. Reference is also made to olive oil as a distinguishing food in the MetDiet with claimed health benefits, which have been proposed to rely, at least in part, on its characteristic polyphenols, which are different to those present in wine.

2. Polyphenols as Key Components of Mediterranean Diets

Plant phenolic compounds, commonly referred to as polyphenols, are widespread in the diet, and are nowadays considered, at least in part, responsible for the health protective effects of fruit and vegetable-rich diets. They can be classified in two major classes: flavonoids and non-flavonoids, including phenolic acids (i.e., hydroxybenzoic and hydroxycinnamic acids and their derivatives), stilbenes, and lignans (Figure 2), as well as phenolic alcohols and their secoiridoid derivatives.

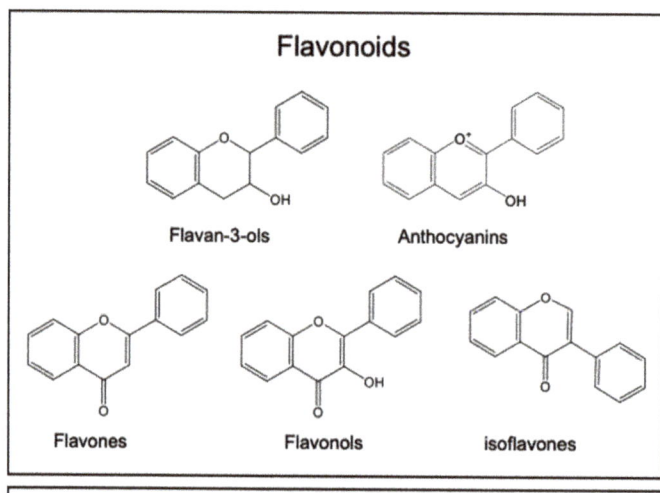

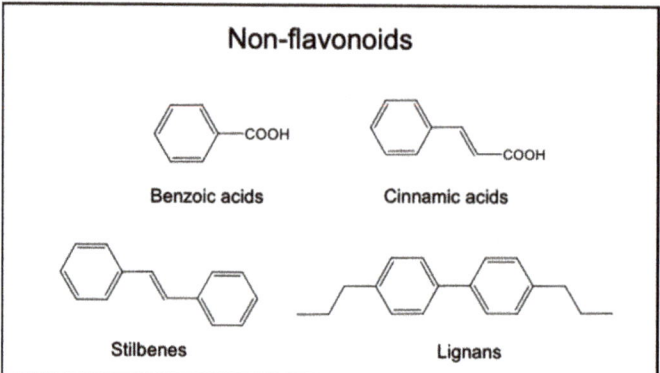

Figure 2. Core structures of the main classes of plant phenolic compounds.

The dietary intake of polyphenols largely varies among individuals, and is estimated to range from a few hundred mg/day to more than 1800 mg/day depending on the region and target population, as well as the methodology used for the assessment [17]. Hydroxycinnamic acid esters, namely caffeoylquinic acids and flavan-3-ols oligo/polymers (i.e., proanthocyanidins), are usually reported as the most important groups of consumed polyphenols, followed by anthocyanins and flavonols [17]. In general, the contribution of phenolic acid derivatives and flavonoids tends to be equilibrated, although there are differences across countries and population groups as a function of their dietary habits. For example, there are higher proportions of flavonoids in Mediterranean regions, while phenolic acids would predominate in non-Mediterranean countries [18–21]. The main food sources for individual polyphenols tend to be similar among individuals, with coffee, tea, and fruits as major items, and vegetables and red wine in a second range [17]. It is suggested that moderate red wine drinkers consume polyphenols at levels well above the population average [6].

Despite the fact that the antioxidant capacity of polyphenols is well-substantiated in vitro and has been recurrently associated in the literature to their health effects, the little bioavailability and large biotransformation of most polyphenols in the organism raise doubts that this activity can have a primary role on their in vivo effects [17]. Although this possibility might not be discarded for particular compounds or situations, nowadays, other alternatives are considered to contribute to the in vivo effects of polyphenols. For example, they could act as modulators of gene expression and intracellular signaling cascades involved in cell function and protection [22,23]. There is also increasing evidence about the crucial role of the interactions between polyphenols and gut microbiota as a mainstay to explain the health benefits of their consumption. A vast majority of the consumed polyphenols reach the large intestine unaltered, where they can be catabolized by the colonic microflora to a variety of metabolites [24,25]. Some of these metabolites can be biologically active, and be responsible for the activity associated with their parent polyphenols. Among others, this would be the case of tyrosols, produced from oleuropein and related phenolics from olive oil, with putative effects against some types of cancer [26]; urolithins, involved in the lipid-lowering effects and improvement in the cardiovascular risk biomarkers of ellagitannins [27]; or estrogenic S-equol, enterodiol, and enterolactone, derived from soy isoflavones [28] and lignans [29], respectively. The role of other metabolites, such as phenolic acids and aldehydes resulting from the bacterial breakdown of flavonoids, is still uncertain, although they might be expected to contribute to a part of their effects, both at the local and systemic level. Additionally, unabsorbed polyphenols and phenolic metabolites can also have an impact on the composition of the gut microbiota, acting as prebiotic-like compounds. For instance, they have been suggested to be able to decrease the Firmicutes/Bacteroidetes ratio [30,31], linked to obesity trends in humans [32], and increase the abundance of beneficial *Bifidobacteria* and *Lactobacilli* spp. [30,33–35], while producing a reduction in the levels of Bacteroides, Streptococci, Enterobacteriacae, or Clostridia [36,37]. In the end, several mechanisms might be involved in the biological effects of polyphenols and contribute to their health benefits. This is a current active field of research that is rapidly progressing, so that advances are expected in coming years [38].

Most of the available information on the biological activity and effects of the phenolic compounds has been obtained from in vitro, ex vivo, and animal studies, whereas data directly obtained in humans are scarce, and restricted, in general, to short-term intervention trials on a reduced number of people. Some attempts have been made in Mediterranean cohorts, whose results support the role of polyphenol-rich foods to the health benefits of the Mediterranean diet [16,19,39,40]. Nevertheless, assessing the precise contribution of dietary polyphenols to those benefits remains complex, owing to the fact that the same food sources are also rich in other bioactives, such as vitamins, minerals, dietary fiber, or other antioxidants, which should also contribute to the health effects [17].

3. Olive Oil

Olive oil, and especially virgin olive oil (VOO), is one of the products most usually associated with the health properties of the MedDiet. Its regular consumption has been claimed to provide benefits against a number of disease conditions, such as atherosclerosis, diabetes mellitus, obesity, cancer, or neurodegenerative diseases [41]. It is well-known that olive oil is very rich in monounsaturated fatty acids—mainly oleic acid, accounting for up to 80% of its total fatty acids—with acknowledged positive effects on the profiles of plasmatic lipoproteins, triglycerides, and platelet aggregation [42,43], which has been linked to protection against cardiovascular and neurodegenerative diseases [44]. Actually, the EFSA has approved health claims regarding the positive effects of "monounsaturated fatty acids (mainly oleic acid)", "oleic acid", and "extra virgin olive oil" in the maintenance of normal blood LDL-cholesterol concentrations and the maintenance of normal (fasting) blood concentrations of triglycerides, when replacing saturated fatty acids (SFAs) in foods or diets [8].

In addition to its fatty acid profile, VOO also contains a series of biologically active polyphenols, in a concentration that oscillates within a large range from 50 to 1000 mg/kg, depending on the olive cultivar and ripening stage, environmental factors (climate, altitude, agricultural practices), extraction techniques, storage conditions, and time [45]. It has been estimated that they may account for up to around 2% of total olive oil weight, contributing not only to olive oil's health properties, but also to its taste and fatty acid stability against oxidation [46].

VOO possesses a unique phenolic composition mainly consisting of secoiridoid derivatives, the most abundant one being oleuropein, the glucosylated form of 3,4-dihydroxyphenylethanol-elenolic acid (3,4-DHPEA-EA). Oleuropein is considered the main compound contributing to the bitterness of olives. Other related secoiridoids are the ligstroside aglycone (p-HPEA-EA) and the dialdehydic form of elenolic acid linked to either hydroxytyrosol (3,4-DHPEA-EDA; oleacein) or tyrosol (p-HPEA-EDA; oleocanthal), both existing as aglycones and glucosyl derivatives. Besides, VOO also contains phenolic alcohols such as tyrosol (p-HPEA) and hydroxytyrosol (3,4-DHPEA), mostly derived from their se-coiridoid precursors. The structures of these polyphenols are depicted in Figure 3. Other phenolic compounds also reported in lower amounts in VOO include lignans (pinoresinol, 1-acetoxypinoresinol, and 1-hydroxypinoresinol), verbascoside (i.e., caffeoylrhamnosyl-glucoside linked to hydroxytyrosol), some phenolic acids (vanillic, gallic, coumaric, caffeic acids) and flavonoids (especially flavonols derived from apigenin, luteolin, or quercetin) [46,47].

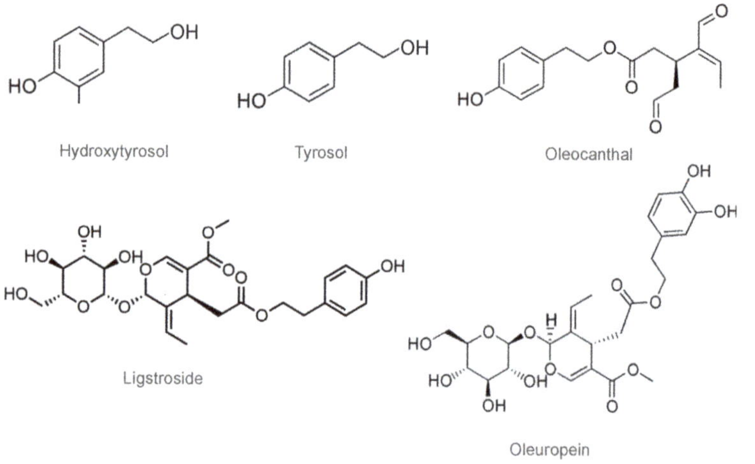

Figure 3. Representative polyphenols present in virgin olive oils.

Olive oil phenolics have been extensively studied for their potential to counteract the onset and progression of a variety of chronic and aging-related diseases, and is attributed to hypoglycemic, anti-obesity, cardioprotective, neuroprotective, antimicrobial, and anti-cancer properties [47–49]. Several in vitro and in vivo studies have associated the health-promoting effects of olive oil phenolics to their antioxidant and anti-inflammatory potential as related to their ability to modulate a series of molecular pathways. Thus, they have been reported to be able to activate AMPK (AMP-activated protein kinase) with subsequent inhibition of the mTOR signaling pathway [22], which is involved in the regulation of adipose tissue functions, such as adipogenesis, thermogenesis, and lipid metabolism. It also modulates processes like mitochondrial biogenesis and functionality, hypoxia signaling, autophagy, and cell cycle progression [50]. In intervention studies, VOO-rich Mediterranean diets were deemed effective in reducing several inflammatory markers, such as C-reactive protein, TNF-α, interleukin-6 (IL6), endothelial adhesion molecules (VCAM-1, ICAM), or chemokines like MCP-1, which has been related to their polyphenol content [40,51]. A compound that demonstrated strong in vitro anti-inflammatory properties is oleocanthal, with a structure that resembles ibuprofen, which was shown to cause a dose-dependent inhibition of cyclooxygenase enzymes COX-1 and COX-2 [52]. Similarly, hydroxytyrosol was able to inhibit TNF-α, iNOS, and COX-2 in LPS-challenged human monocytic cell lines [53]. Additionally, in vitro and animal studies have reported that oleuropein and hydroxytyrosol may reduce fat tissue accumulation by downregulating the expression of adipogenesis-related genes like PGC-1α, lipoprotein lipase, acetyl CoA carboxylase-1, and carnitine palmitoyltransferase-1 [54]. Recent reviews can be consulted for further information on olive oil phenolic effects and mechanisms of action [44,47,49,55,56].

The beneficial effects of phenolic compounds from olives and olive oil (i.e., hydroxytyrosol and oleuropein complex) were recognized by the European Food Safety Authority (EFSA), which authorized health claims in relation to polyphenols in olives and the protection of LDL particles from oxidative damage, the maintenance of normal blood HDL-cholesterol concentrations, the maintenance of normal blood pressure, and "anti-inflammatory properties". It also recognized their contribution to upper respiratory tract health, body defences against external agents, and the maintenance of a normally functioning gastrointestinal tract [57].

Within the PREDIMED study (http://www.predimed.es, accessed on 1 September 2021), a large Spanish trial on the primary prevention of chronic diseases through the Mediterranean Diet carried out in subjects at cardiovascular risk followed since 2013, it was estimated that olive oil and olives may provide about approximately 11% of the total polyphenol intake in a typical MedDiet, representing an important differential contribution to the profile of phenolic compounds consumed by Mediterranean populations [19]. Less optimistic calculations have been made by other authors. Thus, Parkinson and Cicerale [56], assuming a mean VOO intake of 30–50 g/day in Mediterranean countries, estimated that the amount of polyphenols ingested from VOO consumption would not exceed 9 mg/day. Whatever the dietary intake, at present there is not enough evidence to confirm that the consumption of olive phenolic compounds isolated by or as components of the VOO can be healthy [58]. Most of the in vivo studies with olive oil polyphenols have been carried out using supraphysiological concentrations that are difficult to extrapolate to a dietary context, while the number and variety of randomized clinical trials (RCT)—providing the highest level of scientific evidence—are very limited and insufficient to confirm their beneficial effects on humans, except for some markers of cardiovascular risk. Actually, the strongest piece of evidence has been obtained for the ability of VOO polyphenols to protect lipoproteins from oxidation and to reduce systolic blood pressure in hypertensive individuals [56]. Extensive RCT in different population groups with distinct disorders and at phenolic levels adjusted to usual VOO consumptions are, therefore, necessary to achieve high quality scientific evidence before nutritional recommendations can be given [56,58].

The health benefits attributed to olive oil could also be supposed for table olives. Nevertheless, the phenolic composition of table olives differs from that of olive oil, as they are influenced not only by the cultivar and harvesting time (green or fully ripened), but also by the processing conditions used for making them edible, which lead to chemical transformations in the polyphenols [59,60]. Thus, under the alkaline conditions used for the debittering of fruits in Spanish-style olives, oleuropein is hydrolyzed to practical disappearance. Moreover, in Greek-style black olives, in which the fruits are collected fully ripened and directly put into brine, an acid hydrolysis of oleuropein occurs, and orthodiphenols are oxidized and polymerized during the darkening step [60]. Tyrosol and hydroxytyrosol and their acetates have been identified as the most representative phenolic compounds in table olives, with concentrations of total polyphenols ranging between 200 mg/kg to 1200 mg/kg, depending on the cultivar and processing method, with oxidized olives containing the lowest levels. A further decrease of phenolic content is produced in pitted olives due to their loss in the washing liquids, which reduce their concentration to almost half that of the nonpitted fruits [60].

Besides polyphenols, olives also contain other bioactive compounds in the unsaponifiable fraction, such as pentacyclic triterpenoids like maslinic acid and oleanolic acid (Figure 4). A range of biological activities have been shown for maslinic acid, mostly from in vitro studies, such as anti-inflammatory, antiproliferative, antioxidant, and antidiabetic properties. In regard to oleanolic acid, hepatoprotective, antitumor, and antiviral properties have been reported [60–62]. These compounds are not lost during processing, and they are present in table olives and olive-pomace oil, a byproduct from olive oil extraction submitted to a refining process that leads to the complete loss of polyphenols. Table olives may contain more than 1300 mg/kg (dw) of maslinic acid, which is considered its richest food source [63]. Other dietary sources are spinach and eggplant, aromatic herbs, legumes, and to a lesser extent, some fruits like mandarin and pomegranate. Actually, plant-based diets including olives and olive oil, like the MedDiet, could provide a constant supply of maslinic acid, which might partly contribute to their health-enhancing properties [61].

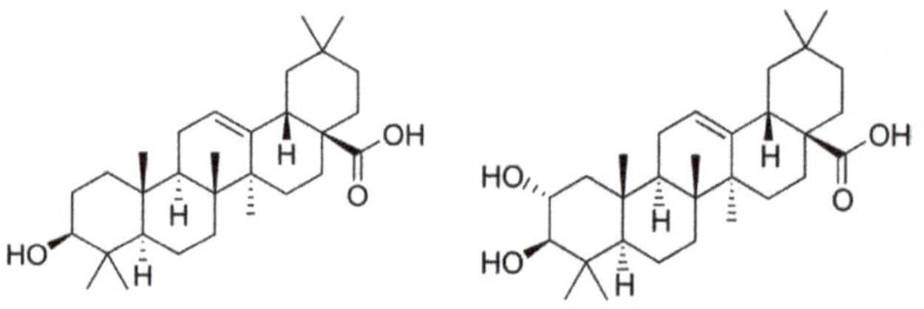

Figure 4. Structures of oleanolic and maslinic acids.

4. Wine in the Context of the Mediterranean Diet

Wine is considered another distinguishing food of the Mediterranean diet contributing to its health benefits [44]. Nevertheless, it should not be forgotten that in several countries and regions that follow typical Mediterranean dietary patterns, alcohol, and therefore wine, is excluded for religious reasons.

Since the early St. Leger et al. [64] and Framingham studies [65], a lot of epidemiological evidence has accumulated, pointing to the existence of inverse relationships between light to moderate alcohol consumption—especially wine—and incidences and mortality of cardiovascular diseases (see, e.g., [66–69]), as well as of other chronic disorders like type 2 diabetes [70–73] or dementia and cognitive decline in old age [74,75]. The relationship has been described as a U- or J-shaped curve [76], with a minimum situated at a level of consumption around 10 to 30 g of alcohol/day. These studies are not free from debate, as they have been attributed to suffer from methodological limitations, which may have led to misinterpretations or biased conclusions [77–80]. Nevertheless, despite possible bias, many authors agree that when confounding factors are specifically adjusted, epidemiological trials still continue to be remarkably consistent regarding the beneficial effects from low to moderate alcohol/wine intake on CVD morbidity and mortality, as well as diabetes, osteoporosis, and neurological disorders [81–83].

A point of discussion is whether the purported wine benefits are due to ethanol or to other components. It is known that ethanol itself is able to increase HDL-cholesterol, prevent platelet aggregation, and enhance fibrinolysis, which may have positive effects on the cardiovascular system [84]. However, when differentiation among drinks is made, it is generally concluded that wine provides superior health benefits to other alcoholic drinks—especially spirits—either regarding protection against CVD [85–88], type 2 diabetes [73], or dementia [89]. This perception has also been supported by the results obtained in human clinical studies [90–94] and observations over Mediterranean cohorts [19,39,95].

The intended superior benefits of wine have been related to its phenolic compounds, which are absent or in very low concentrations in other alcoholic drinks. Wine contains a variable mixture of flavonoid and non-flavonoid compounds, extracted from the grape during winemaking. Phenolic contents in red wine is usually above 1 g/L—concentrations that are higher than those that can be found in most fruits and vegetables—while in white wine, it does not commonly exceed a few hundred mg/L, due to the fact that it is not normally submitted to maceration with grape solids during winemaking [96]. The majority phenolic fraction in red wine is constituted by flavonoids (>85%), especially procyanidins (i.e., flavan-3-ol oligo/polymers; condensed tannins). Actually, red wine is one of the richest dietary sources of procyanidins [97], a type of compound recognized to possess a range of biological activities, and that is related with the disease preventive properties of plant-based diets [98,99]. Red wine is also rich in anthocyanins (especially young red wine) and flavonols, with acknowledged biological activities, including antioxidant, anti-inflammatory, antiproliferative, or gene modulating abilities [100], which are also considered to contribute to the health protective effects of fruits and vegetables. Hydroxycinnamic acids and their tartaric esters are the most important phenolic compounds in white wine, while other phenolics, like hydroxybenzoic acids, stilbenes (e.g., resveratrol), lignans, or dihydroflavonols are usually present in low concentrations in either type of wine, usually not exceeding a few mg/L [96].

Polyphenols, and especially flavonoids, have been proposed to be the main vasoactive components in red wine. They have been reported to be able to modulate the plasmatic lipid profile to a healthy shape, reducing triglyceride and LDL-cholesterol circulating levels [90,101,102]. They may also improve both systolic and diastolic blood pressure, stimulate endothelial-dependent vasodilation by enhancing nitric oxide (NO) generation, decrease platelet aggregation, and inhibit the activity of inflammatory enzymes and the production of several types of proinflammatory and oxidant mediators [103–105]. Many recent reports have been published dealing with the putative health effects of polyphenols, either from wine or other plant sources, and their possible mechanisms of action (see, e.g., [17,106–111]), and thus it does not seem necessary to insist herein.

In addition to polyphenols, other bioactive phenolic and non-phenolic components can also be present in wine that might contribute to the putative health effects and that are usually less considered. Thus, during must fermentation, yeasts catabolize aromatic amino acids—such as tyrosine, tryptophan, and phenylalanine—to their respective aromatic alcohols, tyrosol, tryptophol, and phenyl ethanol, which also possess bioactive properties and are also associated with some of the beneficial effects of moderate wine consumption [112]. Tyrosol has been indicated to be the second most abundant non-hydroxycinnamate phenolic in many wines, with concentrations that may reach up to 95 mg/L. Its antioxidant and anti-inflammatory properties were suggested to contribute to the beneficial effects attributed to a moderate consumption of wine [113,114]. Among others, tyrosol was found to be able to inhibit the LPS-induced production of pro-inflammatory cytokines tumor necrosis, like factor alpha (TNF-α), and interleukins IL-1β and IL-6 in human peripheral blood mononuclear cells at nanomolar concentrations, either alone or in synergy with caffeic acid [113,114]. Hydroxytyrosol is also present in wine in levels under 10 mg/L [115–117], but it can also be formed in the human organism from hydroxylation of tyrosol. De la Torre et al. [118] found that the consumption of moderate doses of wine or olive oil by healthy subjects led to a higher increase in urinary concentrations of hydroxytyrosol in the wine group, despite the fact that the amount of hydroxytyrosol administered was fivefold greater in the olive oil group (1.7 mg vs. 0.35 mg). This was explained by the biotransformation of tyrosol to hydroxytyrosol; besides, the alcohol could help to increase the bioavailability of the tyrosol present in the wine. The authors indicated that a single glass of wine was at least equivalent to 25 mL (22 g) of virgin olive oil in its capacity to increase hydroxytyrosol concentrations in the body, leading to similar beneficial effects. The same group found that there was a direct association between wine consumption and the urinary concentrations of tyrosol and hydroxytyrosol determined in individuals at cardiovascular risk included in the PREDIMED study [119], suggesting that the endogenous formation of hydroxytyrosol might explain part of the cardiovascular benefits associated with light-to-moderate wine consumption.

Another bioactive compound that may contribute to the health benefits of wine is melatonin (*n*-acetyl-5-methoxytryptamine). This is a neurohormone secreted from the pineal gland, with well-characterized antioxidant, anti-inflammatory, and immune-modulating properties. It also contributes to the regulation of the circadian rhythms and has been attributed to tumor inhibitory activities and positive effects on the cardiovascular system, lipid, glucose metabolism, and neuroprotection [120,121]. It is present in grapes and can also be formed in wine from tryptophan metabolism by yeasts [122]. Actually, its content in wine is mostly influenced by the fermentation process, where the yeast strain and the fermentation time are the most influential factors [122]. It has been shown that blood levels of melatonin and total antioxidant capacity in plasma increased after the dietary intake of food containing it [123–125]. Melatonin concentrations ranging from a few µg/L to more than 150 µg/L have been reported in wine [126], which is higher than those found in most fruits and vegetables. Moreover, most fruits and vegetables are usually situated in the low ng/g level, with only a few products, such as mushrooms, coffee beans, or some berries showing contents in the µg/g range [120]. Therefore, wine can be considered a significant source of dietary melatonin, though it is not unlikely that it could be a contributor to the beneficial effects associated with wine consumption [121].

5. What about Resveratrol?

A phenolic compound that has been frequently associated with the putative beneficial effects of wine is the stilbene resveratrol (3,4′,5-trihydroxy-trans-stilbene), a phytoalexin that can be found in grape skin and is extracted into wine during winemaking. The average contents of resveratrol in wine does not usually exceed a few mg/L [96]. Since white wine is not usually submitted to maceration with grape solids, it possesses lower resveratrol concentrations than red wine.

Dietary sources of resveratrol are scarce and, in addition to grapes, they include rhubarb, peanuts, or berries, though they are always present in low levels. Actually, grapes and wine are considered the most relevant food sources for humans [127]. Stilbenes are synthetized by plants in response to biotic or abiotic stress, so that exposure to UV radiation can induce the formation of resveratrol in grapes, increasing its concentration by up to tenfold [128]. Post-harvest UV irradiation has been employed as a strategy to increase resveratrol levels so as to "functionalize" grapes [129].

The presence of resveratrol in wine was firstly described in 1992 [130], suggesting that it might be an active component in the lowering effects of serum lipids associated with wine consumption. Since then, a high number of studies have been published reporting a diversity of bioactivities and multiple potential health outcomes for stilbene, including antioxidant, anti-inflammatory, anti-obesity, chemopreventive, glucose-modulating, cardiovascular protective, or calorie restriction mimicking effects [131]. A departure point in resveratrol research could be established in the study by Jang et al. [132], reporting its ability to inhibit the enzymatic activity of both forms of cyclooxygenase (COX1 and COX2), suggesting that it may behave as an anti-inflammatory and anticarcinogenic agent. Further studies showed that it was able to enhance stress resistance and extend lifespan in various model organisms, including *Saccharomyces cerevisiae*, *Caenorhabditis elegans*, *Drosophila melanogaster*, fish, and mice [133–135]. Those effects were related to the activation of Sir2 proteins (sirtuins), a family of NAD^+-dependent deacetylases and mono-ADP-ribosyltransferases involved in key regulation processes, such as glucose and insulin production, fat metabolism, the regulation of the p53 tumour suppressor, and cell survival [136].

Later on, several authors have also explored the effects of resveratrol on obesity, brain function, and visual performance. The results obtained in a number of studies in cell, animal, and human trials revealed that resveratrol and related stilbenes were able to inhibit adipocyte differentiation and proliferation, decrease lipogenesis, and promote lipolysis and fatty acid beta-oxidation [137], pointing out that it may be used as an anti-obesity agent. Regarding brain function, Kennedy et al. [138] found that the oral administration of a single dose of resveratrol (250 or 500 mg) to healthy adults increased cerebral blood flow during task performance in a dose-dependent way without affecting cognitive function. Furthermore, Evans et al. [139] reported that daily consumption of 150 mg of resveratrol for 14 weeks enhanced verbal memory and overall cognitive performance in postmenopausal women. Another study in postmenopausal women concluded that supplementation with 75 mg of trans-resveratrol twice a day for a year improved overall cognitive performance and cerebrovascular responsiveness to cognitive stimuli, which was also associated with a reduction of fasting blood glucose [140]. By contrast, a nutritional intervention with 200 mg/day of resveratrol failed to show significant improvements in verbal memory after 26 weeks in healthy elderly individuals [141]. Moreover, in a meta-analysis on the results obtained from four randomized clinical trials, Farzaei et al. [142] did not conclude significant effects on memory and cognitive performance assessed by auditory verbal learning test. Similarly, Marx et al. [143] concluded that, despite the fact that resveratrol supplementation might improve cognitive performance, the results obtained among clinical trials are limited and inconsistent. As for visual performance, studies carried out in different retinal cell lines found that resveratrol at micromolar concentrations was able to protect them from damage caused by oxidative stress and hyperglycemia-induced low-grade inflammation, suggesting that it might contribute to preventing age-related ocular disorders like cataracts, glaucoma, or macular degeneration [144–146]. Additionally, oral administration of resveratrol (5 to 200 mg/kg for 5 days) to mice was seen to prevent endotoxin-induced uveitis by inhibiting oxidative damage, leading authors to propose that supplementation with resveratrol is a possible strategy to treat ocular inflammation [147].

However, despite the range of evidence on the potential benefits of resveratrol obtained in model and preclinical studies, attempts have failed to come to clear and consistent outcomes in cohort and clinical trials [148,149]. It must also be highlighted that the available studies have been performed using relatively high doses of resveratrol, which are unlikely to be provided by the diet when taking into account the scarcity of food sources and the very low concentrations at which stilbenes are present. It does not seem that Mediterranean diets, either with or without wine, can represent further improvements in this sense. Thus, it should not be expected that resveratrol may have a relevant contribution to the beneficial health effects associated with Mediterranean diets or any other type of diet. Supplementation or therapeutic approaches might, therefore, be the way to take advantage of its potential benefits. Nonetheless, much work seems still required in this respect. As recently reviewed by Ren et al. [148], poor pharmacokinetics and low potency—as well as possible toxicity issues, including gastrointestinal disorders, headache, rash, or nephrotoxicity [131,148]—seem the main bottlenecks to overcome for its nutritional or therapeutical application. The development of more potent analogues and/or novel resveratrol formulations to enhance its bioavailability may be promising strategies to take it from bench to people [148].

6. The Social Context

Polyphenols are not the only reason that has been argued to support the beneficial effects associated with wine consumption, but socioeconomical and contextual factors also matter and could be even more important. Indeed, when interpreting the relationship between wine consumption and health, the underlying lifestyle and dietary patterns have to be considered, as they can be as influential on the health outcome as the type of drink. Mediterranean diets are themselves considered to constitute healthy dietary and lifestyle behaviour, making it difficult to extract the contribution of wine; otherwise, they might counteract the negative impact of alcohol on the organism.

It has been claimed that the MedDiet involves a "Mediterranean way of drinking", that is, a regular, moderate wine intake mainly consumed with meals [6]. When consumed with meals, wine tends to be sipped more slowly as compared to other alcoholic drinks, which may provide metabolic advantages. Among others, the concomitant presence of food in the stomach slows down gastric emptying and subsequent ethanol absorption which favours hepatic metabolism and clearance, lowering the peak of alcohol concentration in the blood [150]. It has been reported that, when consumed within meals, alcohol intake is associated with a lower risk of acute myocardial infarctions [151]. The concurrent presence of food might also reduce the amount of alcohol available to the oral microbiota, which has the capacity to metabolize ethanol to acetaldehyde, a compound associated with the tumorigenic effects of ethanol in the upper gastrointestinal tract [152]. It has also been observed that when wine is consumed with food, the onset of the plasma uric acid elevation coincides with the period of postprandial oxidative stress produced after a meal, which may contribute to the wine's protective effects [153]. Moreover, the presence of alcohol may improve the bioavailability of polyphenols in the food bolus, which would thus be more easily assimilated [154].

Studies in countries where wine is not the traditional alcoholic drink have also supported that a preference for wine is associated with healthy outcomes and more favourable dietary patterns [155]. Burke et al. [156], in a health screening on middle-aged men in Australia, found that a preference for wine was related to a greater consumption of fruit, vegetables, and bread, as compared to people that preferred beer. In a survey in Finland, Mannisto et al. [157] observed that wine drinkers had significantly higher intakes of antioxidants in their diet, indicating a greater consumption of fruit and vegetables than groups with other drink preferences. A higher intake of fruits, salads, cooked vegetables, fish, and olive oil was also found by Tjonneland et al. [158] in those that preferred wine, as compared with other alcoholic drinks, in a cross-sectional study conducted in Denmark. Similarly, Sluik et al. [159], in a representative sample of people from the Netherlands, found that wine drinkers consumed less energy and more vegetables and fruit juices, while the choice of beer was associated with a higher intake of meat, soft drinks, margarine, and snacks. All those behaviours associated with wine choice result in diets closer to the MedDiet, supporting the idea that it is not only wine, but the associated dietary and lifestyle patterns which contribute to healthier outcomes. Interestingly, this type of association has not been found in studies performed in some Mediterranean countries, as was the case of some Italian [160] or Spanish cohorts [161,162], where no significant correlation between wine consumption and healthier dietary habits was observed in relation to non-drinkers or consumers of other alcoholic beverages.

7. Risks of Wine Consumption

Despite the fact that moderate consumption may have health benefits, it is also well-known that alcohol, even at a low level of consumption, has some risks. It is well-known that there is a causal relationship between alcohol intake and the incidence of a variety of pathologies—particularly liver diseases—which, in their more severe form, such as the alcoholic hepatitis, lead to a mortality rate exceeding 50% in three months. Other manifestations, like steatosis of alcoholic cirrhosis, are initially less severe, although in advanced cirrhosis, the median of survival is situated around 1–2 years [163]. In addition, there are also well-established relationships between alcohol intake and incidence of pancreatitis and diverse types of cancer, as well as some infectious diseases and non-intentional injuries.

A comprehensive report on alcohol-attributable deaths was released in 2018 within the frame of the Global Burden of Diseases, Injuries, and Risk Factors Study 2016 [164]. For that, a meta-analysis of relative risks for 23 health outcomes associated with alcohol use was made using 694 data sources of individual and population-level alcohol consumption, along with 592 prospective and retrospective studies on the risk of alcohol use. The study used 195 locations and a time span from 1990 to 2016, including people aged above 15 of both sexes. It was concluded that alcohol use was a leading risk factor for the global disease burden worldwide, causing substantial health loss from many causes and accounting for nearly 10% of global deaths among people aged 15–49 years. The risk of all-cause mortality, and of cancers specifically, raised with increasing levels of consumption, with no level of consumption that can be considered free of risks [164].

The International Agency for Research on Cancer (IARC) classifies alcohol as a Group 1 carcinogen, causally associated with the development of cancers of the upper digestive tract and liver, and has sufficient evidence to be positively associated with colorectum and female breast cancer, without differences among the type of alcoholic drink [165]. The existence of a high association between alcohol intake and the increased risk of different types of cancers was confirmed in many prospective studies. In a meta-analysis carried out on 156 epidemiological studies, Corrao et al. [166] concluded that the risk for all types of cancer significantly increased for ethanol intakes of above 25 g/day. Also, a highly significant association was found for liver cirrhosis and essential hypertension, although, for coronary heart disease and ischemic stroke, a reduction in the risk was observed with a minimum consumption of 20 g alcohol/day [66].

An aspect to notice is that observational studies on alcohol and health usually consider average alcohol consumption, which may hide risky drinking behaviours, such as irregular binge drinking, that always involves higher health risks and mortality rates [167,168]. A pattern of irregular heavy drinking is associated with pathophysiological mechanisms that increase the risk of sudden cardiac death, hypertension, atrial or ventricular fibrillation, and cardiomyopathy, even if the average consumption is comparable to moderate consumption [169]. Heavy drinking during pregnancy is known to produce foetal alcohol syndrome, leading to abnormalities and mental retardation. Nevertheless, there is also evidence that prenatal exposure to light to moderate levels of alcohol could affect foetal development and result in decreased body weight, neurodevelopmental deficits, and long-term effects on the growth of children [170,171]. All in all, there is no level of alcohol that can be considered safe during pregnancy. As a result, its consumption must be avoided by pregnant women, as well as during the period of breastfeeding. Similarly, alcohol must be avoided by younger people: adolescent alcohol use shows clear positive relationships with total mortality and is associated with an increased risk for development of chronic alcohol use disorders in adulthood [172].

It has been suggested that the detrimental effects of ethanol might be partly counterbalanced by the polyphenols contained in wine and other foods that play a part in the MedDiet, like extra-virgin olive oil [173], although this may be more of a perception that is not supported by consistent studies in humans. In a recent position paper on Dietary Guidelines for the Spanish Population [174], the Spanish Society of Community Nutrition (SENC) established that the consumption of alcoholic beverages is not encouraged or recommended in any case. Nevertheless, taking into account the prevalence of the Mediterranean uses and customs in Spain, an optional consumption of wine in limited amounts (no more than 40 g alcohol/day for men and no more than 20 g alcohol/day for women) and with meals is suggested only for adults who so desire and are not subject to contraindication due to a health condition or medication use. The SENC also highlighted that people who do not use alcoholic beverages should not start drinking because of its potential beneficial effects, and that equivalent results can be achieved through an adequate diet without the potential risks of alcohol.

8. Concluding Remarks

The Mediterranean diet has been associated with beneficial health outcomes in the prevention of chronic degenerative disorders, including cardiovascular diseases, type-2 diabetes, cognitive decline, or cancers. Its benefits were recognized by the UNESCO, which in 2010 inscribed the Mediterranean diet as an Intangible Cultural Heritage of Humanity. A feature of the MedDiet that has been related to its health benefits is that it contributes significant amounts of antioxidants, and especially polyphenols, whose regular intake is related to beneficial effects on the lipids profile, blood pressure, glucose metabolism, adiposity, and inflammatory processes. Virgin olive oil and moderate wine consumption have been indicated as two distinctive hallmarks of the MedDiet, contributing to its health benefits [44]. Indeed, olive oil represents a differential Mediterranean product, with a peculiar phenolic composition based on secoiridoids and derived phenolic alcohols, described to be able to improve the blood lipidic profile, maintain blood pressure, and provide anti-inflammatory properties, as recognized by the EFSA with a health claim.

On the other hand, a moderate consumption of wine, especially red wine, has been proposed to provide some degree of protection against cardiovascular diseases, diabetes mellitus, or cognitive decline, which has been related to its polyphenol content. The available studies in this respect are, however, limited by their observational nature, and there is a lack of randomized clinical trials that may prove a causal relationship. Furthermore, wine contains alcohol, which even at moderate consumption increases the risks of liver disorders and several types of cancers, among other diseases, Although the Mediterranean habit of drinking wine with meals may delay ethanol absorption and favour its more rapid clearance, at the same time that it may contribute to a decrease in postprandial oxidative stress produced after a meal. Furthermore, although polyphenols present in wine are also found in fruits and vegetables that lack the risks associated with alcohol, the concomitant presence of ethanol in the food bolus might make wine polyphenols more bioavailable. Some authors have, however, highlighted that a high wine and total alcohol intake, particularly by men, can represent a problematic aspect of the Mediterranean diet that may have not been critically evaluated [175]. Indeed, the potential risks of wine consumption, even at moderate doses, may have been overlooked or undervalued by many authors, which inadvertently may have disclosed a confusing message, although not only restricted to the context of the Mediterranean diets. Certainly, it does not seem wise to think of wine or any other alcoholic drink as an element for health promotion, but the risks of alcohol should always be considered in the first place. Releasing any message that might induce people to drink in the hope of gaining health benefits could likely have more harmful than beneficial consequences.

All in all, it is not easy to give a simple answer to the question of whether wine should be considered a key food contributing to the beneficial health outcomes of the MedDiet. Despite the fact that it is excluded from the diet in many Mediterranean areas for religious reasons, we do think that it definitely constitutes a distinguishing feature of many Mediterranean cultures, and plays an undeniable part of their historical legacy. In those regions, wine can be a relevant contributor to polyphenol intake and could be considered a side element in the beneficial health effects of the MedDiet, provided that it is consumed in the 'traditional' way, that is, light to moderate regular consumption with meals. In our opinion, wine has to be regarded as a fruitive food, to be enjoyed responsibly and in moderation, in a convivial environment and in the context of an adequate diet. In this case, it may constitute another element of a healthy lifestyle, provided that there are no reasons that advise against their intake.

Author Contributions: Conceptualization, C.S.-B.; methodology, C.S.-B., S.G.-M. and A.M.G.-P.; resources, C.S.-B. and A.M.G.-P.; writing—original draft preparation, C.S.-B.; writing—review and editing, C.S.-B., S.G.-M. and A.M.G.-P.; project administration, C.S.-B. and A.M.G.-P.; funding acquisition, C.S.-B. and A.M.G.-P. All authors have read and agreed to the published version of the manuscript.

Funding: The GIP-USAL is funded by the Spanish Ministerio de Ciencia e Innovación (Project PID2019-106167RB-I00), Consejería de Educación de la Junta de Castilla y León (Project SA093P20), and Strategic Research Programs for Units of Excellence from Junta de Castilla y León (ref CLU-2018-04).

Conflicts of Interest: The authors declare no conflict of interest.

Sample Availability: Samples of the compounds are not available from the authors.

References

1. Keys, A. Coronary heart disease in seven countries. *Circulation* **1970**, *41*, 186–195. [CrossRef]
2. Knoops, K.T.; de Groot, L.C.P.G.M.; Kromhout, D.; Perrin, A.E.; Moreiras-Varela, O.; Menotti, A.; van Staveren, W.A. Mediterranean diet; lifestyle factors; and 10-year mortality in elderly European men and women: The HALE project. *JAMA* **2004**, *292*, 1433–1439. [CrossRef]
3. Dinu, M.; Pagliai, G.; Casini, A.; Sofi, F. Mediterranean diet and multiple health outcomes: An umbrella review of meta-analyses of observational studies and randomised trials. *Eur. J. Clin. Nutr.* **2018**, *72*, 30–43. [CrossRef]
4. Serra-Majem, L.; Roman, B.; Estruch, R. Scientific evidence of interventions using the mediterranean diet: A systematic review. *Nutr. Rev.* **2006**, *64*, S27–S47. [CrossRef]
5. Davis, C.; Bryan, J.; Hodgson, J.; Murphy, K. Definition of the Mediterranean Diet: A Literature Review. *Nutrients* **2015**, *7*, 9139–9153. [CrossRef]
6. Giacosa, A.; Barale, R.; Bavaresco, L.; Faliva, M.A.; Gerbi, V.; La Vecchia, C.; Negri, E.; Opizzi, A.; Perna, S.; Pezzotti, M.; et al. Mediterranean way of drinking and longevity. *Crit. Rev. Food Sci. Nutr.* **2016**, *56*, 635–640. [CrossRef] [PubMed]
7. Román, G.C.; Jackson, R.E.; Gadhia, R.; Román, A.N.; Reis, J. Mediterranean diet: The role of long-chain ω-3 fatty acids in fish; polyphenols in fruits; vegetables; cereals; coffee; tea; cacao and wine; probiotics and vitamins in prevention of stroke; age-related cognitive decline; and Alzheimer disease. *Rev. Neurol.* **2019**, *175*, 724–741. [CrossRef] [PubMed]
8. EFSA Panel on Dietetic Products; Nutrition and Allergies (NDA). Scientific Opinion on the substantiation of health claims related to oleic acid intended to replace saturated fatty acids (SFAs) in foods or diets and maintenance of normal blood LDL-cholesterol concentrations (ID 673; 728; 729; 1302; 4334) and maintenance of normal (fasting) blood concentrations of triglycerides (ID 673; 4334) pursuant to Article 13(1) of Regulation (EC) No 1924/2006. *EFSA J.* **2011**, *9*, 2043.
9. Saura-Calixto, F.; Goñi, I. Definition of the mediterranean diet based on bioactive compounds. *Crit. Rev. Food Sci. Nutr.* **2009**, *49*, 145–152. [CrossRef]
10. Grosso, G.; Buscemi, S.; Galvano, F.; Mistretta, A.; Marventano, S.; La Vela, V.; Drago, F.; Gangi, S.; Basile, F.; Biondi, A. Mediterranean diet and cancer: Epidemiological evidence and mechanism of selected aspects. *BMC Surg.* **2013**, *13*, 1–9. [CrossRef]
11. Mentella, M.C.; Scaldaferri, F.; Ricci, C.; Gasbarrini, A.; Miggiano, G.A.D. Cancer and Mediterranean Diet: A Review. *Nutrients* **2019**, *11*, 2059. [CrossRef] [PubMed]
12. Ruhee, R.T.; Suzuki, K. The Integrative role of sulforaphane in preventing inflammation; oxidative stress and fatigue: A review of a potential protective phytochemical. *Antioxidants* **2020**, *9*, 521. [CrossRef]
13. Cannataro, R.; Fazio, A.; La Torre, C.; Caroleo, M.C.; Cione, E. Polyphenols in the Mediterranean Diet: From Dietary Sources to microRNA Modulation. *Antioxidants* **2021**, *10*, 328. [CrossRef] [PubMed]
14. Chiva-Blanch, G.; Badimon, L. Effects of polyphenol intake on metabolic syndrome: Current evidences from human trials. *Oxid. Med. Cell Longev.* **2017**, *2017*, 5812401. [CrossRef]
15. Del Bo, C.; Bernardi, S.; Marino, M.; Porrini, M.; Tucci, M.; Guglielmetti, S.; Cherubini, A.; Carrieri, B.; Kirkup, B.; Kroon, P.; et al. Systematic review on polyphenol intake and health outcomes: Is there sufficient evidence to define a health-promoting polyphenol-rich dietary pattern? *Nutrients* **2019**, *11*, 1355.
16. Tresserra-Rimbau, A.; Rimm, E.B.; Medina-Remon, A.; Martínez-González, M.A.; de la Torre, R.; Corella, D.; Salas-Salvadó, J.; Gómez-Garcia, E.; Lapetra, J.; Arós, F.; et al. Inverse association between habitual polyphenol intake and incidence of cardiovascular events in the PREDIMED study. *Nutr. Metab. Cardiovasc. Dis.* **2014**, *24*, 639–647. [CrossRef]
17. Santos-Buelga, C.; González-Paramás, A.M.; Oludemi, T.; Ayuda-Durán, B.; González-Manzano, S. Plant phenolics as functional food ingredients. *Adv. Food Nutr. Res.* **2019**, *90*, 183–257.
18. Godos, J.; Marventano, S.; Mistretta, A.; Galvano, F.; Grosso, G. Dietary sources of polyphenols in the Mediterranean healthy Eating; Aging and Lifestyle (MEAL) study cohort. *Int. J. Food Sci. Nutr.* **2017**, *68*, 750–756. [CrossRef] [PubMed]
19. Tresserra-Rimbau, A.; Medina-Remón, A.; Pérez-Jiménez, J.; Martínez-González, M.A.; Covas, M.I.; Corella, D.; Salas-Salvadó, J.; Gómez-Gracia, E.; Lapetra, J.; Arós, F.; et al. Dietary intake and major food sources of polyphenols in a Spanish population at high cardiovascular risk: The PREDIMED study. *Nutr. Metab. Cardiovasc. Dis.* **2013**, *23*, 953–959. [CrossRef]
20. Vitale, M.; Masulli, M.; Rivellese, A.A.; Bonora, E.; Cappellini, F.; Nicolucci, A. Dietary intake and major food sources of polyphenols in people with type 2 diabetes: The TOSCA.IT Study. *Eur. J. Nutr.* **2018**, *57*, 679–688. [CrossRef] [PubMed]
21. Zamora Ros, R.; Knaze, V.; Rothwell, J.A.; Hémon, B.; Moskal, A.; Overvad, K.; Tjønneland, A.; Kyrø, C.; Fagherazzi, G.; Boutron-Ruault, M.-C.; et al. Dietary polyphenol intake in Europe: The European Prospective Investigation into Cancer and Nutrition (EPIC) study. *Eur. J. Nutr.* **2016**, *55*, 1359–1375. [CrossRef]
22. Barrajón-Catalán, E.; Herranz-López, M.; Joven, J.; Segura-Carretero, A.; Alonso-Villaverde, C.; Menéndez, J.A.; Micol, V. Molecular promiscuity of plant polyphenols in the management of age-related diseases: Far beyond their antioxidant properties. *Adv. Exp. Med. Biol.* **2014**, *824*, 141–159.
23. Joven, J.; Micol, V.; Segura-Carretero, A.; Alonso-Villaverde, C.; Menéndez, J.A.; for the Bioactive Food Components Platform. Polyphenols and the modulation of gene expression pathways: Can we eat our way out of the danger of chronic disease? *Crit. Rev. Food Sci. Nutr.* **2014**, *54*, 985–1001. [CrossRef] [PubMed]
24. Aura, A.M. Microbial metabolism of dietary phenolic compounds in the colon. *Phytochem. Rev.* **2008**, *7*, 407–429. [CrossRef]

25. Selma, M.V.; Espín, J.C.; Tomás-Barberán, F.A. Interaction between phenolics and gut microbiota: Role in human health. *J. Agric. Food Chem.* **2009**, *57*, 6485–6501. [CrossRef] [PubMed]
26. Karkovic Markovic, A.; Toric, J.; Barbaric, M.; Jakobušic Brala, C. Hydroxytyrosol, tyrosol and derivatives and their potential effects on human health. *Molecules* **2019**, *24*, 2001. [CrossRef] [PubMed]
27. González-Sarrías, A.; García-Villalba, R.; Romo-Vaquero, M.; Alasalvar, C.; Örem, A.; Zafrilla, P.; Tomás-Barberán, F.A.; Selma, M.V.; Espín, J.C. Clustering according to urolithin metabotype explains the interindividual variability in the improvement of cardiovascular risk biomarkers in overweight-obese individuals consuming pomegranate: A randomized clinical trial. *Mol. Nutr. Food Res.* **2017**, *61*, 1600830. [CrossRef] [PubMed]
28. Setchell, K.D.; Brown, N.M.; Lydeking-Olsen, E. The clinical importance of the metabolite equol-a clue to the effectiveness of soy and its isoflavones. *J. Nutr.* **2002**, *132*, 3577–3584. [CrossRef] [PubMed]
29. Adlercreutz, H. Lignans and human health. *Crit. Rev. Clin. Lab. Sci.* **2007**, *44*, 483–525. [CrossRef]
30. Etxeberria, U.; Arias, N.; Boqué, N.; Macarulla, M.T.; Portillo, M.P.; Martínez, J.A.; Milagro, F.I. Reshaping faecal gut microbiota composition by the intake of trans-resveratrol and quercetin in high-fat sucrose diet-fed rats. *J. Nutr. Biochem.* **2015**, *26*, 651–660. [CrossRef]
31. Jin, G.; Asou, Y.; Ishiyama, K.; Okawa, A.; Kanno, T.; Niwano, Y. Proanthocyanidin-rich grape seed extract modulates intestinal microbiota in ovariectomized mice. *J. Food Sci.* **2018**, *83*, 1149–1152. [CrossRef]
32. Cox, L.M.; Blaser, M.J. Pathways in microbe-induced obesity. *Cell Metab.* **2013**, *17*, 883–894. [CrossRef] [PubMed]
33. Cardona, F.; Andrés-Lacueva, C.; Tulipani, S.; Tinahones, F.J.; Queipo-Ortuño, M.I. Benefits of polyphenols on gut microbiota and implications in human health. *J. Nutr. Biochem.* **2013**, *24*, 1415–1422. [CrossRef]
34. Hervert-Hernández, D.; Pintado, C.; Rotger, R.; Goñi, I. Stimulatory role of grape pomace polyphenols on Lactobacillus acidophilus growth. *Int. J. Food Microbiol.* **2009**, *136*, 119–122. [CrossRef]
35. Pozuelo, M.J.; Agis-Torres, A.; Hervert-Hernández, D.; López-Oliva, M.E.; Muñoz-Martínez, E.; Rotger, R.; Goñi, I. Grape antioxidant dietary fiber stimulates Lactobacillus growth in rat cecum. *J. Food Sci.* **2012**, *77*, H59–H62. [CrossRef] [PubMed]
36. Fiesel, A.; Gessner, D.K.; Most, E.; Eder, K. Effects of dietary polyphenol-rich plant products from grape or hop on pro-inflammatory gene expression in the intestine; nutrient digestibility and faecal microbiota of weaned pigs. *BMC Vet. Res.* **2014**, *10*, 196. [CrossRef] [PubMed]
37. Kafantaris, I.; Kotsampasi, B.; Christodoulou, V.; Kokka, E.; Kouka, P.; Terzopoulou, Z.; Gerasopoulos, K.; Stagos, D.; Mitsagga, C.; Giavasis, I.; et al. Grape pomace improves antioxidant capacity and faecal microflora of lambs. *J. Anim. Physiol. Anim. Nutr.* **2017**, *101*, 108–121. [CrossRef]
38. Zorraquín, I.; Sánchez-Hernández, E.; Ayuda-Durán, B.; Silva, M.; González-Paramás, A.M.; Santos-Buelga, C.; Moreno-Arribas, M.V.; Bartolomé, B. Current and future experimental approaches in the study of grape and wine polyphenols interacting gut microbiota. *J. Sci. Food Agric.* **2020**, *100*, 3789–3802. [CrossRef] [PubMed]
39. Zamora-Ros, R.; Serafini, M.; Estruch, R.; Lamuela-Raventós, R.M.; Martínez-González, M.A.; Salas-Salvadó, J.; Fiol, M.; Lapetra, J.; Arós, F.; Covas, M.I.; et al. Mediterranean diet and non-enzymatic antioxidant capacity in the PREDIMED study: Evidence for a mechanism of antioxidant tuning. *Nutr. Metab. Cardiovasc. Dise.* **2013**, *23*, 1167–1174. [CrossRef] [PubMed]
40. Medina-Remón, A.; Casas, R.; Tresserra-Rimbau, A.; Ros, E.; Martínez-González, M.A.; Fitó, M.; Corella, D.; Salas-Salvadó, J.; Lamuela-Raventós, R.M.; Estruch, R.; et al. Polyphenol intake from a Mediterranean diet decreases inflammatory biomarkers related to atherosclerosis: A substudy of the PREDIMED trial. *Br. J. Clin. Pharmacol.* **2017**, *83*, 114–128. [CrossRef]
41. Covas, M.I.; de la Torre, R.; Fitó, M. Virgin olive oil: A key food for cardiovascular risk protection. *Br. J. Nutr.* **2015**, *113*, S19–S28. [CrossRef]
42. Mata, P.; Garrido, J.A.; Ordovás, J.M.; Blázquez, E.; Alvarez-Sala, L.A.; Rubio, M.J.; Alonso, R.; de Oya, M. Effect of dietary monounsaturated fatty acids on plasma lipoproteins and apolipoproteins in women. *Am. J. Clin. Nutr.* **1992**, *56*, 77–83. [CrossRef]
43. Smith, R.D.; Kelly, C.N.M.; Fielding, B.A.; Hauton, D.; Silva, K.D.R.R.; Nydahl, M.C.; Miller, G.J.; Williams, C.M. Long-term monounsaturated fatty acid diets reduce platelet aggregation in healthy young subjects. *Br. J. Nutr.* **2007**, *90*, 597–606. [CrossRef]
44. Ditano-Vázquez, P.; Torres-Peña, J.D.; Galeano-Valle, F.; Pérez-Caballero, A.I.; Demelo-Rodríguez, P.; López-Miranda, J.; Katsiki, N.; Delgado-Lista, J.; Alvarez-Sala-Walther, L.A. The fluid aspect of the Mediterranean diet in the prevention and management of cardiovascular disease and diabetes: The role of polyphenol content in moderate consumption of wine and olive oil. *Nutrients* **2019**, *11*, 2833. [CrossRef]
45. Ramírez-Tortosa, M.C.; Granados, S.; Quiles, J.L. Chemical composition; types and characteristics of olive oil. In *Olive Oil Health*; CABI Publishing: Oxford, UK, 2006; pp. 45–61.
46. Servili, M.; Esposto, S.; Fabiani, R.; Urbani, S.; Taticchi, A.; Mariucci, F.; Selvaggini, R.; Montedoro, G.F. Phenolic compounds in olive oil: Antioxidant, health and organoleptic activities according to their chemical structure. *Inflammopharmacology* **2009**, *17*, 76–84. [CrossRef] [PubMed]
47. Rodríguez-López, P.; Lozano-Sánchez, J.; Borrás-Linares, I.; Emanuelli, T.; Menéndez, J.A.; Segura-Carretero, A. Structure-biological activity relationships of extra-virgin olive oil phenolic compounds: Health properties and bioavailability. *Antioxidants* **2020**, *9*, 685. [CrossRef] [PubMed]
48. Covas, M.I.; Nyyssonen, K.; Poulsen, H.E.; Kaikkonen, J.; Zunft, H.J.; Kiesewetter, H.; Gaddi, A.; de la Torre, R.; Mursu, J.; Bäumler, H.; et al. The effect of polyphenols in olive oil on heart disease risk factors: A randomized trial. *Ann. Intern. Med.* **2006**, *145*, 333–341. [CrossRef] [PubMed]

49. Bucciantini, M.; Leri, M.; Nardiello, P.; Casamenti, F.; Stefani, M. Olive Polyphenols: Antioxidant and anti-inflammatory properties. *Antioxidants* **2021**, *10*, 1044. [CrossRef]
50. Cai, Y.; Yang, L.; Hu, G.; Chen, X.; Niu, F.; Yuan, L.; Liu, H.; Xiong, H.; Arikkath, J.; Buch, S. Regulation of morphine-induced synaptic alterations: Role of oxidative stress, ER stress, and autophagy. *J. Cell Biol.* **2016**, *215*, 245–258. [CrossRef]
51. Urpi-Sardá, M.; Casas, R.; Chiva-Blanch, G.; Romero-Mamani, E.S.; Valderas-Martínez, P.; Arranz, S.; Andrés-Lacueva, C.; Llorach, R.; Medina-Remón, A.; Lamuela-Raventós, R.M.; et al. Virgin olive oil and nuts as key foods of the Mediterranean diet effects on inflammatory biomarkers related to atherosclerosis. *Pharmacol. Res.* **2012**, *65*, 577–583. [CrossRef]
52. Beauchamp, G.K.; Keast, R.S.; Morel, D.; Lin, J.; Pika, J.; Han, Q.; Lee, C.H.; Smith, A.B.; Breslin, P.A. Phytochemistry: Ibuprofen-like activity in extra-virgin olive oil. *Nature* **2005**, *437*, 45–46. [CrossRef]
53. Zhang, X.; Cao, J.; Zhong, L. Hydroxytyrosol inhibits proinflammatory cytokines, iNOS, and COX-2 expression in human monocytic cells. *Naunyn-Schmiedeberg's Arch. Pharmacol.* **2009**, *379*, 581–586. [CrossRef]
54. Finicelli, M.; Squillaro, T.; Di Cristo, F.; Di Salle, A.; Beatrice Melone, M.A.; Galderisi, U.; Peluso, G. Metabolic syndrome, Mediterranean diet, and polyphenols: Evidence and perspectives. *J. Cell. Physiol.* **2019**, *234*, 5807–5826. [CrossRef]
55. Emma, M.R.; Augello, G.; Di Stefano, V.; Azzolina, A.; Giannitrapani, L.; Montalto, G.; Cervello, M.; Cusimano, A. Potential uses of olive oil secoiridoids for the prevention and treatment of cancer: A narrative review of preclinical studies. *Int. J. Mol. Sci.* **2021**, *22*, 1234. [CrossRef] [PubMed]
56. Parkinson, L.; Cicerale, S. The health benefiting mechanisms of virgin olive oil phenolic compounds. *Molecules* **2016**, *16*, 1734. [CrossRef] [PubMed]
57. EFSA Panel on Dietetic Products; Nutrition and Allergies (NDA). Scientific Opinion on the substantiation of health claims related to polyphenols in olive and protection of LDL particles from oxidative damage (ID 1333; 1638; 1639; 1696; 2865); maintenance of normal blood HDL-cholesterol concentrations (ID 1639); maintenance of normal blood pressure (ID 3781); "anti-inflammatory properties" (ID 1882); "contributes to the upper respiratory tract health" (ID 3468); "can help to maintain a normal function of gastrointestinal tract" (3779); and "contributes to body defences against external agents" (ID 3467) pursuant to Article 13(1) of Regulation (EC) No 1924/2006. *EFSA J.* **2011**, *9*, 203.
58. Castellano, J.M.; Perona, J.S. Effects of virgin olive oil phenolic compounds on health: Solid evidence or just another fiasco? *Grasas Y Aceites* **2021**, *72*, e404. [CrossRef]
59. Romero, C.; Brenes, M.; Yousfi, K.; García, P.; García, A.; Garrido, A. Effect of cultivar and processing method on the contents of polyphenols in table olives. *J. Agric. Food Chem.* **2004**, *52*, 479–484. [CrossRef] [PubMed]
60. Juan, M.E.; Planas, J.M.; Ruiz-Gutierrez, V.; Daniel, H.; Wenzel, U. Antiproliferative and apoptosis-inducing effects of maslinic and oleanolic acids, two pentacyclic triterpenes from olives, on HT-29 colon cancer cells. *Br. J. Nutr.* **2008**, *100*, 36–43. [CrossRef]
61. Lozano-Mena, G.; Sánchez-González, M.; Juan, M.E.; Planas, J.M. Maslinic acid, a natural phytoalexin-type triterpene from olives. A promising nutraceutical? *Molecules* **2014**, *19*, 11538–11559. [CrossRef]
62. Nagai, N.; Yagyu, S.; Hata, A.; Nirengi, S.; Kotani, K.; Moritani, T.; Sakane, N. Maslinic acid derived from olive fruit in combination with resistance training improves muscle mass and mobility functions in the elderly. *J. Clin. Biochem. Nutr.* **2019**, *64*, 224–230. [CrossRef]
63. Romero, C.; García, A.; Medina, E.; Ruiz-Méndez, M.V.; de Castro, A.; Brenes, M. Triterpenic acids in table olives. *Food Chem.* **2010**, *118*, 670–674. [CrossRef]
64. St Leger, A.S.; Cochrane, A.L.; Moore, F. Factors associated with cardiac mortality in developed countries with particular reference to the consumption of wine. *Lancet* **1979**, *313*, 1017–1020. [CrossRef]
65. Gordon, T.; Kannell, W.B. Drinking habits and cardiovascular disease: The Framingham study. *Am. Heart J.* **1983**, *105*, 667–673. [CrossRef]
66. Corrao, G.; Rubbiati, L.; Bagnardi, V.; Zambon, A.; Poikolainen, K. Alcohol and coronary heart disease: A meta-analysis. *Addiction* **2000**, *95*, 1505–1523. [CrossRef] [PubMed]
67. Di Castelnuovo, A.; Costanzo, S.; Bagnardi, V.; Donati, M.B.; Iacoviello, L.; de Gaetano, G. Alcohol dosing and total mortality in men and women: An updated meta-analysis of 34 prospective studies. *Arch. Intern. Med.* **2006**, *166*, 2437–2445. [CrossRef] [PubMed]
68. Larsson, S.C.; Wallin, A.; Wolk, A. Alcohol consumption and risk of heart failure: Metaanalysis of 13 prospective studies. *Clin. Nutr.* **2018**, *37*, 1247–1251. [CrossRef]
69. Reynolds, K.; Lewis, B.; Nolen, J.D.; Kinney, G.L.; Sathya, B.; He, J. Alcohol consumption and risk of stroke: A meta-analysis. *JAMA* **2003**, *289*, 579–588. [CrossRef] [PubMed]
70. Carlsson, S.; Hammar, N.; Grill, V. Alcohol consumption and type 2 diabetes Metaanalysis of epidemiological studies indicates a U-shaped relationship. *Diabetologia* **2005**, *48*, 1051–1054. [CrossRef] [PubMed]
71. Koppes, L.L.J.; Dekker, J.M.; Hendriks, H.F.J.; Bouter, L.M.; Heine, R.J. Moderate alcohol consumption lowers the risk of type 2 diabetes: A meta-analysis of prospective observational studies. *Diabetes Care* **2005**, *28*, 719–725. [CrossRef] [PubMed]
72. Djousse, L.; Biggs, M.L.; Mukamal, K.J.; Siscovick, D.S. Alcohol consumption and type 2 Diabetes among older adults: The Cardiovascular Health Study. *Obesity* **2007**, *15*, 1758–1765. [CrossRef]
73. Huang, J.; Wang, X.; Zhang, Y. Specific types of alcoholic beverage consumption and risk of type 2 diabetes: A systematic review and meta-analysis. *J. Diabetes Invest.* **2017**, *8*, 56–68. [CrossRef]

74. Letenneur, L. Risk of dementia and alcohol and wine consumption: A review of recent results. *Biol. Res.* **2004**, *37*, 189–193. [CrossRef]
75. Peters, R.; Peters, J.; Warner, J.; Beckett, N.; Bulpitt, C. Alcohol, dementia and cognitive decline in the elderly: A systematic review. *Age Ageing* **2008**, *37*, 505–512. [CrossRef]
76. Marmot, M.G.; Shipley, M.J.; Rose, G.; Thomas, B. Alcohol and mortality: A U-shaped curve. *Lancet* **1981**, *315*, 580–583. [CrossRef]
77. Fillmore, K.; Stockwell, T.; Chikritzhs, T.; Bostrom, A.; Kerr, W. Moderate alcohol use and reduced mortality risk: Systematic error studies and new hypotheses. *Ann. Epidemiol.* **2007**, *17*, 16–23. [CrossRef] [PubMed]
78. Roerecke, M.; Rehm, J. Alcohol consumption, drinking patterns, and ischemic heart disease: A narrative review of meta-analyses and a systematic review and meta-analysis of the impact of heavy drinking occasions on risk for moderate drinkers. *BMC Med.* **2014**, *12*, 1–11. [CrossRef]
79. Naimi, T.S.; Stockwell, T.; Zhao, J.; Xuan, Z.; Dangardt, F.; Saitz, R.; Liang, W.; Chikritzhs, T. Selection biases in observational studies affect associations between 'moderate' alcohol consumption and mortality. *Addiction* **2017**, *112*, 207–214. [CrossRef]
80. Naimi, T.S.; Stadtmueller, L.A.; Chikritzhs, T.; Stockwell, T.; Zhao, J.; Britton, A.; Saitz, R.; Sherk, A. Alcohol, age, and mortality: Estimating selection bias due to premature death. *J. Stud. Alcohol Drugs* **2019**, *80*, 63–68. [CrossRef] [PubMed]
81. Hansel, B.; Thomas, F.; Pannier, B.; Bean, K.; Kontush, A.; Chapman, M.J.; Bruckert, E. Relationship between alcohol intake, health and social status and cardiovascular risk factors in the urban Paris-Ile-De-France Cohort: Is the cardioprotective action of alcohol a myth. *Eur. J. Clin. Nutr.* **2010**, *64*, 561–568. [CrossRef] [PubMed]
82. Rehm, J.; Roerecke, M. Cardiovascular effects of alcohol consumption. *Trends Cardiov. Med.* **2017**, *27*, 534–538. [CrossRef]
83. Zhao, J.; Stockwell, T.; Roemer, A.; Naimi, T.; Chikritzhs, T. Alcohol consumption and mortality from coronary heart disease: An updated meta-analysis of cohort studies. *J. Stud. Alcohol Drugs* **2017**, *78*, 375–386. [CrossRef] [PubMed]
84. Covas, M.I.; Gambert, P.; Fitó, M.; de la Torre, R. Wine and oxidative stress: Up-to-date evidence of the effects of moderate wine consumption on oxidative damage in humans. *Atherosclerosis* **2010**, *208*, 297–304. [CrossRef] [PubMed]
85. Gronbaek, M.; Deis, A.; Sorensen, T.I.A.; Becker, U.; Schnohr, P.; Jensen, G. Mortality associated with moderate intakes of wine, beer, or spirits. *BMJ* **1995**, *310*, 1165–1169. [CrossRef]
86. Haseeb, S.; Alexander, B.; Baranchuk, A. Wine and Cardiovascular Health. *Circulation* **2017**, *136*, 1434–1448. [CrossRef]
87. Liberale, L.; Bonaventura, A.; Montecucco, F.; Dallegri, F.; Carbone, F. Impact of red wine consumption on cardiovascular health. *Cur. Med. Chem.* **2019**, *26*, 3542–3566. [CrossRef]
88. Snopek, L.; Mlcek, J.; Sochorova, L.; Baron, M.; Hlavacova, I.; Jurikova, T.; Kizek, R.; Sedlackova, E.; Sochor, J. Contribution of red wine consumption to human health protection. *Molecules* **2018**, *23*, 1684. [CrossRef] [PubMed]
89. Pinder, R.M.; Sandler, M. Alcohol, wine and mental health: Focus on dementia and stroke. *J. Psychopharm.* **2004**, *18*, 449–456. [CrossRef]
90. Chiva-Blanch, G.; Urpi-Sardá, M.; Ros, E.; Valderas-Martínez, P.; Casas, R.; Arranz, S.; Guillén, M.; Lamuela-Raventós, R.M.; Llorach, R.; Andrés-Lacueva, C.; et al. Effects of red wine polyphenols and alcohol on glucose metabolism and the lipid profile: A randomized clinical trial. *Clin. Nutr.* **2013**, *32*, 200–206. [CrossRef]
91. Droste, D.W.; Iliescu, C.; Vaillant, M.; Gantenbein, M.; De Bremaeker, N.; Lieunard, C.; Velez, T.; Meyer, M.; Guth, T.; Kuemmerle, A.; et al. A daily glass of red wine associated with lifestyle changes independently improves blood lipids in patients with carotid arteriosclerosis: Results from a randomized controlled trial. *Nutr. J.* **2013**, *12*, 147. [CrossRef]
92. Estruch, R.; Sacanella, E.; Mota, F.; Chiva-Blanch, G.; Antúnez, E.; Casals, E.; Urbano-Marquez, A. Moderate consumption of red wine, but not gin, decreases erythrocyte superoxide dismutase activity: A randomised cross-over trial. *Nutr. Metab. Cardiovasc. Dis.* **2011**, *21*, 46–53. [CrossRef]
93. Toth, A.; Sandor, B.; Papp, J.; Rabai, M.; Botor, D.; Horvath, Z.; Kenyeres, P.; Juricskay, I.; Toth, K.; Czopf, L. Moderate red wine consumption improves hemorheological parameters in healthy volunteers. *Clin. Hemorheol, Microc.* **2014**, *56*, 13–23. [CrossRef] [PubMed]
94. Vázquez-Fresno, R.; Llorach, R.; Perera, A.; Mandal, R.; Feliz, M.; Tinahones, F.J.; Wishart, D.S.; Andrés-Lacueva, C. Clinical phenotype clustering in cardiovascular risk patients for the identification of responsive metabotypes after red wine polyphenol intake. *J. Nutr. Biochem.* **2016**, *28*, 14–20. [CrossRef]
95. Gea, A.; Bes-Rastrollo, M.; Toledo, E.; García-López, M.; Beunza, J.J.; Estruch, R.; Martinez-Gonzalez, M.A. Mediterranean alcohol-drinking pattern and mortality in the SUN (Seguimiento Universidad de Navarra) Project: A prospective cohort study. *Br. J. Nutr.* **2014**, *111*, 1871–1880. [CrossRef] [PubMed]
96. Waterhouse, A.L. Wine phenolics. *Ann. N. Y. Acad. Sci.* **2002**, *957*, 21–36. [CrossRef] [PubMed]
97. Manach, C.; Scalbert, A.; Morand, C.; Rémésy, C.; Jiménez, L. Polyphenols: Food sources and bioavailability. *Am. J. Clin. Nutr.* **2004**, *79*, 727–747. [CrossRef]
98. Rasmussen, S.E.; Frederiksen, H.; Krogholm, K.S.; Poulsen, L. Dietary proanthocyanidins: Occurrence, dietary intake, bioavailability, and protection against cardiovascular disease. *Mol. Nutr. Food Res.* **2005**, *49*, 159–174. [CrossRef]
99. Santos-Buelga, C.; Scalbert, A. Proanthocyanidins and tannin-like compounds—Nature, occurrence, dietary intake and effects on nutrition and health. *J. Sci. Food Agric.* **2000**, *80*, 1094–1117. [CrossRef]
100. Santos-Buelga, C.; González-Paramás, A.M. Flavonoids: Functions, metabolism and biotechnology. In *Industrial Biotechnology of Vitamins, Pigments, and Antioxidants*; John Wiley & Sons, Inc.: Weinhein, Germany, 2016; pp. 469–496.

101. Frankel, E.; Kanner, J.; German, J.; Parks, E.; Kinsella, J. Inhibition of oxidation of human low-density lipoprotein by phenolic substances in red wine. *Lancet* **1993**, *341*, 454–457. [CrossRef]
102. Rifler, J.-P.; Lorcerie, F.; Durand, P.; Delmas, D.; Ragot, K.; Limagne, E.; Mazué, F.; Riedinger, J.-M.; d'Athis, P.; Hudelot, B. A moderate red wine intake improves blood lipid parameters and erythrocytes membrane fluidity in post myocardial infarct patients. *Mol. Nutr. Food Res.* **2012**, *56*, 345–351. [CrossRef] [PubMed]
103. Araim, O.; Ballantyne, J.; Waterhouse, A.L.; Sumpio, B.E. Inhibition of vascular smooth muscle cell proliferation with red wine and red wine polyphenols. *J. Vasc. Surg.* **2002**, *35*, 1226–1232. [CrossRef]
104. Diebolt, M.; Bucher, B.; Andriantsitohaina, R. Wine polyphenols decrease blood pressure, improve NO vasodilatation, and induce gene expression. *Hypertension* **2001**, *38*, 159–165. [CrossRef]
105. Zenebe, W.; Pechanova, O.; Andriantsitohaina, R. Red wine polyphenols induce vasorelaxation by increased nitric oxide bioactivity. *Physiol. Res.* **2003**, *52*, 425–432. [PubMed]
106. Del Rio, D.; Rodríguez-Mateos, A.; Spencer, J.P.; Tognolini, M.; Borges, G.; Crozier, A. Dietary (poly) phenolics in human health: Structures, bioavailability, and evidence of protective effects against chronic diseases. *Antiox. Redox Signal.* **2013**, *18*, 1818–1892. [CrossRef]
107. Cueva, C.; Gil-Sánchez, I.; Ayuda-Durán, B.; González-Manzano, S.; González-Paramás, A.M.; Santos-Buelga, C.; Bartolomé, B.; Moreno-Arribas, M.V. An integrated view of the effects of wine polyphenols and their relevant metabolites on gut and host health. *Molecules* **2017**, *22*, 99. [CrossRef]
108. Fernandes, I.; Pérez-Gregorio, R.; Soares, S.; Mateus, N.; de Freitas, V. Wine Flavonoids in health and disease prevention. *Molecules* **2017**, *22*, 292. [CrossRef] [PubMed]
109. Williamson, G.; Kay, C.D.; Crozier, A. The bioavailability, transport, and bioactivity of dietary flavonoids: A review from a historical perspective. *Comp. Rev. Food Sci. Food Saf.* **2018**, *17*, 1054–1112. [CrossRef] [PubMed]
110. Fraga, C.G.; Croft, K.D.; Kennedy, D.O.; Tomás-Barberán, F.A. The effects of polyphenols and other bioactives on human health. *Food Funct.* **2019**, *10*, 514. [CrossRef]
111. González-Paramás, A.M.; Ayuda-Durán, B.; Martínez, S.; González-Manzano, S.; Santos-Buelga, C. The Mechanisms behind the Biological Activity of Flavonoids. *Cur. Med. Chem.* **2019**, *26*, 6976–6990. [CrossRef] [PubMed]
112. Mas, A.; Guillamón, J.M.; Torija, M.J.; Beltrán, G.; Cerezo, A.B.; Troncoso, A.M.; García-Parrilla, M.C. Bioactive compounds derived from the yeast metabolism of aromatic amino acids during alcoholic fermentation. *BioMed Res. Int.* **2014**, *2014*. [CrossRef]
113. Bertelli, A.A.E.; Migliori, M.; Panichi, V.; Longoni, B.; Origlia, N.; Ferretti, A.; Cuttano, M.G.; Giovannini, L. Oxidative stress and inflammatory reaction modulation by white wine. *Ann. N. Y. Acad. Sci.* **2002**, *957*, 295–301. [CrossRef] [PubMed]
114. Bertelli, A.; Migliori, M.; Bertelli, A.A.E.; Origlia, N.; Filippi, C.; Panichi, V.; Falchi, M.; Giovannini, L. Effect of some white wine phenols in preventing inflammatory cytokine release. *Drugs Exp. Clin. Res.* **2002**, *28*, 11–15.
115. Bordiga, M.; Lorenzo, C.; Pardo, F.; Salinas, M.R.; Travaglia, F.; Arlorio, M.; Garde-Cerdán, T. Factors influencing the formation of histaminol, hydroxytyrosol, tyrosol, and tryptophol in wine: Temperature; alcoholic degree, and amino acids concentration. *Food Chem.* **2016**, *197*, 1038–1045. [CrossRef] [PubMed]
116. Piñeiro, Z.; Cantos-Villar, E.; Palma, M.; Puertas, B. Direct liquid chromatography method for the simultaneous quantification of hydroxytyrosol and tyrosol in red wines. *J. Agric. Food Chem.* **2011**, *59*, 11683–11689. [CrossRef] [PubMed]
117. Rocchetti, G.; Gatti, M.; Bavaresco, L.; Lucini, L. Untargeted metabolomics to investigate the phenolic composition of Chardonnay wines from different origins. *J. Food Comp. Anal.* **2018**, *71*, 87–93. [CrossRef]
118. De La Torre, R.; Covas, M.I.; Pujadas, M.A.; Fitó, M.; Farré, M. Is dopamine behind the health benefits of red wine? *Eur. J. Nutr.* **2006**, *45*, 307–310. [CrossRef]
119. Pérez-Mañá, C.; Farré, M.; Rodríguez-Morató, J.; Papaseit, E.; Pujadas, M.; Fitó, M.; Robledo, P.; Covas, M.I.; Cheynier, V.; Meudec, E.; et al. Moderate consumption of wine, through both its phenolic compounds and alcohol content, promotes hydroxytyrosol endogenous generation in humans. A randomized controlled trial. *Mol. Nutr. Food Res.* **2015**, *59*, 1213–1216. [CrossRef]
120. Meng, X.; Li, Y.; Li, S.; Zhou, Y.; Gan, R.Y.; Xu, D.P.; Li, H.B. Dietary sources and bioactivities of melatonin. *Nutrients* **2017**, *9*, 367. [CrossRef]
121. Iriti, M.; Varoni, E.M. Cardioprotective effects of moderate red wine consumption: Polyphenols vs ethanol. *J. Appl. Biomed.* **2014**, *12*, 193–202. [CrossRef]
122. Fernández-Cruz, E.; Cerezo, A.B.; Cantos-Villar, E.; Troncoso, A.M.; García-Parrilla, M.C. Time course of l-tryptophan metabolites when fermenting natural grape musts: Effect of inoculation treatments and cultivar on the occurrence of melatonin and related indolic compounds. *Aust. J. Grape Wine Res.* **2019**, *25*, 92–100. [CrossRef]
123. Aguilera, Y.; Rebollo-Hernanz, M.; Herrera, T.; Cayuelas, L.T.; Rodríguez-Rodríguez, P.; de Pablo, Á.L.; Arribas, S.M.; Martin-Cabrejas, M.A. Intake of bean sprouts influences melatonin and antioxidant capacity biomarker levels in rats. *Food Funct.* **2016**, *7*, 1438–1445. [CrossRef]
124. González-Flores, D.; Gamero, E.; Garrido, M.; Ramírez, R.; Moreno, D.; Delgado, J.; Valdés, E.; Barriga, C.; Rodríguez, A.B.; Paredes, S.D. Urinary 6-sulfatoxymelatonin and total antioxidant capacity increase after the intake of a grape juice cv. Tempranillo stabilized with HHP. *Food Funct.* **2012**, *3*, 34–39. [CrossRef]
125. Reiter, R.J.; Manchester, L.C.; Tan, D.X. Melatonin in walnuts: Influence on levels of melatonin and total antioxidant capacity of blood. *Nutrition* **2003**, *21*, 579–588. [CrossRef] [PubMed]

126. Rodríguez-Naranjo, M.I.; Torija, M.J.; Mas, A.; Cantos-Villar, E.; García-Parrilla, M.C. Production of melatonin by Saccharomyces strains undergrowth and fermentation conditions. *J. Pineal Res.* **2012**, *53*, 219–224. [CrossRef]
127. Benbouguerra, N.; Hornedo-Ortega, R.; Garcia, F.; El Khawand, T.; Saucier, C.; Richard, T. Stilbenes in grape berries and wine and their potential role as anti-obesity agents: A review. *Trends Food Sci. Technol.* **2021**, *112*, 362–381. [CrossRef]
128. Triska, J.; Houska, M. Physical methods of resveratrol induction in grapes and grape products—A review. *Czech J. Food Sci.* **2012**, *30*, 489–502. [CrossRef]
129. Cantos, E.; Espín, J.C.; Tomás-Barberán, F.A. Postharvest induction modeling method using UV irradiation pulses for obtaining resveratrol-enriched table grapes: A new "functional" fruit? *J. Agric. Food Chem.* **2001**, *49*, 5052–5058. [CrossRef] [PubMed]
130. Siemann, E.H.; Creasy, L.L. Concentration of the phytoalexin resveratrol in wine. *Am. J. Enol. Vitic.* **1992**, *43*, 49–52.
131. Cottart, C.H.; Nivet-Antoine, V.; Beaudeux, J.L. Review of recent data on the metabolism, biological effects, and toxicity of resveratrol in humans. *Mol. Nutr. Food Res.* **2014**, *58*, 7–21. [CrossRef]
132. Jang, M.; Cai, L.; Udeani, G.O.; Slowing, K.V.; Thomas, C.F.; Beecher, C.W.; Fong, H.H.; Farnsworth, N.R.; Kinghorn, A.D.; Mehta, R.G.; et al. Cancer chemopreventive activity of resveratrol; A natural product derived from grapes. *Science* **1997**, *275*, 218–220. [CrossRef]
133. Baur, J.A.; Pearson, K.J.; Price, N.L.; Jamieson, H.A.; Lerin, C.; Kalra, A.; Prabhu, V.V.; Allard, J.S.; Lopez-Lluch, G.; Lewis, K.; et al. Resveratrol improves health and survival of mice on a high-calorie diet. *Nature* **2006**, *444*, 337–342. [CrossRef] [PubMed]
134. Howitz, K.T.; Bitterman, K.J.; Cohen, H.Y.; Lamming, D.W.; Lavu, S.; Wood, J.G.; Zipkin, R.E.; Chung, P.; Kisielewski, A.; Zhang, L.L.; et al. Small molecule activators of sirtuins extend Saccharomyces cerevisiae lifespan. *Nature* **2003**, *425*, 191–196. [CrossRef] [PubMed]
135. Valenzano, D.R.; Terzibasi, E.; Genade, T.; Cattaneo, A.; Domenico, L.; Cellerino, A. Resveratrol prolongs lifespan and retards the onset of age-related markers in a short-lived vertebrate. *Curr. Biol.* **2006**, *16*, 296–300. [CrossRef]
136. Baur, J.A.; Sinclair, D.A. Therapeutic potential of resveratrol: The in vivo evidence. *Nat. Rev.* **2006**, *5*, 493–506. [CrossRef] [PubMed]
137. Wang, S.; Moustaid-Moussa, N.; Chen, L.; Mo, H.; Shastri, A.; Su, R.; Bapat, P.; Kwun, I.; Shen, C.L. Novel insights of dietary polyphenols and obesity. *J. Nutr. Biochem.* **2014**, *25*, 1–18. [CrossRef] [PubMed]
138. Kennedy, D.O.; Wightman, E.L.; Reay, J.L.; Lietz, G.; Okello, E.J.; Wilde, A.; Haskell, C.F. Effects of resveratrol on cerebral blood flow variables and cognitive performance in humans: A double-blind; placebo-controlled, crossover investigation. *Am. J. Clin. Nutr.* **2010**, *91*, 1590–1597. [CrossRef]
139. Evans, H.M.; Howe, P.R.; Wong, R.H. Effects of resveratrol on cognitive performance, mood and cerebrovascular function in post-menopausal women; a 14-week randomised placebo-controlled intervention trial. *Nutrients* **2017**, *9*, 27. [CrossRef]
140. Thaung Zaw, J.J.; Howe, P.R.C.; Wong, R.H.X. Sustained cerebrovascular and cognitive benefits of resveratrol in postmenopausal women. *Nutrients* **2020**, *12*, 828. [CrossRef]
141. Huhn, S.; Beyer, F.; Zhang, R.; Lampe, L.; Grothe, J.; Kratzsch, J.; Willenberg, A.; Breitfeld, J.; Kovacs, P.; Stumvoll, M.; et al. Effects of resveratrol on memory performance; hippocampus connectivity and microstructure in older adults–A randomized controlled trial. *Neuroimage* **2018**, *174*, 177–190. [CrossRef]
142. Farzaei, M.H.; Rahimi, R.; Nikfar, S.; Abdollahi, M. Effect of resveratrol on cognitive and memory performance and mood: A meta-analysis of 225 patients. *Pharmacol. Res.* **2018**, *128*, 338–344. [CrossRef]
143. Marx, W.; Kelly, J.T.; Marshall, S.; Cutajar, J.; Annois, B.; Pipingas, A.; Tierney, A.; Itsiopoulos, C. Effect of resveratrol supplementation on cognitive performance and mood in adults: A systematic literature review and meta-analysis of randomized controlled trials. *Nutr. Rev.* **2018**, *76*, 432–443. [CrossRef] [PubMed]
144. Losso, J.N.; Truax, R.E.; Richard, G. Trans-resveratrol inhibits hyperglycemia-induced inflammation and connexin downregulation in retinal pigment epithelial cells. *J. Agric. Food Chem.* **2010**, *58*, 8246–8252. [CrossRef]
145. Pintea, A.; Rugina, D.; Pop, R.; Bunea, A.; Socaciu, C.; Diehl, H.A. Antioxidant effect of trans-resveratrol in cultured human retinal pigment epithelial cells. *J. Ocul. Pharmacol. Ther.* **2011**, *27*, 315–321. [CrossRef] [PubMed]
146. Sheu, S.J.; Liu, N.C.; Chen, J.L. Resveratrol protects human retinal pigment epithelial cells from acrolein-induced damage. *J. Ocul. Pharmacol. Ther.* **2010**, *26*, 231–236. [CrossRef] [PubMed]
147. Kubota, S.; Kurihara, T.; Mochimaru, H.; Satofuka, S.; Noda, K.; Ozawa, Y.; Oike, Y.; Ishida, S.; Tsubota, K. Prevention of ocular inflammation in endotoxin-induced uveitis with resveratrol by inhibiting oxidative damage and nuclear factor-kappaB activation. *Investig. Ophthalmol. Vis. Sci.* **2009**, *50*, 3512–3519. [CrossRef]
148. Ren, B.; Kwah, M.X.; Liu, C.; Ma, Z.; Shanmugam, M.K.; Ding, L.; Xiang, X.; Ho, P.C.; Wang, L.; Ong, P.S.; et al. Resveratrol for cancer therapy: Challenges and future perspectives. *Cancer Let.* **2021**, *515*, 63–72. [CrossRef]
149. Visioli, F. The resveratrol fiasco. *Pharmacol. Res.* **2014**, *90*, 87. [CrossRef]
150. Jones, A.W.; Jönsson, K.A.; Kechagias, S. Effect of high-fat, high-protein, and high-carbohydrate meals on the pharmacokinetics of a small dose of ethanol. *Br. J. Clin. Pharmacol.* **1997**, *44*, 521–526. [CrossRef] [PubMed]
151. Mukamal, K.J.; Conigrave, K.M.; Mittleman, M.A.; Camargo, C.A.; Stampfer, M.J.; Willett, W.C.; Rimm, E.B. Roles of drinking pattern and type of alcohol consumed in coronary heart disease in men. *N. Engl. J. Med.* **2003**, *348*, 109–118. [CrossRef]
152. Homann, N.; Jousimies-Somer, H.; Jokelainen, K.; Heine, R.; Salaspuro, M. High acetaldehyde levels in saliva after ethanol consumption: Methodological aspects and pathogenetic implications. *Carcinogenesis* **1997**, *18*, 1739–1743. [CrossRef]

153. Boban, M.; Stockley, C.; Teissedre, P.; Restani, P.; Fradera, U.; Stein-Hammer, C.; Ruf, J. Drinking pattern of wine and effects on human health: Why should we drink moderately and with meals? *Food Funct.* **2016**, *7*, 2937–2942. [CrossRef]
154. Rifler, J.-P. Is a meal without wine good for health? *Diseases* **2018**, *6*, 105. [CrossRef] [PubMed]
155. Sluik, D.; Jankovic, N.; O'Doherty, M.G.; Geelen, A.; Schöttker, B.; Rolandsson, O.; Kiefte-de Jong, J.; Ferrieres, J.; Bamia, C.; Fransen, H.P.; et al. Alcoholic beverage preference and dietary habits in elderly across Europe: Analyses within the consortium on health and ageing: Network of cohorts in Europe and the United States (CHANCES) Project. *PLoS ONE* **2016**, *11*, e0161603. [CrossRef] [PubMed]
156. Burke, V.; Puddey, I.B.; Beilin, L.J. Mortality associated with wines, beers, and spirits. Australian data suggest that choice of beverage relates to lifestyle and personality. *BMJ* **1995**, *311*, 1166. [CrossRef] [PubMed]
157. Männistö, S.; Uusitalo, K.; Roos, E.; Fogelholm, M.; Pietinen, P. Alcohol beverage drinking; diet and body mass index in a cross-sectional survey. *Eur. J. Clin. Nutr.* **1997**, *51*, 326–332. [CrossRef] [PubMed]
158. Tjønneland, A.; Grønbaek, M.; Stripp, C.; Overvad, K. Wine intake and diet in a random sample of 48763 Danish men and women. *Am. J. Clin. Nutr.* **1999**, *69*, 49–54. [CrossRef] [PubMed]
159. Sluik, D.; van Lee, L.; Geelen, A.; Feskens, E.J. Alcoholic beverage preference and diet in a representative Dutch population: The Dutch national food consumption survey 2007–2010. *Eur. J. Clin. Nutr.* **2014**, *68*, 287–294. [CrossRef]
160. Chatenoud, L.; Negri, E.; La Vecchia, C.; Volpato, O.; Franceschi, S. Wine drinking and diet in Italy. *Eur. J. Clin. Nutr.* **2000**, *54*, 177–179. [CrossRef]
161. Alcácera, M.A.; Marques-Lopes, I.; Fajó-Pascual, M.; Foncillas, J.P.; Carmona-Torre, F.; Martínez-González, M.A. Alcoholic beverage preference and dietary pattern in Spanish university graduates: The SUN cohort study. *Eur. J. Clin. Nutr.* **2008**, *62*, 1178–1186. [CrossRef]
162. Carmona-Torre, F.A.; García-Arellano, A.; Marques-Lopes, I.; Basora, J.; Corella, D.; Gómez-Gracia, E.; Fiol, M.; Covas, M.I.; Aros, F.; Conde, M.; et al. Relationship of alcoholic beverage consumption to food habits in a Mediterranean population. *Am. J. Health. Promot.* **2008**, *23*, 27–30. [CrossRef]
163. World Health Organization. *Global Status Report on Alcohol and Health 2018*; World Health Organization: Geneva, Switzerland, 2018.
164. GBD 2016 Alcohol Collaborators. Alcohol use and burden for 195 countries and territories, 1990–2016: A systematic analysis for the Global Burden of Disease Study 2016-ClinicalKey. *Lancet* **2018**, *392*, 1015–1035. [CrossRef]
165. International Agency for Research on Cancer (IARC). *IARC Monographs on the Evaluation of Carcinogenic Risks to Humans. Volume 96—Alcohol Consumption and Ethyl Carbamate*; International Agency for Research on Cancer: Lyon, France, 2010.
166. Corrao, G.; Bagnardi, V.; Zambon, A.; La Vecchia, C. A meta-analysis of alcohol consumption and the risk of 15 diseases. *Prev. Med.* **2004**, *38*, 613–619. [CrossRef]
167. Rehm, J.; Greenfield, T.K.; Rogers, J.D. Average volume of alcohol consumption, patterns of drinking, and all-cause mortality: Results from the US National Alcohol Survey. *Am. J. Epidemiol.* **2001**, *153*, 64–71. [CrossRef] [PubMed]
168. Nordqvist, C.; Holmqvist, M.; Nilsen, P.; Bendtsen, P.; Lindqvist, K. Usual drinking patterns and non-fatal injury among patients seeking emergency care. *Public Health* **2006**, *120*, 1064–1073. [CrossRef]
169. De Lange, D.W. From red wine to polyphenols and back: A journey through the history of the French Paradox. *Thromb. Res.* **2007**, *119*, 403–406. [CrossRef] [PubMed]
170. Day, N.L.; Zuo, Y.; Richardson, G.A. Prenatal alcohol use and offspring size at 10 years of age. *Alcohol. Clin. Exp. Res.* **1999**, *23*, 863–869. [CrossRef]
171. Olson, H.C.; Streissguth, A.P.; Sampson, P.D. Association of prenatal alcohol exposure with behavioural and learning problems in early adolescence. *J. Am. Acad. Child Adol. Psych.* **1997**, *36*, 1187–1194. [CrossRef]
172. Anderson, P.; Baumberg, B. *Alcohol in Europe: A Report for the European Commission*; Institute of Alcohol Studies: London, UK, 2006.
173. Fiore, M.; Messina, M.P.; Petrella, C.; D'Angelo, A.; Greco, A.; Ralli, M.; Ferraguti, G.; Tarani, L.; Vitali, M.; Ceccanti, M. Antioxidant properties of plant polyphenols in the counteraction of alcohol abuse induced damage: Impact on the Mediterranean diet. *J. Funct. Foods* **2020**, *71*, 104012. [CrossRef]
174. Aranceta-Bartrina, J.; Partearroyo, T.; López-Sobaler, A.M.; Ortega, R.M.; Varela-Moreiras, G.; Serra-Majem, L.; Pérez-Rodrigo, C. The Collaborative Group for the Dietary Guidelines for the Spanish Population (SENC). Updating the Food-Based Dietary Guidelines for the Spanish Population: The Spanish Society of Community Nutrition (SENC) Proposal. *Nutrients* **2019**, *11*, 2675. [CrossRef]
175. Stamler, J. Toward a modern Mediterranean diet for the 21st century. *Nutr. Metab. Cardiovasc. Dis.* **2013**, *23*, 1159–1162. [CrossRef]

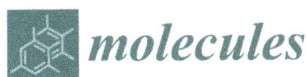

Review

Wine Intake in the Framework of a Mediterranean Diet and Chronic Non-Communicable Diseases: A Short Literature Review of the Last 5 Years

Simona Minzer [1], Ramon Estruch [2,3] and Rosa Casas [2,3,*]

1. El Pino Hospital, Avenida Padre Hurtado, San Bernardo, 13560 Santiago de Chile, Chile; simona.minzer@gmail.com
2. Department of Internal Medicine, Hospital Clinic, Institut d'Investigació Biomèdica August Pi i Sunyer (IDIBAPS), University of Barcelona, Villarroel, 170, 08036 Barcelona, Spain; restruch@clinic.cat
3. Center for Biomedical Research Network (CIBER) 06/03, Fisiopatología de la Obesidad y la Nutrición, Instituto de Salud Carlos III, 28029 Madrid, Spain
* Correspondence: rcasas1@clinic.cat; Tel.: +34-93-2275745; Fax: +34-93-2275758

Academic Editor: Paula Silva
Received: 5 October 2020; Accepted: 28 October 2020; Published: 30 October 2020

Abstract: Dietary habits are a determining factor of the higher incidence and prevalence of chronic non-communicable diseases (NCDs). In the aim to find a possible preventive and intervention strategy, the Mediterranean diet (MedDiet) has been proposed as an effective approach. Within the MedDiet, moderate wine consumption with meals is a positive item in the MedDiet score; however, recent studies have reported a dose-response association between alcohol consumption and higher risk of a large number of NCDs. This review aimed to evaluate the association between NCDs and wine consumption in the framework of the MedDiet, with a simple review of 22 studies of the highest-level literature published over the last five years. We found that the information regarding the effects of wine in different health outcomes has not varied widely over the past five years, finding inconclusive results among the studies evaluated. Most of the literature agrees that light to moderate wine intake seems to have beneficial effects to some extent in NCDs, such as hypertension, cancer, dyslipidemia and dementia, but no definitive recommendations can be made on a specific dose intake that can benefit most diseases.

Keywords: Mediterranean diet; wine intake; cardiovascular disease; cancer; dementia

1. Introduction

Lifestyle, including dietary habits, is a determining factor of the high incidence and prevalence of chronic non-communicable diseases (NCDs), such as cardiovascular disease (CVD), diabetes and dementia [1]. Several studies have shown that non-smokers, the practice of physical activity, having an adequate body mass index (BMI) and a healthy diet pattern (rich in vegetables, fruits, legumes and fish, and limited in red meat), with moderate alcohol consumption, are factors associated with a lower risk of mortality by all causes and CVD (≥65%) compared to subjects who have an unhealthy lifestyle [2–4]. Moreover, the adoption of a healthy lifestyle is associated with a longer life expectancy free of the main NCDs (cancer, CVD and type 2 diabetes [T2DM] [5].

In this sense, the Mediterranean diet (MedDiet), one of the most widely evaluated dietary patterns throughout different clinical trials, and prospective cohort studies and has been proposed as an effective approach for CVD prevention and intervention [6–8]. This healthy dietary pattern is recommended by the American Heart Association and has been included in the 2015–2020 Dietary Guidelines for Americans [6,9]. The MedDiet has been associated with better long-term weight control, blood pressure

(BP), lipid profile, glucose metabolism and insulin resistance, inflammation, endothelial dysfunction, the presence of arrhythmia, and gut microbiome [6,8], and a significant reduction in all-cause mortality (8–10%), and the risk of CVD (10%) and neoplasias (4%) for every two-point increment in adherence to the Mediterranean diet pattern (MDP) [10,11].

The MedDiet is characterized by a high consumption of plant foods, that mainly comprises fruits and vegetables, whole-grain cereals and breads, nuts and seeds; locally grown, fresh and seasonal, unprocessed foods; primarily extra-virgin olive oil as a main source of healthy fat for cooking and dressing meals; moderate amounts of dairy products; small amounts of red meat, moderate amounts of fish; and light-to-moderate intake of red wine often during the main meals [12].

Although moderate consumption of wine with meals (≤1 and ≤2 drinks/day for women and men, respectively) is a positive item in the MedDiet score, results from recent studies have reported that there is a dose-response association between alcohol consumption and a high risk of a large number of NCDs [13,14]. Specifically, a certain association has been observed between alcohol consumption and the risk of developing different types of cancer, regardless of the amount consumed [15]. On the other hand, some authors have reported that alcohol consumption is associated with a decreased incidence of cancer because of its stilbenoid content [16–22].

According to the World Health Organization (WHO), the amount and pattern of alcohol consumption plays a key role in the appearance of detrimental effects on health [14]. Excessive alcohol consumption is not only linked to an increased risk of traffic accidents and deaths, child abuse, spousal violence and suicide [23] but also to the development of cancer and liver disease [24]. In 2016, the WHO reported that CVD death was directly associated with excessive alcohol consumption, accounting for 19% of deaths [14]. In addition, other determining factors on the harmful effects of alcohol on health are gender (male or female), inter-individual variability, type of alcoholic beverage consumed (fermented or distilled), amount (low, moderate, high, excessive) and duration of consumption, drinking patterns (occasional, daily, compulsive), as well as socioeconomic factors [23,25–27]. Furthermore, a systematic review and meta-analysis analyzing 2865 participants performed by Roerecke et al. [28] reported that participants who alcohol intake >6 drinks/day leads to reduction of BP in a dose-dependent manner with an apparent threshold effect at 2 drinks/day. Drinkers (≤2 drinks/day) did not report significant reduction in BP after reducing their consumption near abstinence. The same authors in a new systematic review and meta-analysis of cohort studies [29], including 361,254 participants and 90,160 incident cases of hypertension, concluded that the risk of hypertension was increased for any alcohol consumption in men, in contrast to women who showed no greater risk with a daily consumption of 1 to 2 drinks or higher. According to results reported by Wood et al. [30], in high-income countries, among current alcohol drinkers, 100 g of alcohol per week, showed a lower risk threshold for all-cause mortality. In addition, exploratory analysis showed among alcoholic beverages that beer or spirits drinkers and binge drinkers have a higher risk of all-cause mortality. Nonetheless, wine, a fermented drink, consumed during meals and in the context of a MDP, has shown favorable effects on the prevention of CVD. These cardio-protective mechanisms involve not only an increase of high-density lipoprotein cholesterol (HDL-C) levels and the regulation of blood lipids but also improvement in glucose metabolism and endothelial function, decreasing inflammation and platelet aggregation as well as exerting antioxidant effects [31–33]. Moreover, wine consumption in the context of a healthy diet, such as the MedDiet, has shown positive effects against cancer risk. Results of a meta-analysis with an overall population of 2,130,753 subjects [34] reported that moderate wine consumption in the framework of a MDP has a higher protective effect (relative risk (RR) 0.89; 95% CI: 0.85–0.93) compared to the rest of its components (fruit, vegetable and whole grain intake).

Wine is an alchemy with unique properties, having a rich and original composition in terms of known polyphenols and antioxidants [35–39]. The alcohol content varies among different types of wines, being 14% for red wine and 11% for white wine, a much lower content than spirits (approximately 35%) [40–43]. In addition to ethanol, the polyphenol content in wine can provide a greater protective effect on health [44–46]. While red wine has a high concentration of bioactive compounds, the content in white wine is lower and is practically negligible in distilled beverages (liquors and spirits) [40]. Resveratrol, anthocyanins (ANC), catechins, and tannins (proanthocyanidins and ellagitannins) are the main polyphenols in wine [35,47]. Since alcoholic beverages present a different molecular composition, different health effects are to be expected. Besides wine, other bioactive components from the MedDiet, such as polyphenolic compounds and phytosterols in olive oil (hydroxytyrosol, tyrosol, oleocanthal), and nuts, fruits and vegetables (flavonoids, mainly), can also contribute to increasing this cardioprotective effect through different synergic mechanisms [47].

1.1. Moderate Alcohol Consumption

According to the WHO and the US National Institute on Alcohol Abuse and Alcoholism, the measure most frequently used in studies is a standard drink, which is defined as the amount of alcohol an average adult can metabolize in 1 h [40,48,49]. While in the United Kingdom and Iceland a standard drink is defined as an alcoholic beverage that contains 8 g of pure alcohol (10 mL), other countries such as Australia, France, the Netherlands or Spain consider a standard drink as 10 g of pure alcohol (12.5 mL), and the United States considers it as 14 g of pure alcohol (17.5 mL) [50]. In lay terms, these amounts can be translated into 330 mL of beer (~5% ethanol), 125 mL of table wine (~12% ethanol), or 40 mL of distilled spirits or liquor (~40% ethanol) [50,51]. Moreover, the alcohol content in wine can vary from 5% to 15% according to the different formulations [40].

The definition of moderate alcohol consumption may vary depending the country referred, as may the amount of alcohol content in an alcoholic drink. The American Dietary Guidelines Advisory Committee [52] consider a moderate alcohol intake by adults of legal drinking age as a daily amount consumed $\leq$10 g of ethanol ($\leq$1 drink) for women and $\leq$20 g of ethanol ($\leq$2 drinks) for men. However, other guidelines consider a low-risk pattern as a daily consumption of 10 g up to 42 g of alcohol (1 to 3 drinks) for women or 10 g to 56 g for men (1 to 4 drinks).

Furthermore, besides the amount of alcohol consumed, other aspects such as age (young people engage in more heavy drinking episodes than older individuals), sex (women are more sensitive to the toxic effects of alcohol), ethnicity, genetics, type of alcoholic beverage consumed (wine, beer, distilled), drinking frequency (heavy or binge, occasional, daily, weekend, etc.) and socioeconomic level, account for the inter-individual variability of the adverse effects of alcohol on health [23,25,27,51,53].

1.2. Wine Polyphenols in Human Health

Wine matrix composition is complex and mainly constituted by water (86%), ethanol (8–15%), glycerol and polysaccharides or other trace elements (1%), different types of acids (0.5%), and a volatile fraction (0.5%) [54]. The wine matrix contains several hundred compounds that are found in very low concentrations, and they have been found to play an important role in the evolution and quality of wine, as well as in the protection against NCDs [55].

Among the minority compounds, wine contains a large variety of phenolic compounds (range from 2000 to 6000 mg/L in red wines), also called polyphenols, which are responsible for special organoleptic features of wine (color, flavor, smell) [52,55]. Currently, there is a great interest in the volatile fraction of wine as these compounds are closely related to beverage flavor [56]. These volatile organic compounds (VOC) include alcohols, esters, aldehydes, ketones, acids, terpenes, phenols, and sulfur compounds in a great variety of concentrations that are secondary metabolites produced in grape plants as a defense mechanism [57]. The perception of aroma and flavor are a result of a complex interaction between the volatile (which includes flavor and aroma compounds) and nonvolatile (ethanol, polyphenolic compounds, proteins, and carbohydrates) fractions in wine [57,58]. It is estimated that wine contains more than a thousand volatile compounds, whose concentrations range between mg/L to ng/L [58]. Wine flavor is obtained by varietal aroma, grape variety, pre-fermentative (during alcoholic and malolactic fermentations) and post-fermentative aroma (during conservation and aging of wine) [54,59]. Wine aroma is quantitatively produced by higher alcohols, acids and esters, which are important for the sensory properties as quality of wine, intrinsic factors that influence consumer acceptance [54,60]. While the higher amount of alcohol is directly associated with wine quality (higher amounts, less wine quality), the amount of esters (generally ≤100 mg/L) is associated with wine odor (higher amounts, strong odor) [54,61]. Wine oligosaccharides (complex carbohydrate molecules) have been associated with significant physicochemical properties beneficial to consumers' health. So, some oligosaccharides such as arabinoxylan-, fructo-, gluco-, galacto-, isomalto-, mannan-, xylo-, soyo-oligosaccharides and others can be fermented, exerting benefits on the intestinal microbiota (prebiotic effect) [62,63]. In addition, it has been suggested pectin-derived acidic oligosaccharides and arabinoxylooligosaccharides may have anti-cancer [64] and antioxidant effects [65,66]. Similarly, it has been suggested that polysaccharides could also have a significant antioxidant effect in wine [63]. In addition, some of these VOCs are sesquiterpenes and monoterpenes, which have been shown to have potential health benefits, such as decreased risk of chronic diseases. These compounds have been associated with anti-inflammatory, antioxidant, anti-carcinogenic and anti-bacterial properties [67–70], contributing to wine's health effects.

During the red winemaking process the contact with grape skins and seeds is longer, and therefore, red wines tend to have a higher polyphenol content (six-fold greater) than white wines. It is estimated that the polyphenolic compound content in red wine varies from 1800 to 3000 mg/L [71]. Polyphenols, especially flavonoids such as flavonols (quercetin and myricetin), flavanols (catechin and epicatechin) and ANC, and non-flavonoids, which include phenolic acids (hydroxybenzoic acids and hydroxycinnamic acids) and stilbenes (trans-resveratrol), have been related to beneficial effects on human health due to their protective properties, antioxidant activity and capacity to delete reactive oxygen species (ROS) caused by exercise, food metabolism and environmental factors, such as exposure to air pollutants. These free radicals can lead to aging, cardiovascular and neurodegenerative diseases and even cancer by the reduction of cell proliferation, which can be used for potential cancer therapy [36,55,71].

Even though the alcoholic fraction of wine (ethanol) has been associated with pro-oxidant effects, the phenolic content (polyphenols) seems to counteract the potential pro-oxidant effect of ethanol [38]. The antioxidant capacity of wines is only associated to its phenolic content or the action of a single phenolic compound but within the total polyphenol content (synergistic antioxidant effect) [55].

To date, the main biological effects attributed to phenolic acids (gallic acid or caffeic acid) are their antioxidant, anti-mutagenic, anti-proliferative and antimicrobial properties [36]. In addition, in vitro studies have reported vasodilator activity of phenolic acids [36,71]. However, Mudnic et al. [72] found a negative correlation between antioxidant activity and vasodilatory capacity after testing nine different phenolic acids. Moreover, caffeic acid has been associated with neuroprotective activity [73] and inhibition of peroxynitrite-induced neuronal injury, and ferulic acid is considered to have antidiabetic properties [74] because of its capacity to reduce blood glucose levels through increasing plasma insulin concentrations.

Flavonols (quercetin, mainly) found in red wine have an approximate concentration of 50 mg/L [75]. The beneficial effects of dietary flavonol on human health have been related to the inhibition of low-density lipoprotein cholesterol (LDL-C) oxidation and a reduction of oxidative stress through decreases in BP, which are primary risk factors for the development of atheroma plaque [71,76]. This flavonol is able to reduce oxidative stress through an upregulation of nitric oxide synthase (NOS) expression, as well as an activation and modulation of antioxidant mechanisms. In addition, quercetin has been associated with decreased inflammation, reduction of the expression of Toll-like receptors (TLR2 and TLR4) by the inhibition of nuclear factor kappa-B's (NF-κB) translocation to the nucleus. Quercetins can inhibit cell proliferation, which leads to an attenuation of the progression of cancer [55]. Besides their anti-hypertensive and anti-atherogenic effects, flavonols have been inversely related to aging, obesity and the occurrence of neurodegenerative diseases, CVD and several specific types of cancer such as breast, pancreatic, uterine, prostate or urinary tract cancer, among others [36,55,77–81].

It has also been demonstrated that ANC are beneficial to human health. Their concentration in red wine is approximately 500 mg/L [82]. ANC are strong antioxidants and have the capacity of inhibiting cancer cell growth, inflammation, neuro-inflammation and oxidative stress, as well as preventing obesity [83–87]. Finally, stilbenes are bioactive compounds with concentrations in red wine of approximately 20 mg/L [88]. The main function of stilbenes in plants is to protect them against pathogens and fungi, and therefore, they present a strong antifungal and antimicrobial capacity [89]. The most important stilbene is trans-resveratrol, as it presents multiple relevant pharmacological effects on health. These compounds (resveratrol, mainly) present anti-inflammatory, anti-oxidative and anti-aggregatory effects, as well as a high capacity for modulating lipoproteins and inhibit the initiation, promotion and progression of tumors. Therefore, their biological activity has frequently been related to atherosclerosis, cancer, CVD or neurodegenerative diseases (e.g., Alzheimer's disease) [71,90–93]. In addition, resveratrol is associated with a lower risk of coronary heart disease (CHD) and myocardial infarction [94], and several clinical studies and meta-analyses have found a significant reduction of systolic BP (SBP) with resveratrol intake. Therefore stilbenes might have an protective role against hypertension, as well as diabetes and diabetes-related complications [95–99].

There is noteworthy information suggesting that the potential benefits of wine intake on NCDs such as dyslipidemia, hypertension, MetS, CVD and T2DM, are dependent on the bioavailability of polyphenols [55]. Phenolic compounds' bioavailability can be affected by different factors such as environmental, dietary factors (fibers and fats that help or reduce absorption), possible interactions with others compounds of similar mechanisms of absorption. Moreover, thermal treatments, storage, cooking techniques, food matrix, chemical structure, amount of polyphenols in food could contribute to their bioavility. Therefore, others intrinsic factors such as age, gender and genetic differences, enzyme activity, transporters, intestinal microflora, health status, among others may influence [36,100,101]. So not all polyphenols are absorbed with equal efficacy, only between 5 to 10% of the total polyphenol intake may be directly absorbed in the small intestine [102,103].

This review aimed to evaluate the association between NCD (hypertension, T2DM, dyslipidemia, cancer and dementia) and wine consumption within the framework of a MDP and its underlying mechanisms of protection, with a simple review of the highest-level literature (randomized control trials (RCT) and meta-analyses) published in the last five years, evaluating humans, adults (>18 years), addressing wine intake or specifically red wine polyphenols. The bibliographic search was performed through PubMed, ScienceDirect, and Google Scholar from June 2020 to August 2020.

2. Results

A total of 22 studies were selected for the final evaluation; seven studies evaluating hypertension as an outcome, eight studies on T2DM, four studies on dyslipidemia, four studies on cancer and one study on dementia. Some of the studies evaluated two or more outcomes, thus overlapping in the results. The study characteristics are summarized in Table 1.

Table 1. Summary of study characteristics, outcomes and main results of studies included in the analysis.

Reference	Design, Subjects (n), Follow-up	Population	Intervention/Dose	Outcomes	Main Results
Y. Gepner et al. [104]	Randomized controlled trial, n = 54, 6 months	Adults, T2D, alcohol abstainers	150 mL water, white wine, or red wine	BP (24-h ABPM)	Moderate daily red wine intake (150 mL) had no effect on mean daily BP, but showed transient hypotensive response at midnight (3–4 h after ingestion), decreasing SBP −10.6 mmHg (95% CI −14.1 to −0.6; $p = 0.03$) and DBP −7.7 mmHg (−11.8 to 0.9; $p = 0.076$).
T.A. Mori et al. [105]	Randomized controlled trial, cross-over design, n = 28, 16 weeks	Adults, T2DM, men and post-menopausal women, regular drinkers	Red wine or DRW 230 mL/day for women and 300 mL/d for men, or water.	Effect of wine consumption on 24 h ambulatory BP, heart rate and other markers	Red wine significantly increased awake SBP (2.5 ± 1.2 mmHg; $p = 0.033$) and DBP (1.9 ± 0.7 mmHg; $p = 0.008$) compared to water and decreased DBP overnight (2.0 ± 0.8 mmHg; $p = 0.016$) compared to DRW. Nonetheless, there was no significant overall effect of red wine on mean 24 h SBP or DBP. Red wine had no effect on TC, TG, HDL-C, LDL-C, fasting glucose and insulin levels, or HOMA-IR score.
S. McDonagh et al. [106]	Randomized, crossover trial, n = 12, 2 weeks	Healthy normotensive men	175 mL red wine, vodka or water	BP response to NO_3^- rich salad and red wine	Red wine and NO_3^- rich salad lowered SBP at 2 h (−5 mmHg) and 5 h (−4 mmHg) and DBP (2–4 mmHg) after intake.
I. Roth et al. [107]	Randomized controlled trial, cross-over design, n = 38, 10 weeks	Adults, men, T2DM or ≥3 cardiovascular risk factors	30g ethanol from white wine or gin	Effect of white wine on BP and plasma NO concentration	White wine decreased SBP (−4.91 mmHg, 95% CI −9.41 to −0.42; $p = 0.033$) and DBP (−2.90, 95% CI −5.50 to −0.29; $p = 0.030$) significantly compared to gin ($p < 0.040$); and significantly increased plasma NO concentrations (27.86, 95% CI −6.86 to 62.59; $p = 0.013$).
M.T. García-Conesa et al. [108]	Meta-analysis of 128 human randomized controlled trials (n = 5538)	Adults, distributed over five continents	250 to 400 mL red wine	Association between intake of wine and other foods on different biomarkers of cardio-metabolic	Anthocyanin rich products (wine/red grapes) reduced systolic (−3.31 mmHg; $p = 0.014$) and diastolic (−1.50 mmHg; $p = 0.002$) BP, but increased Hb1Ac (+0.26; $p = 0.026$)

Table 1. Cont.

Reference	Design, Subjects (n), Follow-up	Population	Intervention/Dose	Outcomes	Main Results
S. Weaver et al. [109]	Meta-analysis, 37 studies	Adults, healthy or T2DM/obesity/MS	RWP supplementation (dose ND)	Effect of RWP on vascular health	RWP significantly improved SBP (−2.6 mmHg, 95% CI −4.8 to −0.4; $p = 0.010$), especially in at risk population (−3.2 mmHg, 95% CI −5.7 to −0.8; $p = 0.010$)
J. Ye et al. [110]	Meta-analysis, 9 studies, N/D	Adults, T2DM	Red wine 120–360 mL/d	Effect of wine intake on BP, glucose parameters and lipid profile in T2DM	Red wine intake significantly reduced DBP (MD 0.10, 95% CI 0.01–0.20; $p = 0.03$). No significant differences in glucose or lipid parameters.
Y. Gepner et al. [111]	Randomized controlled trial, n = 224 2 years	Adults, 40–75 years with T2DM	150 mL of red wine or white wine	Changes in lipid profile (HDL-C, apolipoprotein (a), TC/HDL-C ratio) and glycemic control (FPG, HOMA-IR)	Red wine intake increased HDL-C (2.9 mg/dL, 95% CI 1.6–2.2 mg/dL; $p < 0.001$) and apolipoprotein (a) (0.03 g/L, 95% CI 0–0.06 g/L; $p = 0.05$), and decreased TC/HDL-C ratios (0.27, 95% CI −0.52 to −0.01; $p = 0.039$). White wine decreased FPG (−17.2 mg/dL, 95% CI −28.9 to −5.5 mg/dL; $p = 0.004$) and HOMA-IR score (−1.2, 95% CI −2.1 to −0.2; $p = 0.019$)
K. Abraham et al. [112]	Randomized controlled trial, n = 9, 2 weeks	Adults, T2DM and pre-diabetic	263 mL red wine or water	Acute effect of red wine in glycemic control	Greater insulin iAUC response after wine intake (50%; $p < 0.05$), but no change in glucose iAUC ($p = 0.82$)
J. Huang et al. [113]	Meta-analysis, 13 prospective studies, 397,296 subjects	Adults, T2DM or healthy	Stratified in 0–10 g/day, 10–20 g/day or >20 g/day	Risk of T2DM	Wine intake was associated with 15% reduction in T2DM risk (RR 0.85, 95% CI 0.80–0.89), with a peak risk reduction at 20–30g/d
J. Woerdeman et al. [114]	Randomized controlled trial, n = 30, 8 weeks	Adults, obese (BMI ≥30 kg/m^2), white ethnicity, healthy	RWP extract 600 mg/d or placebo	Effect of supplementation of RWP on insulin sensitivity in obese adults	RWP supplementation did not alter insulin sensitivity nor lipid profile compared to placebo (M-value (mg/kg/min) 3.3, CI 2.4–4.8 vs. 2.9, CI 2.8–5.9; $p = 0.65$, respectively)
R. Golan et al. [115]	Randomized controlled trial, n = 224, 2 years	Adults, T2DM, abstainers	16.9 g of ethanol from dry red wine (150 mL), or 15.8 g from white wine (150 mL)	Effect of moderate wine intake in atherosclerosis	Moderate wine intake was associated with no progression in carotid total plaque volume (−1.2 mm^3, SD 16.9, CI −3.8 to 6.2; $p = 0.6$ for white wine; −1.3, mm^3, SD 17.6, CI −3.4 to 6.0; $p = 0.5$ for red wine) and with a small regression among those with higher carotid plaque burden at baseline (mean −0.11; $p = 0.04$)

Table 1. Cont.

Reference	Design, Subjects (n), Follow-up	Population	Intervention/Dose	Outcomes	Main Results
M. Taborsky et al. [116]	Randomized controlled trial, n 157, 12 months	Adults, healthy, mild to moderate cardiovascular risk	Red or white wine, 0.2 L/day in women <70 kg and 0.3 L/d in women <70 kg and men	Effect of regular red and wine intake in HDL-C and other markers of atherosclerosis	HDL-C significantly decreased at 6 months in the white wine group (−0.14 (SD 0.41); $p = 0.005$), no changes for red wine. LDL-C significantly decreased in both groups at 6 months (−0.39 (0.74); $p < 0.001$ for white wine and −0.27 (0.68); $p < 0.001$ for red wine) and at 12 months (−0.24 (0.73); $p = 0.003$ for white wine and −0.24 (0.78); $p = 0.013$ for red wine) compared with baseline. A significant reduction in TC was observed at 6 months in both groups (−0.32 (1.13); $p = 0.017$ for white wine and −0.33 (0.82); $p = 0.001$ for red wine), but only for red wine at 12 months (−0.24 (0.82); $p = 0.016$).
L. di Renzo et al. [117]	Randomized controlled trial, n 55, 1 day	Healthy adults	30 g of ethanol from red wine, white wine or vodka	Effect of ethanol and polyphenols present in alcoholic beverages on oxidative status when eating an antioxidant meal	Red wine intake during a HFM significantly reduced Ox-LDL-C levels (−4.97 ± 33.18; $p < 0.05$) compared with HFM alone. Red wine significantly up-regulated CAT gene expression (fold change 4.04)
Fang et al. [118]	Meta-analysis, 76 observational studies, n = 6,316,385 subjects, 11.4 years (3.3–30y)	Adults, general population	Dose ND	Association between gastric cancer and dietary factors	Alcohol consumption increased gastric cancer risk (RR 1.15, 95% CI 1.01–1.31), nonetheless wine did not significantly increase this risk (RR 1.02, 95% CI 0.77–1.34).
J.Y. Chen et al. [119]	Meta-analysis, 26 observational studies, n = 18,106 subjects	Adult women with breast cancer	1 drink or 12.5 g of ethanol	Association between wine dose and breast cancer risk	Wine intake increased breast cancer risk (RR 1.36; 95% CI 1.20–1.54; $p < 0.001$), with a dose-response association, showing a 0.59% increase for each increment of 1g/day of ethanol from wine. However, risk decreased in women consuming <80g/day of wine (10g ethanol), with lowest risk at 40g/day of wine (5g/day ethanol).
M.D. Vartolomei et al. [120]	Meta-analysis, 174 studies, n = 455,413 subjects	Adults, overall population	Moderate red wine intake (ND)	Effect of red wine on prostate cancer development	Moderate red wine consumption was associated with lower risk of prostate cancer (RR 0.88, 95% CI 0.78–0.999; $p = 0.047$)

Table 1. Cont.

Reference	Design, Subjects (n), Follow-up	Population	Intervention/Dose	Outcomes	Main Results
W. Xu et al. [121]	Meta-analysis, 17 observational studies, n = 12,110 subjects	Adults, general population	Stratified in non-drinkers plus occasional drinkers (<0.5 drinks/day), light to moderate drinker (<2 drinks/day) and heavy drinkers (≥2 drinks/day)	Effects of wine intake on colorectal cancer risk	Any wine consumption did not affect colorectal cancer risk versus nondrinkers (RR 0.99, 95% CI 0.89–1.10). No difference among men and women (0.88, CI 0.66–1.18 and 0.83, CI 0.67–1.03, respectively), red or white wine (0.98, CI 0.68–1.40, and 0.95, CI 0.69–1.32, respectively) nor drinking category (light to moderate 0.93, CI 0.80–1.08, and heavy drinking 1.00, CI 0.86–1.16).
L. Schwingshackl et al. [34]	Meta-analysis, 83 prospective studies, n = 2,130,753 subjects	Adults, overall population	Moderate red wine intake in a Mediterranean diet (ND)	Cancer risk and cancer mortality risk	Inverse association for moderate alcohol intake and cancer risk (RR 0.89, 95% CI 0.85–0.93)
W. Xu et al. [122]	Meta-analysis, 16 observational studies, 3–25 years	Adults, general population	Stratified in light (<7 drinks/week), light-to-moderate (<14 drinks/week), moderate (7–14 drinks/week) and moderate-to-heavy (>7 drinks/week) and heavy drinkers (>14 drinks/week)	Association between quantity of alcohol intake and risk of dementia	U-shaped association between alcohol consumption and risk of dementia. Wine showed a trend towards a protective effect for dementia, for current drinkers versus never drinkers (RR 0.67, 95% CI 0.48–0.94; $p = 0.2$) or light-to-moderate drinker versus non-drinkers (RR 0.58, 95% CI 0.39–0.87; $p = 0.196$).

24-h ABPM: ambulatory blood pressure measurement; BMI: body mass index; BP: blood pressure; CAT: catalase; CI: confidence interval; DBP: diastolic blood pressure; DRW: dealcoholized rec wine; FPG: fasting plasma glucose; Hb1Ac: glycated hemoglobin; HDL-C: high-density lipoprotein cholesterol; HFM: high-fat meal; HOMA-IR: Homeostatic Model Assessment for Insulin Resistance; iAUC: incremental blood glucose area under the curve; LDL-C: low-density lipoprotein cholesterol; MS: metabolic syndrome; ND: non-defined; NO: nitric oxide; NO_3^-: nitrate; Ox-LDL-C: Oxidized low-density lipoprotein cholesterol; RR: relative ratio; RWP: Red wine polyphenols; SPB: systolic blood pressure; T2DM: type 2 diabetes mellitus; TC: total cholesterol; TG: trygliceride.

2.1. Hypertension

Alcohol intake has been associated with BP levels in a J-shaped form, in which low to moderate intake contributes to lower BP levels, and higher intakes increase these levels [40,49]. A RCT by Gepner et al. evaluated the effect of moderate red wine intake on BP in individuals with T2DM who abstained from alcohol intake. After a 6-month intervention, reductions in BP were observed in the red wine group at midnight (SBP −10.6 mmHg, 95% confidence interval (CI) −14.1 to −0.6; $p = 0.03$ and diastolic (DBP) −7.7 mmHg, 95% CI −11.8 to 0.9; $p = 0.076$) and at 7 to 9 am (SBP −6.2 mmHg, 95% CI −17.3 to −0.8; $p = 0.014$), but no long-term effects in the mean 24-h BP were found [104]. Other studies using ambulatory BP monitoring have described a biphasic BP pattern after alcohol intake, showing lower levels after acute ingestion but higher levels after 13–23 h [123]. In 2016, Mori et al. published a RCT that evaluated the effects of red wine (24–31g of alcohol/day) over four weeks on BP levels in 24 adults with T2DM. The authors described that red wine significantly increased awake SBP and DBP compared to water (2.5 ± 1.2 mmHg vs 1.9 ± 0.7 mmHg; $p = 0.033$ and $p = 0.008$ respectively), but decreased DBP during sleep (2.0 ± 0.8 mmHg; $p = 0.016$), resulting in a non-significant overall effect on the mean 24-h SBP and DBP [105].

Within the MDP, high intakes of green leafy vegetables are recommended. Dietary nitrate (NO_3^-) and nitrite (NO_2^-) intake, present in vegetables, can affect BP levels by increasing plasma nitric oxide (NO) production and help reduce BP in a dose-dependent manner [106,107]. NO can reduce vascular oxidative stress and act as a natural vasodilator. It has been described that red wine intake along with NO_3^- or NO_2^- promotes NO formation, attributing this phenomenon to its polyphenol content [106,124]. In 2018, McDonagh et al. published a RCT evaluating the response to a NO_3^- rich meal associated with red wine (175 mL), compared to vodka or water intake, in 12 healthy normotensive males. Results showed that compared with the controls SBP decreased at 2 h after consumption of red wine (111 ± 7 mmHg vs. 116 ± 6 mmHg; $p < 0.05$) and at 5 h (115 ± 8 mmHg versus 119 ± 7 mmHg), and DBP was also significantly reduced after consumption of red wine (1h: −3 mmHg, 2h: −4 mmHg) compared with baseline and also compared with controls (1h: 59 ± 5; 2h 58 ± 4 mmHg vs. 1h: 62 ± 5, 2h: 61 ± 6 mmHg; $p < 0.05$). Moreover, the mean arterial pressure was reduced 2 h after intake of the NO_3^- rich meal alongside red wine (76 ± 4 mmHg) compared with baseline (80 ± 6 mmHg) and controls (80 ± 6 mmHg; $p < 0.05$) and also at 3 h (77 ± 6 mmHg) compared with controls (81 ± 7 mmHg). Even though vodka was also effective in reducing BP, the magnitude of the SBP reduction was consistently higher after red wine intake [106]. Another crossover trial by Roth et al. evaluated the effects of short-term white wine and gin intake (21 days) on BP and plasma NO in 41 adult men (55 to 80 years) with cardiovascular risk factors. All participants presented low to moderate alcohol consumption, quantified around 30 g ethanol per day. After the intervention, white wine intake showed a significant mean reduction in SBP (−4.91 mmHg, 95% CI −9.41 to −0.42; $p = 0.033$) and DBP (−2.90, 95% CI −5.50 to −0.29; $p = 0.030$), and this reduction was also significant when compared to gin intake ($p < 0.040$). Moreover, plasma NO concentrations significantly increased after white wine intake (27.86, 95% CI −6.86 to 62.59; $p = 0.013$), but no differences were observed between the two groups. The authors suggested that the hypotensive effects of white wine evaluated in this study could be attributed to non-alcohol compounds found in this beverage [107].

It has been described that the phenolic content of wine contributes to its BP lowering effect. In vitro studies in human endothelial cells have described that wine polyphenols inhibit nicotinamide adenine dinucleotide phosphate (NADPH) oxidase activity and increase calcium intracellular concentrations and NO synthesis, contributing to the vasorelaxant effect attributed to wine [125,126]. Red wine is a rich source of ANC, an important type of polyphenols. Multiple cardio-metabolic components can be altered in response to ANC food products, and their intake has been associated with a lower risk of CVD [108]. Studies evaluating the effects of ANC and other polyphenols on cardio-metabolic risk factors (i.e., serum lipids, blood glucose levels, insulin resistance, hypertension, among others) show inconsistent results, depending on various factors, such as the health status of the participants, sources of bioactive compounds, type and dose of polyphenols supplied, their bioavailability, and host characteristics. A meta-analysis by García-Contesa et al. studied the association between various food sources of ANC, including red wine, with different biomarkers of cardio-metabolic risk. The study included 128 human RCTs, with a total of 5538 participants. The authors found that the intake of specific sources of ANC significantly reduced SBP (-3.31; $p = 0.014$) and DBP (1.50; $p = 0.002$), specifically red wine; nonetheless red wine did not reduce total cholesterol or glycated hemoglobin (HbA1c) [108].

Another important polyphenol present in wine is resveratrol, which has been widely studied. A meta-analysis published by Weaver et al. evaluated the effects of red wine polyphenols, especially resveratrol, on vascular health. Supplementation with red wine polyphenols significantly decreased SBP (-2.62 mmHg, 95% CI -4.81 to -0.44; $p = 0.010$), but group analysis showed this effect only in at-risk populations (-3.2 mmHg, 95% CI -5.7 to -0.8; $p = 0.010$) and not in healthy cohorts (0.7 mmHg, 95% CI -2.5 to 3.8; $p = 0.673$). When analyzing resveratrol-only studies, this significant mean difference was maintained (-3.7 mmHg, 95% CI -7.3 to -0.0; $p = 0.047$) but was not seen in the non-resveratrol group. No significant effects were found for DBP (-1.0 mmHg, 95% CI -2.2 to 0.3; $p = 0.139$). The authors suggested that the non-significant effect on DBP could be attributed to the small changes seen in DBP in clinical hypertension [109]. Nonetheless, these findings are consistent with previous studies on resveratrol [95]. Moreover, Ye et al. published a meta-analysis of 9 randomized intervention studies evaluating the effects of wine intake on BP, glucose parameters and the lipid profile of T2DM patients. The results showed no significant differences in SBP (weighted mean difference (WMD) 0.12, 95% CI -0.05 to 0.28; $p = 0.17$)), yet a reduction was seen in DBP levels (WMD 0.10, 95% CI: 0.01 to -0.20; $p = 0.03$). These findings were attributed to the fact that the results were pooled as an average, rather than evaluated at individual hours [110].

These studies published over the last five years indicate that, overall, wine intake helps reduce BP. Even though this effect could be different depending on the time of day and time after intake, the general conclusion in most studies is that wine and its polyphenol supplementation help reduce SBP and DBP when taken in light to moderate quantities.

2.2. Type 2 Diabetes Mellitus

Epidemiological studies suggest that the risk of T2DM is decreased in moderate alcohol drinkers [111,112]. Alcohol, especially wine, has been associated with enhanced glycemic control [127,128]. A RCT study by Gepner et al. recruited 224 alcohol-abstaining adults 40 to 75 years of age with T2DM. The subjects were randomized to consume mineral water, white wine or red wine (150 mL) and were followed during 24 months. The authors described that both types of wine tended to improve glucose metabolism, yet only white wine significantly decreased fasting plasma glucose (-17.2 mg/dL, 95% CI -28.9 to -5.5 mg/dL; $p = 0.004$) and the Homeostatic Model Assessment for Insulin Resistance (HOMA-IR) score by 1.2 (95% CI -2.1 to -0.2; $p = 0.019$) compared with the water group. Red wine did not significantly decrease these measures. No changes were observed in HbA1c% for either type of wine. The authors suggested that the effect of wine seen on glycemic control was mainly due to alcohol [111].

It has been suggested that the glucose lowering effect of alcohol may be mediated by the incretin effect (glucose-dependent insulinotropic polypeptide (GIP) and glucagon-like peptide 1 (GLP-1)). Abraham et al. carried out an interventional study evaluating if acute red wine intake affects glycemic control during an oral glucose tolerance test and the potential involvement of incretins in the augmentation of insulin response after alcohol intake. Nine diabetic or pre-diabetic subjects consuming 263 mL of water or red wine were evaluated in a randomized crossover study. After 15 min, a higher rate of increase in glucose was observed in the wine group (0.15 ± 0.01 vs. 0.11 ± 0.01 mmol/L/min; $p < 0.001$), yet the incremental blood glucose area under the curve (iAUC) was similar in both groups (917 ± 88 vs. 904 ± 79 mmol/L/min for water and wine, respectively; $p = 0.82$). The iAUC for insulin was 50% greater after wine than after water intake ($14{,}837 \pm 4759$ vs. 9885 ± 2686 µU/mL/min; $p < 0.05$), as GIP iAUC increased 25% after wine treatment (7729 ± 1548 vs. 6191 ± 1049 pmol/L/min; $p < 0.05$), with no difference in GLP-1 iAUC. The authors suggested that the higher insulin secretion after wine intake may be partially defined by an increase in GIP levels. Nonetheless, wine did not alter glucose iAUC, and therefore, glycemic control, which could be explained by the basal insulin resistance of the subjects [112].

Huang et al. carried out a meta-analysis of 13 prospective studies to evaluate the association between specific types of alcoholic beverages (wine, beer, spirits) and the risk of T2DM. Alcohol consumption was categorized into three groups of intake, low (0–10 g/day), moderate (10–20 g/day) and high (>20 g/day). The results showed that wine consumption reduced the risk of T2DM by 15% (RR 0.85, 95% CI 0.80 to 0.89). Moreover, all three categories of intake significantly decreased the risk of T2DM, showing a U-shaped relationship. For wine, all levels of consumption <80 g/day were associated with a decreased risk of T2DM, with the lowest risk at 20–30 g/day (pooled RR of moderate and high intake category 0.83, 95% CI 0.76 to 0.91). Beer consumption showed a slightly lower risk of T2DM (RR 0.96, 95% CI 0.92 to 1.0), and spirits intake did not have a significant effect on reducing the risk of diabetes (RR 0.95, 95% CI 0.89 to 1.03). The authors suggested that the greater effect of wine in the reduction of T2DM risk could be attributed to the polyphenols present in wine, especially resveratrol [113].

In the literature, moderate wine consumption has been associated with a decreased risk of metabolic syndrome and CVDs [129]. These effects have been attributed to the polyphenols present in wine, as seen in animal studies [130]. Unfortunately, these findings have been difficult to consistently observe in human studies. Woerdeman et al. performed a RCT to evaluate the effects of an 8-week supplementation with red wine polyphenols on insulin sensitivity in obese subjects (body mass index ≥30 kg/m^2). The authors described that high dose red wine polyphenols (600 mg per day) did not alter insulin sensitivity measured by a hyperinsulinemic-euglycemic clamp, the Matsuda index and HOMA-IR, compared with placebo. The authors attributed these findings to the healthy state of the participants, the small sample size and the unknown bioavailability of the polyphenols in the study subjects [114].

The previously cited meta-analysis by García-Contesa et al. also studied the association between various food sources of ANC on HbA1c, finding that this parameter was increased (+0.97; $p = 0.038$) [108]. In a similar study by Mori et al., adults with T2DM consumed red wine, dealcoholized red wine and water during four weeks, over a three-period cross-over study. The authors described that red wine had no significant impact on home blood glucose monitoring or the HOMA-IR score, relative to dealcoholized red wine or water [105]. Moreover, in a RCT by Golan et al., 224 diabetic subjects were studied to observe if moderate wine consumption, as part of a MedDiet, would decrease their metabolic risk. After two years, the subjects assigned to white or red wine consumption showed a non-significant reduction in carotid total plaque volume (TPV) (−1.2 mm^3, 95% CI −3.8 to 6.2; $p = 0.6$ and −1.3 mm^3, 95% CI −3.4 to 6.0; $p = 0.5$, respectively). Among participants with the highest tertile of baseline carotid TPV, those assigned to wine consumption showed a significant regression in carotid plaque compared to baseline levels (mean −0.11; $p = 0.04$). The authors concluded that moderate wine consumption was associated with no progression in carotid plaque or de novo formation, and that a small regression could be seen in subjects with a higher baseline burden. They speculated that MedDiet counseling could have contributed to this result [115]. Finally, in a similar meta-analysis by Ye et al., the nine interventional studies evaluated showed no significant differences in fasting glucose (WMD −0.00, 95% CI −0.58 to 0.59; $p = 1.00$), fasting insulin (weighted mean difference (WMD) −0.22, 95% CI −2.09 to 1.65; $p = 0.82$) or HbA1C% (WMD −0.16, 95% CI −0.40 to 0.07; $p = 0.17$) [110].

Most studies evaluated in this review suggest that acute or long-term wine intake has little or no effects on blood glucose markers. Nonetheless, one meta-analysis did show that the overall T2DM risk decreased with wine intake [113]. More information is needed in order to provide definitive recommendations.

2.3. Dyslipidemia

It has been widely studied that the beneficial effects of alcohol on cardiovascular health are mainly due to its ability to raise HDL-C levels [131]. In the previously mentioned study by Gepner et al., HDL-C levels significantly increased in the red wine group (2.0 mg/dL, 95% CI 1.6 to 2.2 mg/dL; $p < 0.001$) compared to water, and both types of wine decreased triglyceride levels. The authors suggested that red wine may be superior in improving lipid variables, which may be attributed to the synergistic effect between alcohol and non-alcoholic wine compounds [104].

Red wine has also been associated with a protective effect against LDL-C for its higher antioxidant capacity compared to white wine [132]. Taborsky et al. published a RCT in 2017 in which they evaluated the long-term effects (12 months) of red and white wine intake (0.2–0.3 L per day) on biomarkers of atherosclerosis in 157 healthy subjects with mild to moderate CVD risk. They observed that HDL-C levels significantly decreased at six months in the white wine group compared to baseline (-0.14 ± 0.41; $p = 0.005$) with a significant reduction in LDL-C in both groups at 6 (-0.39 ± 0.74; $p < 0.001$ and -0.27 ± 0.68; $p = 0.001$ for white and red wine respectively) and 12 months (-0.24 ± 0.68; $p = 0.003$ and -0.24 ± 0.78; $p = 0.013$ for white and red wine respectively) compared to baseline. Total cholesterol showed a significant reduction in both groups at 6 months (-0.33 ± 0.99; $p < 0.001$ and -0.33 ± 0.82; $p = 0.001$ for white and red wine respectively), but only for red wine at the 12-month evaluation (-0.24 ± 0.82; $p = 0.016$). Triglyceride levels were not significantly altered. The authors could not confirm any clinically important differences in biomarkers of atherosclerosis between the two types of wine, and they attributed this partially to the prospective long-term design of the trial [116].

Previous studies have evidenced that red wine can modulate the inflammatory response caused by different types of meals [133]. Di Renzo et al. published a RCT in which they evaluated the effects of different types of beverages (red wine, white wine and vodka) on the oxidative status of 55 healthy subjects after a Mediterranean or high-fat meal. They found significant differences in oxidized low-density lipoprotein cholesterol (oxLDL-C) levels between the Mediterranean meal and the high-fat diet (-1.32 ± 20.43 vs. $21.29 \pm 29.93\%$; $p \leq 0.05$, respectively) and between the high-fat diet alone versus the high-fat diet plus red wine intake (21.29 ± 29.93 vs. $-4.97 \pm 33.18\%$; $p \leq 0.05$, respectively). Moreover, a significant up-regulation was observed in catalase levels after red wine intake (4.04-fold change in gene expression). No other differences were observed. It was speculated that the fat profile found in the high fat meal could explain the higher levels of oxLDL-C observed, and that these could be reduced by the presence of the antioxidant molecules found in red wine. The authors also suggested that ethanol may play a role in the bioavailability of polyphenols during digestion [117].

In a similar meta-analysis by Ye et al., the intervention studies evaluated showed a significant reduction in total cholesterol following wine intake in T2DM patients (WMD -0.16, 95% CI 0.02 to 0.31; $p = 0.03$). Moreover, no significant associations were found for measures of LDL-C, HDL-C or triglycerides. The authors associated these results with the wine dose, trial duration and the study populations evaluated in the different studies [110].

The most recent studies evaluating the effect of wine on the lipid profile have shown different and inconsistent results. Even though the most accepted effect is the rising of HDL-C, one RCT and a meta-analysis failed to support this outcome. Nonetheless, oxLDL-C was lowered, contributing to the healthier cardiovascular profile attributed to wine intake within a MedDiet.

2.4. Cancer

It has been widely described that only 5 to 10% of all cancers can be attributed to genetic predisposition, leaving 90 to 95% of cases to be associated with lifestyle factors [134]. Among these factors, diet and more specifically, alcohol consumption have been studied as an important modifiable risk factor. Alcohol has been described to show different effects on cancer risk depending on location. A meta-analysis by Fang et al. published in 2015 evaluated the association between gastric cancer and a diversity of dietary factors, with alcohol being among them. Among the 76 prospective studies revised (n = 6,316,385 subjects and 32,758 incident gastric cancer cases), the authors found a strong effect of alcohol on gastric cancer risk (RR 1.15, 95% CI 1.01 to 1.31) when comparing the highest reported intake with the lowest, but not of wine intake (RR 1.02, 95% CI 0.77 to 1.34). The authors suggested that these findings could be associated with the protective substances found in wine [118].

Another meta-analysis by Chen et al. evaluated the dose-response association between wine intake and the risk of breast cancer. They included 26 prospective studies with a total of 18,106 breast cancer cases and found an increased risk of breast cancer (RR 1.36, 95% CI 1.20 to 1.54; $p < 0.001$) when comparing the highest versus the lowest category of wine drinking. Furthermore, a dose-response analysis showed that greater wine intake could lead to a higher risk of breast cancer, with a 0.59% of non-significant risk increase for every 1g of ethanol per day derived from wine (RR 1.0059, 95% CI 0.9670 – 1.0464; $p = 0.6156$). Moreover, the lowest risk was observed in women who consumed <40 g of wine per day (<5 g of ethanol) [119].

Vartolomei et al. published a meta-analysis in 2018 in which they studied the effect of moderate wine consumption on prostate cancer. They included 17 studies and found a pooled RR for prostate cancer risk of 0.98 (95% CI 0.92 to 1.05; $p = 0.57$). When evaluating each type of wine, the authors described that moderate white wine intake increased the risk of prostate cancer (pooled RR 1.26, 95% CI 1.10 to 1.43; $p = 0.001$) and moderate red wine consumption decreased this risk (pooled RR 0.88, 95% CI 0.78 to 0.999; $p = 0.047$). Nonetheless, it must be taken into account that this study is based in non-randomized observational studies, implying possible bias [120]. Another meta-analysis by Xu et al. evaluated the effects of wine intake on the risk of colorectal cancer in 17 observational studies (12,110 colorectal cancer cases). The risk of developing colorectal cancer due to wine consumption was RR 0.99 (95% CI 0.89 to 1.10) compared to non-drinkers. The authors did not find any associations for red wine consumption or white wine consumption [standardized rate ratio (SRR) 0.98, 95% CI 0.68 to 1.40 and SRR 0.95, 95% CI 0.69 to 1.32, respectively]. When evaluating the amount of intake, light to moderate drinkers (<2 drinks per day) showed a lower risk (SRR 0.93, 95% CI 0.80 to 1.08) than heavy drinkers (≥2 drinks per day) (SRR 1.00, 95% CI 0.86 to 1.16). Overall, no association could be found between wine consumption and the risk of colorectal cancer [121].

Finally, a meta-analysis by Schwingshackl et al. was aimed at evaluating the association between a MedDiet and the risk of cancer in 83 prospective studies. Among other components of the MedDiet, the authors found an inverse association between moderate alcohol intake and the risk of developing cancer (RR 0.89, 95% CI 0.85 to 0.93), when compared to higher intakes. The authors of this study stated that even though red wine contains beneficial compounds that may play a role in cancer, to date it is impossible to certify the effects of alcohol on tumor pathogenesis, and therefore it should not be recommended to abstinent individuals [34].

When evaluating the risk of cancer, it appears that dose and type of beverage are two main factors that affect this risk. Alcohol by itself, at high doses, seems to increase the risk of cancer, and the same seems to happen with wine intake. A recent review showed that alcohol intake at low doses does not increase the risk of cancer, with the exception of breast and prostate cancer [135]. However, red wine seems to have a more protective effect when compared to other alcoholic beverages.

2.5. Dementia

Dementia is a progressive neurodegenerative disorder and is a major cause of disability worldwide. Modifiable lifestyle factors, including diet and specific foods, have been addressed as risk factors for this disease with inconclusive results [136,137]. A meta-analysis published by Xu et al. in 2017 evaluated the association between alcohol intake and dementia in order to better define the quantity of alcohol that could significantly increase the risk of this disease. A U-shaped association was observed between alcohol consumption and the risk of dementia, in which light, light-to-moderate and moderate intake showed an inverse association, while heavier doses showed higher risk, even though there was no statistical significance. Moreover, only wine showed a trend towards a protective effect for dementia when comparing current drinkers with never drinkers (RR 0.67, 95% CI 0.48 to 0.94; $p = 0.2$) or light-to-moderate drinker versus none (RR0.58, 95% CI 0.39 to 0.87; $p = 0.196$), among other types of alcoholic beverages. Furthermore, the authors identified the dose of alcohol intake to be associated with the lowest risk of dementia, revealing that intake ≤ 12.5 g/day decreased the risk. The authors concluded that a modest quantity of alcohol consumption might help decrease the risk of dementia, mainly due to its higher polyphenolic content [122].

3. Conclusions

The information regarding the effects of wine on different health outcomes has not varied widely over the last five years. Inconclusive and contradictory studies remain an important part of the available information, mainly because of the different populations, alcohol dosage, and study design used in the analyses. For now, light to moderate wine intake seems to have some beneficial effects on NCD, such as hypertension, cancer, dyslipidemia and dementia. We can agree that high doses of any alcohol intake, including wine, are harmful and should be avoided. Nonetheless, there is still a long way to go before definitive recommendations on wine intake can be made.

Author Contributions: Conceptualization, R.C. and R.E.; methodology, S.M. and R.C.; investigation, R.C. and S.M.; writing—original draft preparation, S.M. and R.C.; writing—review and editing, R.E. and R.C.; visualization, R.E. and R.C.; supervision, R.C. All authors approved the final version of the manuscript.

Funding: This research was funded by the Instituto de Salud Carlos III, Spain, grant number PIE14/00045; by the Instituto de Salud Carlos III, Spain, grant number PI044504; and the Sociedad Española de Medicina Interna (SEMI), Spain, grant number DN40585.

Acknowledgments: This research was funded by the Instituto de Salud Carlos III, Spain, grant number PIE14/00045. CIBER OBN is an initiative of the Instituto de Salud Carlos III, Spain.

Conflicts of Interest: R.E. reports serving on the board of and receiving lecture fees from the Research Foundation on Wine and Nutrition (FIVIN); serving on the boards of the Beer and Health Foundation and the European Foundation for Alcohol Research (ERAB); receiving lecture fees from Cerveceros de España and Sanofi-Aventis; and receiving grant support through his institution from Novartis. No other potential conflict of interest relevant to this article was reported.

References

1. Bruins, M.J.; Van Dael, P.; Eggersdorfer, M. The Role of Nutrients in Reducing the Risk for Noncommunicable Diseases during Aging. *Nutrients* **2019**, *11*, 85. [CrossRef] [PubMed]
2. Ford, E.S.; Bergmann, M.M.; Boeing, H.; Li, C.; Capewell, S. Healthy lifestyle behaviors and all-cause mortality among adults in the United States. *Prev. Med.* **2012**, *55*, 23–27. [CrossRef] [PubMed]
3. Loef, M.; Walach, H. The combined effects of healthy lifestyle behaviors on all cause mortality: A systematic review and meta-analysis. *Prev. Med.* **2012**, *55*, 163–170. [CrossRef] [PubMed]
4. Zhu, N.; Yu, C.; Guo, Y.; Bian, Z.; Han, Y.; Yang, L.; Chen, Y.; Du, H.; Li, H.; Liu, F.; et al. Adherence to a healthy lifestyle and all-cause and cause-specific mortality in Chinese adults: A 10-year prospective study of 0.5 million people. *Int. J. Behav. Nutr. Phys. Act.* **2019**, *16*, 98–113. [CrossRef] [PubMed]
5. Li, Y.; Schoufour, J.; Wang, D.D.; Dhana, K.; Pan, A.; Liu, X.; Song, M.; Liu, G.; Shin, H.J.; Sun, Q.; et al. Healthy lifestyle and life expectancy free of cancer, cardiovascular disease, and type 2 diabetes: Prospective cohort study. *BMJ* **2020**, *368*, l6669. [CrossRef]
6. Mozaffarian, D. Dietary and Policy Priorities for Cardiovascular Disease, Diabetes, and Obesity. *Circulation* **2016**, *133*, 187–225. [CrossRef]
7. Rodríguez González, M.; Loreto, M.; Marcos, T.; Marcos, F.M.; Sadek, I.M.; Roldan, C.C.; Tárraga López, P.J. Efectos de la dieta mediterránea sobre los factores de riesgo cardiovascular (Effects of the Mediterranean diet on the cardiovascular risk factors). *J. Negat. No Posit. Results* **2019**, *4*, 25–51. (In Spanish)
8. Estruch, R.; Ros, E.; Salas-Salvadó, J.; Covas, M.-I.; Corella, D.; Arós, F.; Gómez-Gracia, E.; Ruiz-Gutiérrez, V.; Fiol, M.; Lapetra, J.; et al. Primary Prevention of Cardiovascular Disease with a Mediterranean Diet Supplemented with Extra-Virgin Olive Oil or Nuts. *N. Engl. J. Med.* **2018**, *378*, e34. [CrossRef]
9. Odphp. *2015–2020 Dietary Guidelines for Americans*; Department of Agriculture (USDA) Department of Health and Human Services (HHS) Press: Washington, DC, USA, 2015.
10. Soltani, S.; Jayedi, A.; Shab-Bidar, S.; Becerra-Tomas, N.; Salas-Salvadó, J. Adherence to the Mediterranean Diet in Relation to All-Cause Mortality: A Systematic Review and Dose-Response Meta-Analysis of Prospective Cohort Studies. *Adv. Nutr.* **2019**, *10*, 1029–1039. [CrossRef] [PubMed]
11. Sofi, F.; Macchi, C.; Abbate, R.; Gensini, G.F.; Casini, A. Mediterranean diet and health status: An updated meta-analysis and a proposal for a literature-based adherence score. *Public Heal. Nutr.* **2013**, *17*, 2769–2782. [CrossRef] [PubMed]

12. Martínez-González, M.A.; Gea, A.; Ruiz-Canela, M. The Mediterranean Diet and Cardiovascular Health. *Circ. Res.* **2019**, *124*, 779–798. [CrossRef] [PubMed]
13. Burton, R.; Sheron, N. No level of alcohol consumption improves health. *Lancet* **2018**, *392*, 987–988. [CrossRef]
14. World Health Organization. *Status Report on Alcohol Consumption, Harm and Policy Responses in 30 European Countries 2019*; WHO: Geneva, Switzerland, 2019.
15. Fedirko, V.; Tramacere, I.; Bagnardi, V.; Rota, M.; Scotti, L.; Islami, F.; Negri, E.; Straif, K.; Romieu, I.; La Vecchia, C.; et al. Alcohol drinking and colorectal cancer risk: An overall and dose–response meta-analysis of published studies. *Ann. Oncol.* **2011**, *22*, 1958–1972. [CrossRef] [PubMed]
16. Sharma, A. Tollefsbol Combinatorial Epigenetics Impact of Polyphenols and Phytochemicals in Cancer Prevention and Therapy. *Int. J. Mol. Sci.* **2019**, *20*, 4567.
17. Akinwumi, B.C.; Bordun, K.-A.M.; Anderson, H.D. Biological Activities of Stilbenoids. *Int. J. Mol. Sci.* **2018**, *19*, 792. [CrossRef]
18. Chen, W.; Jia, Z.; Pan, M.-H.; Babu, P.V.A. Natural Products for the Prevention of Oxidative Stress-Related Diseases: Mechanisms and Strategies. *Oxidative Med. Cell. Longev.* **2016**, *2016*, 1–2. [CrossRef] [PubMed]
19. Subedi, L.; Teli, M.K.; Lee, J.H.; Gaire, B.P.; Kim, M.-H.; Do, M.H. A Stilbenoid Isorhapontigenin as a Potential Anti-Cancer Agent against Breast Cancer through Inhibiting Sphingosine Kinases/Tubulin Stabilization. *Cancers* **2019**, *11*, 1947. [CrossRef]
20. Beetch, M.; Harandi-Zadeh, S.; Shen, K.; Stefanska, B. Stilbenoids as dietary regulators of the cancer epigenome. *Nutr. Epigenomics* **2019**, 353–370. [CrossRef]
21. Amor, S.; Châlons, P.; Aires, V.; Delmas, D. Polyphenol Extracts from Red Wine and Grapevine: Potential Effects on Cancers. *Diseases* **2018**, *6*, 106. [CrossRef]
22. Da Costa, D.C.F.; Rangel, L.P.; Martins-Dinis, M.M.D.D.C.; Ferretti, G.D.D.S.; Ferreira, V.F.; Silva, J.L. Anticancer Potential of Resveratrol, β-Lapachone and Their Analogues. *Molecules* **2020**, *25*, 893. [CrossRef]
23. Institute of Medicine. *Health and Behavior: Research, Practice, and P. Health and Behavior*; National Academies Press: Washington, DC, USA, 2001.
24. Matsushita, H.; Takaki, A. Alcohol and hepatocellular carcinoma. *BMJ Open Gastroenterol.* **2019**, *6*, e000260. [CrossRef] [PubMed]
25. Li, Y.; Pan, A.; Wang, D.D.; Liu, X.; Dhana, K.; Franco, O.H.; Kaptoge, S.; Di Angelantonio, E.; Stampfer, M.; Willett, W.C.; et al. Impact of Healthy Lifestyle Factors on Life Expectancies in the US Population. *Circulation* **2018**, *138*, 345–355. [CrossRef] [PubMed]
26. Hernández-Hernández, A.; Gea, A.; Ruíz-Canela, M.; Toledo, E.; Beunza, J.J.; Bes-Rastrollo, M.; Martinez-Gonzalez, M.A. Mediterranean Alcohol-Drinking Pattern and the Incidence of Cardiovascular Disease and Cardiovascular Mortality: The SUN Project. *Nutrients* **2015**, *7*, 9116–9126. [CrossRef]
27. Collins, S.E. Associations Between Socioeconomic Factors and Alcohol Outcomes. *Alcohol Res. Curr. Rev.* **2016**, *38*, 83–94.
28. Roerecke, M.; Kaczorowski, J.; Tobe, S.W.; Gmel, M.G.; Hasan, B.O.S.M.; Rehm, J. The effect of a reduction in alcohol consumption on blood pressure: A systematic review and meta-analysis. *Lancet Public Heal.* **2017**, *2*, e108–e120. [CrossRef]
29. Roerecke, M.; Tobe, S.W.; Kaczorowski, J.; Bacon, S.L.; Vafaei, A.; Hasan, O.S.M.; Krishnan, R.J.; Raifu, A.O.; Rehm, J. Sex-Specific Associations Between Alcohol Consumption and Incidence of Hypertension: A Systematic Review and Meta-Analysis of Cohort Studies. *J. Am. Hear. Assoc.* **2018**, *7*, e008202. [CrossRef]
30. Wood, A.M.; Kaptoge, S.; Butterworth, A.S.; Willeit, P.; Warnakula, S.; Bolton, T.; Paige, E.; Paul, D.S.; Sweeting, M.; Burgess, S.; et al. Risk thresholds for alcohol consumption: Combined analysis of individual-participant data for 599 912 current drinkers in 83 prospective studies. *Lancet* **2018**, *391*, 1513–1523. [CrossRef]
31. Kloner, R.A.; Rezkalla, S.H. To Drink or Not to Drink? That Is the Question. *Circulation* **2007**, *116*, 1306–1317. [CrossRef]
32. Rimm, E.B.; Ellison, R.C. Alcohol in the Mediterranean diet. *Am. J. Clin. Nutr.* **1995**, *61*, 1378S–1382S. [CrossRef]
33. Cavallini, G.; Straniero, S.; Donati, A.; Bergamini, E. Resveratrol requires red wine polyphenols for optimum antioxidant activity. *J. Nutr. Heal. Aging* **2015**, *20*, 540–545. [CrossRef]
34. Schwingshackl, L.; Schwedhelm, C.; Galbete, C.; Hoffmann, G. Adherence to Mediterranean Diet and Risk of Cancer: An Updated Systematic Review and Meta-Analysis. *Nutrients* **2017**, *9*, 1063. [CrossRef] [PubMed]

35. Snopek, L.; Mlček, J.; Sochorova, L.; Baron, M.; Hlavacova, I.; Jurikova, T.; Kizek, R.; Sedlackova, E.; Sochor, J. Contribution of Red Wine Consumption to Human Health Protection. *Molecules* **2018**, *23*, 1684. [CrossRef]
36. Banc, R.; Socaciu, C.; Miere, D.; Filip, L.; Cozma, A.; Stanciu, O.; Loghin, F. Benefits of Wine Polyphenols on Human Health: A Review. *Bull. Univ. Agric. Sci. Vet. Med. Cluj-Napoca Food Sci. Technol.* **2014**, *71*, 79–87. [CrossRef]
37. Latruffe, N.; Rifler, J.P. Wine and Vine Components and Health. *Diseases* **2019**, *7*, 30. [CrossRef] [PubMed]
38. Cordova, A.C.; E Sumpio, B. Polyphenols are medicine: Is it time to prescribe red wine for our patients? *Int. J. Angiol.* **2009**, *18*, 111–117. [CrossRef]
39. Mitrevska, K.; Grigorakis, S.; Loupassaki, S.; Calokerinos, A. Antioxidant Activity and Polyphenolic Content of North Macedonian Wines. *Appl. Sci.* **2020**, *10*, 2010. [CrossRef]
40. Chiva-Blanch, G.; Badimon, L. Benefits and Risks of Moderate Alcohol Consumption on Cardiovascular Disease: Current Findings and Controversies. *Nutrients* **2019**, *12*, 108. [CrossRef] [PubMed]
41. National Institute of Alcohol Abuse and Alcoholism (NIAAA). What Is A Standard Drink? Available online: https://www.niaaa.nih.gov/what-standard-drink (accessed on 27 September 2020).
42. Monico, N. Alcohol by Volume (ABV): Beer, Wine, & Liquor. Available online: https://www.alcohol.org/statistics-information/abv/ (accessed on 24 October 2020).
43. International Agency for Research on Cancer. Personal Habits and Indoor Combustions. Volume 100 E. A review of human carcinogens. In *IARC Monographs on the Evaluation of Carcinogenic Risks to Humans*; International Agency for Research on Cancer: Geneva, Switzerland, 2012; Volume 100 Pt E, pp. 1–538. ISBN 9789283213222.
44. Piano, M.R. Alcohol's Effects on the Cardiovascular System. *Alcohol Res. Curr. Rev.* **2017**, *38*, 219–241.
45. Klatsky, A.L. Alcohol and cardiovascular diseases: Where do we stand today? *J. Intern. Med.* **2015**, *278*, 238–250. [CrossRef] [PubMed]
46. Matsumoto, C.; Miedema, M.D.; Ofman, P.; Gaziano, J.M.; Sesso, H.D. An Expanding Knowledge of the Mechanisms and Effects of Alcohol Consumption on Cardiovascular Disease. *J. Cardiopulm. Rehabil. Prev.* **2014**, *34*, 159–171. [CrossRef]
47. Davis, C.; Bryan, J.; Hodgson, J.M.; Murphy, K.J. Definition of the Mediterranean Diet; A Literature Review. *Nutrients* **2015**, *7*, 9139–9153. [CrossRef] [PubMed]
48. World Health Organization. Global Status Report on Alcohol and Health. 2018. Available online: https://www.who.int/publications/i/item/global-status-report-on-alcohol-and-health-2018 (accessed on 27 September 2020).
49. O'Keefe, E.L.; DiNicolantonio, J.J.; O'Keefe, J.H.; Lavie, C.J. Alcohol and CV Health: Jekyll and Hyde J-Curves. *Prog. Cardiovasc. Dis.* **2018**, *61*, 68–75. [CrossRef]
50. Chiva-Blanch, G.; Arranz, S.; Lamuela-Raventos, R.M.; Estruch, R. Effects of Wine, Alcohol and Polyphenols on Cardiovascular Disease Risk Factors: Evidences from Human Studies. *Alcohol Alcohol.* **2013**, *48*, 270–277. [CrossRef]
51. Antai, D.; Lopez, G.B.; Antai, J.; Anthony, D.S. Alcohol Drinking Patterns and Differences in Alcohol-Related Harm: A Population-Based Study of the United States. *Biomed Res. Int.* **2014**, *2014*, 1–11. [CrossRef] [PubMed]
52. Yoo, Y.J.; Saliba, A.J.; Prenzler, P.D. Should Red Wine Be Considered a Functional Food? *Compr. Rev. Food Sci. Food Saf.* **2010**, *9*, 530–551. [CrossRef]
53. Chaiyasong, S.; Huckle, T.; Mackintosh, A.-M.; Meier, P.; Parry, C.D.H.; Callinan, S.; Cuong, P.V.; Kazantseva, E.; Gray-Phillip, G.; Parker, K.; et al. Drinking patterns vary by gender, age and country-level income: Cross-country analysis of the International Alcohol Control Study. *Drug Alcohol Rev.* **2018**, *37*, S53–S62. [CrossRef] [PubMed]
54. Sumby, K.M.; Grbin, P.R.; Jiranek, V. Microbial modulation of aromatic esters in wine: Current knowledge and future prospects. *Food Chem.* **2010**, *121*, 1–16. [CrossRef]
55. Markoski, M.M.; Garavaglia, J.; Oliveira, A.; Olivaes, J.; Marcadenti, A. Molecular Properties of Red Wine Compounds and Cardiometabolic Benefits. *Nutr. Metab. Insights* **2016**, *9*, 51–57. [CrossRef]
56. Sánchez-Palomo, E.; García-Carpintero, E.G.; Viñas, M.G. Aroma Fingerprint Characterisation of La Mancha Red Wines. *S. Afr. J. Enol. Vitic.* **2015**, *36*, 36. [CrossRef]
57. Villamor, R.R.; Ross, C.F. Wine Matrix Compounds Affect Perception of Wine Aromas. *Annu. Rev. Food Sci. Technol.* **2013**, *4*, 1–20. [CrossRef]
58. Fairbairn, S.; Smit, A.; Jacobson, D.; Prior, B.; Bauer, F. Environmental Stress and Aroma Production During Wine Fermentation. *S. Afr. J. Enol. Vitic.* **2016**, *35*, 168–177. [CrossRef]
59. Zhu, F.; Du, B.; Li, J. Aroma Compounds in Wine. In *Grape and Wine Biotechnology*; IntechOpen: Rijeka, Croatia, 2016.

60. Rapp, A.; Mandery, H. Wine aroma. *Cell. Mol. Life Sci.* **1986**, *42*, 873–884. [CrossRef]
61. Gil, J.; Mateo, J.J.; Jimenez, M.; Pastor, A.; Huerta, T. Aroma Compounds in Wine as Influenced by Apiculate Yeasts. *J. Food Sci.* **1996**, *61*, 1247–1250. [CrossRef]
62. Payling, L.; Fraser, K.; Loveday, S.; Sims, I.; Roy, N.; McNabb, W. The effects of carbohydrate structure on the composition and functionality of the human gut microbiota. *Trends Food Sci. Technol.* **2020**, *97*, 233–248. [CrossRef]
63. Apolinar-Valiente, R.; Williams, P.; Doco, T. Recent advances in the knowledge of wine oligosaccharides. *Food Chem.* **2020**, 128330. [CrossRef] [PubMed]
64. Kapoor, S.; Dharmesh, S.M. Pectic Oligosaccharide from tomato exhibiting anticancer potential on a gastric cancer cell line: Structure-Function relationship. *Carbohydr. Polym.* **2017**, *160*, 52–61. [CrossRef] [PubMed]
65. Coelho, E.; Rocha, M.A.M.; Saraiva, J.A.; Coimbra, M.A. Microwave superheated water and dilute alkali extraction of brewers' spent grain arabinoxylans and arabinoxylo-oligosaccharides. *Carbohydr. Polym.* **2014**, *99*, 415–422. [CrossRef]
66. Kang, O.L.; Ghani, M.; Hassan, O.; Rahmati, S.; Ramli, N. Novel agaro-oligosaccharide production through enzymatic hydrolysis: Physicochemical properties and antioxidant activities. *Food Hydrocoll.* **2014**, *42*, 304–308. [CrossRef]
67. Cincotta, F.; Verzera, A.; Tripodi, G.; Condurso, C. Determination of Sesquiterpenes in Wines by HS-SPME Coupled with GC-MS. *Chromatography* **2015**, *2*, 410–421. [CrossRef]
68. Li, Z.; Howell, K.; Fang, Z.; Zhang, P. Sesquiterpenes in grapes and wines: Occurrence, biosynthesis, functionality, and influence of winemaking processes. *Compr. Rev. Food Sci. Food Saf.* **2019**, *19*, 247–281. [CrossRef]
69. Fernandes, E.S.; Passos, G.F.; Medeiros, R.; Da Cunha, F.M.; Ferreira, J.; Campos, M.M.; Pianowski, L.F.; Calixto, J.B. Anti-inflammatory effects of compounds alpha-humulene and (−)-trans-caryophyllene isolated from the essential oil of Cordia verbenacea. *Eur. J. Pharm.* **2007**, *569*, 228–236. [CrossRef]
70. Tatman, D.; Mo, H. Volatile isoprenoid constituents of fruits, vegetables and herbs cumulatively suppress the proliferation of murine B16 melanoma and human HL-60 leukemia cells. *Cancer Lett.* **2002**, *175*, 129–139. [CrossRef]
71. Giovinazzo, G.; Carluccio, M.A.; Grieco, F. Wine Polyphenols and Health. *Refer. Ser. Phytochem.* **2019**, *2019*, 1135–1155.
72. Mudnic, I.; Modun, D.; Rastija, V.; Vukovic, J.; Brizić, I.; Katalinic, V.; Kozina, B.; Medić-Šarić, M.; Boban, M. Antioxidative and vasodilatory effects of phenolic acids in wine. *Food Chem.* **2010**, *119*, 1205–1210. [CrossRef]
73. Vauzour, D.; Houseman, E.J.; George, T.; Corona, G.; Garnotel, R.; Jackson, K.G.; Sellier, C.; Gillery, P.; Kennedy, O.B.; Lovegrove, J.A.; et al. Moderate Champagne consumption promotes an acute improvement in acute endothelial-independent vascular function in healthy human volunteers. *Br. J. Nutr.* **2009**, *103*, 1168–1178. [CrossRef] [PubMed]
74. Eun, H.J.; Sung, R.K.; In, K.H.; Tae, Y.H. Hypoglycemic effects of a phenolic acid fraction of rice bran and ferulic acid in C57BL/KsJ-db/db mice. *J. Agric. Food Chem.* **2007**, *55*, 9800–9804.
75. Niimi, J.; Parker, M.; Smith, P.A. Flavonol composition of Australian red and white wines determined by high-performance liquid chromatography. *Aust. J. Grape Wine Res.* **2008**, *14*, 153–161. [CrossRef]
76. Guerrero, R.F.; García-Parrilla, M.C.; Puertas, B.; Cantos-Villar, E. Wine, Resveratrol and Health: A Review. *Nat. Prod. Commun.* **2009**, *4*, 635–658. [CrossRef]
77. Russo, M.; Spagnuolo, C.; Tedesco, I.; Bilotto, S.; Russo, G.L. The flavonoid quercetin in disease prevention and therapy: Facts and fancies. *Biochem. Pharm.* **2012**, *83*, 6–15. [CrossRef]
78. Hui, C.; Qi, X.; Qianyong, Z.; Xiaoli, P.; Jundong, Z.; Mantian, M. Flavonoids, Flavonoid Subclasses and Breast Cancer Risk: A Meta-Analysis of Epidemiologic Studies. *PLoS ONE* **2013**, *8*, e54318. [CrossRef]
79. Bo, Y.; Sun, J.; Wang, M.; Ding, J.; Lu, Q.; Yuan, L. Dietary flavonoid intake and the risk of digestive tract cancers: A systematic review and meta-analysis. *Sci. Rep.* **2016**, *6*, 24836. [CrossRef]
80. Wang, X.; Ouyang, Y.Y.; Liu, J.; Zhao, G. Flavonoid intake and risk of CVD: A systematic review and meta-analysis of prospective cohort studies. *Br. J. Nutr.* **2013**, *111*, 1–11. [CrossRef] [PubMed]
81. Kim, Y.; Je, Y. Flavonoid intake and mortality from cardiovascular disease and all causes: A meta-analysis of prospective cohort studies. *Clin. Nutr. Espen* **2017**, *20*, 68–77. [CrossRef] [PubMed]
82. Mateus, N.; Machado, J.M.; De Freitas, V. Development changes of anthocyanins in Vitis vinifera grapes grown in the Douro Valley and concentration in respective wines. *J. Sci. Food Agric.* **2002**, *82*, 1689–1695. [CrossRef]
83. Georgiev, V.; Ananga, A.; Tsolova, V. Recent Advances and Uses of Grape Flavonoids as Nutraceuticals. *Nutrients* **2014**, *6*, 391–415. [CrossRef] [PubMed]

84. Manach, C.; Williamson, G.; Morand, C.; Scalbert, A.; Rémésy, C. Bioavailability and bioefficacy of polyphenols in humans. I. Review of 97 bioavailability studies. *Am. J. Clin. Nutr.* **2005**, *81*, 230S–242S. [CrossRef]
85. Azzini, E.; Giacometti, J.; Russo, G.L. Antiobesity Effects of Anthocyanins in Preclinical and Clinical Studies. *Oxid. Med. Cell. Longev.* **2017**, *2017*, 1–11. [CrossRef]
86. Weisel, T.; Baum, M.; Eisenbrand, G.; Dietrich, H.; Will, F.; Stockis, J.-P.; Kulling, S.; Rüfer, C.; Johannes, C.; Janzowski, C. An anthocyanin/polyphenolic-rich fruit juice reduces oxidative DNA damage and increases glutathione level in healthy probands. *Biotechnol. J.* **2006**, *1*, 388–397. [CrossRef]
87. Erlund, I. Review of the flavonoids quercetin, hesperetin, and naringenin. Dietary sources, bioactivities, bioavailability, and epidemiology. *Nutr. Res.* **2004**, *24*, 851–874. [CrossRef]
88. Forester, S.C.; Waterhouse, A.L. Metabolites Are Key to Understanding Health Effects of Wine Polyphenolics. *J. Nutr.* **2009**, *139*, 1824S–1831S. [CrossRef]
89. Zhu, L.; Zhang, Y.; Lu, J. Phenolic Contents and Compositions in Skins of Red Wine Grape Cultivars among Various Genetic Backgrounds and Originations. *Int. J. Mol. Sci.* **2012**, *13*, 3492–3510. [CrossRef]
90. Berman, A.Y.; Motechin, R.A.; Wiesenfeld, M.Y.; Holz, M.K. The therapeutic potential of resveratrol: A review of clinical trials. *NPJ Precis. Oncol.* **2017**, *1*, 1–9. [CrossRef]
91. Reinisalo, M.; Kårlund, A.; Koskela, A.; Kaarniranta, K.; Karjalainen, R.O. Polyphenol Stilbenes: Molecular Mechanisms of Defence against Oxidative Stress and Aging-Related Diseases. *Oxidative Med. Cell. Longev.* **2015**, *2015*, 1–24. [CrossRef]
92. Potì, F.; Santi, D.; Spaggiari, G.; Zimetti, F.; Zanotti, I. Polyphenol Health Effects on Cardiovascular and Neurodegenerative Disorders: A Review and Meta-Analysis. *Int. J. Mol. Sci.* **2019**, *20*, 351. [CrossRef] [PubMed]
93. Parker, J.A.; Arango, M.; Abderrahmane, S.; Lambert, E.; Tourette, C.; Catoire, H.; Néri, C. Resveratrol rescues mutant polyglutamine cytotoxicity in nematode and mammalian neurons. *Nat. Genet.* **2005**, *37*, 349–350. [CrossRef]
94. Fernández-Mar, M.I.; Mateos, R.; García-Parrilla, M.C.; Puertas, B.; Villar, E.C. Bioactive compounds in wine: Resveratrol, hydroxytyrosol and melatonin: A review. *Food Chem.* **2012**, *130*, 797–813. [CrossRef]
95. Liu, Y.; Ma, W.; Zhang, P.; He, S.; Huang, D. Effect of resveratrol on blood pressure: A meta-analysis of randomized controlled trials. *Clin. Nutr.* **2015**, *34*, 27–34. [CrossRef] [PubMed]
96. Hausenblas, H.A.; Schoulda, J.A.; Smoliga, J.M. Resveratrol treatment as an adjunct to pharmacological management in type 2 diabetes mellitus-systematic review and meta-analysis. *Mol. Nutr. Food Res.* **2014**, *59*, 147–159. [CrossRef] [PubMed]
97. Feringa, H.H.; Laskey, D.A.; Dickson, J.E.; Coleman, C.I. The Effect of Grape Seed Extract on Cardiovascular Risk Markers: A Meta-Analysis of Randomized Controlled Trials. *J. Am. Diet. Assoc.* **2011**, *111*, 1173–1181. [CrossRef] [PubMed]
98. Grosso, G.; Stepaniak, U.; Micek, A.; Kozela, M.; Stefler, D.; Bobak, M.; Pajak, A. Dietary polyphenol intake and risk of type 2 diabetes in the Polish arm of the Health, Alcohol and Psychosocial factors in Eastern Europe (HAPIEE) study. *Br. J. Nutr.* **2017**, *118*, 60–68. [CrossRef]
99. Rienks, J.; Barbaresko, J.; Oluwagbemigun, K.; Schmid, M.; Nöthlings, U. Polyphenol exposure and risk of type 2 diabetes: Dose-Response meta-analyses and systematic review of prospective cohort studies. *Am. J. Clin. Nutr.* **2018**, *108*, 49–61. [CrossRef]
100. D'Archivio, M.; Filesi, C.; Varì, R.; Scazzocchio, B.; Masella, R. Bioavailability of the Polyphenols: Status and Controversies. *Int. J. Mol. Sci.* **2010**, *11*, 1321–1342. [CrossRef] [PubMed]
101. Castro-Barquero, S.; Lamuela-Raventós, R.M.; Doménech, M.; Estruch, R. Relationship between Mediterranean Dietary Polyphenol Intake and Obesity. *Nutrients* **2018**, *10*, 1523. [CrossRef]
102. Corrêa, T.A.F.; Rogero, M.M.; Hassimotto, N.M.A.; Lajolo, F.M. The Two-Way Polyphenols-Microbiota Interactions and Their Effects on Obesity and Related Metabolic Diseases. *Front. Nutr.* **2019**, *6*, 188. [CrossRef]
103. Alldritt, I.; Whitham-Agut, B.; Sipin, M.; Studholme, J.; Trentacoste, A.; Tripp, J.A.; Cappai, M.G.; Ditchfield, P.; Devièse, T.; Hedges, R.E.M.; et al. Metabolomics reveals diet-derived plant polyphenols accumulate in physiological bone. *Sci. Rep.* **2019**, *9*, 1–12. [CrossRef] [PubMed]
104. Gepner, Y.; Henkin, Y.; Schwarzfuchs, D.; Golan, R.; Durst, R.; Shelef, I.; Harman-Boehm, I.; Spitzen, S.; Witkow, S.; Novack, L.; et al. Differential Effect of Initiating Moderate Red Wine Consumption on 24-h Blood Pressure by Alcohol Dehydrogenase Genotypes: Randomized Trial in Type 2 Diabetes. *Am. J. Hypertens.* **2015**, *29*, 476–483. [CrossRef]

105. Mori, T.A.; Burke, V.; Zilkens, R.R.; Hodgson, J.M.; Beilin, L.J.; Puddey, I.B. The effects of alcohol on ambulatory blood pressure and other cardiovascular risk factors in type 2 diabetes. *J. Hypertens.* **2016**, *34*, 421–428. [CrossRef] [PubMed]
106. McDonagh, S.T.; Wylie, L.J.; Morgan, P.T.; Vanhatalo, A.; Jones, A.M. A randomised controlled trial exploring the effects of different beverages consumed alongside a nitrate-rich meal on systemic blood pressure. *Nutr. Heal.* **2018**, *24*, 183–192. [CrossRef] [PubMed]
107. Roth, I.; Casas, R.; Ribó-Coll, M.; Estruch, R. Consumption of Aged White Wine under a Veil of Flor Reduces Blood Pressure-Increasing Plasma Nitric Oxide in Men at High Cardiovascular Risk. *Nutrients* **2019**, *11*, 1266. [CrossRef]
108. García-Conesa, M.T.; Chambers, K.; Combet, E.; Pinto, P.; Garcia-Aloy, M.; Andres-Lacueva, C.; De Pascual-Teresa, S.; Mena, P.; Ristic, A.K.; Hollands, W.J.; et al. Meta-Analysis of the Effects of Foods and Derived Products Containing Ellagitannins and Anthocyanins on Cardiometabolic Biomarkers: Analysis of Factors Influencing Variability of the Individual Responses. *Int. J. Mol. Sci.* **2018**, *19*, 694. [CrossRef]
109. Weaver, S.R.; Rendeiro, C.; McGettrick, H.M.; Philp, A.; Lucas, S.J.E. Fine wine or sour grapes? A systematic review and meta-analysis of the impact of red wine polyphenols on vascular health. *Eur. J. Nutr.* **2020**, *2020*. [CrossRef]
110. Ye, J.; Chen, X.; Bao, L. Effects of wine on blood pressure, glucose parameters, and lipid profile in type 2 diabetes mellitus. *Medicine* **2019**, *98*, e15771. [CrossRef]
111. Gepner, Y.; Golan, R.; Harman-Boehm, I.; Henkin, Y.; Schwarzfuchs, D.; Shelef, I.; Durst, R.; Kovsan, J.; Bolotin, A.; Leitersdorf, E.; et al. Effects of Initiating Moderate Alcohol Intake on Cardiometabolic Risk in Adults With Type 2 Diabetes. *Ann. Intern. Med.* **2015**, *163*, 569–579. [CrossRef]
112. Abraham, K.A.; Kearney, M.L.; Reynolds, L.J.; Thyfault, J.P. Red wine enhances glucose-dependent insulinotropic peptide (GIP) and insulin responses in type 2 diabetes during an oral glucose tolerance test. *Diabetol. Int.* **2015**, *7*, 173–180. [CrossRef] [PubMed]
113. Huang, J.; Wang, X.; Zhang, Y. Specific types of alcoholic beverage consumption and risk of type 2 diabetes: A systematic review and meta-analysis. *J. Diabetes Investig.* **2016**, *8*, 56–68. [CrossRef] [PubMed]
114. Woerdeman, J.; Del Rio, D.; Calani, L.; Eringa, E.C.; Smulders, Y.M.; Serné, E.H. Red wine polyphenols do not improve obesity-associated insulin resistance: A randomized controlled trial. *Diabetes Obes. Metab.* **2017**, *20*, 206–210. [CrossRef] [PubMed]
115. Golan, R.; Shai, I.; Gepner, Y.; Harman-Boehm, I.; Schwarzfuchs, D.; Spence, J.D.; Párraga, G.; Buchanan, D.; Witkow, S.; Friger, M.; et al. Effect of wine on carotid atherosclerosis in type 2 diabetes: A 2-year randomized controlled trial. *Eur. J. Clin. Nutr.* **2018**, *72*, 871–878. [CrossRef]
116. Taborsky, M.; Ostadal, P.; Adam, T.; Moravec, O.; Gloger, V.; Schee, A.; Skála, T. Red or white wine consumption effect on atherosclerosis in healthy individuals (In Vino Veritas study). *Bratisl. Med. J.* **2017**, *118*, 292–298. [CrossRef]
117. Di Renzo, L.; Cioccoloni, G.; Salimei, P.S.; Ceravolo, I.; De Lorenzo, A.; Gratteri, S. Alcoholic Beverage and Meal Choices for the Prevention of Noncommunicable Diseases: A Randomized Nutrigenomic Trial. *Oxidative Med. Cell. Longev.* **2018**, *2018*, 1–13. [CrossRef]
118. Fang, X.; Wei, J.; He, X.; An, P.; Wang, H.; Jiang, L.; Shao, D.; Liang, H.; Li, Y.; Wang, F.; et al. Landscape of dietary factors associated with risk of gastric cancer: A systematic review and dose-response meta-analysis of prospective cohort studies. *Eur. J. Cancer* **2015**, *51*, 2820–2832. [CrossRef]
119. Chen, J.-Y.; Zhu, H.-C.; Guo, Q.; Shu, Z.; Bao, X.-H.; Sun, F.; Qin, Q.; Yang, X.; Zhang, C.; Cheng, H.-Y.; et al. Dose-Dependent Associations between Wine Drinking and Breast Cancer Risk—Meta-Analysis Findings. *Asian Pac. J. Cancer Prev.* **2016**, *17*, 1221–1233. [CrossRef] [PubMed]
120. Vartolomei, M.; Kimura, S.; Ferro, M.; Foerster, B.; Abufaraj, M.; Briganti, A.; Karakiewicz, P.I.; Shariat, S.F. The impact of moderate wine consumption on the risk of developing prostate cancer. *Clin. Epidemiol.* **2018**, *10*, 431–444. [CrossRef]
121. Xu, W.; Fan, H.; Han, Z.; Liu, Y.; Wang, Y.; Ge, Z. Wine consumption and colorectal cancer risk. *Eur. J. Cancer Prev.* **2019**, *28*, 151–158. [CrossRef] [PubMed]
122. Xu, W.; Wang, H.; Wan, Y.; Tan, C.; Li, J.; Tan, L.; Yu, J.-T. Alcohol consumption and dementia risk: A dose–response meta-analysis of prospective studies. *Eur. J. Epidemiol.* **2017**, *32*, 31–42. [CrossRef] [PubMed]
123. Moreira, L.B.; Fuchs, F.D.; Moraes, R.S.; Bredemeier, M.; Duncan, B.B. Alcohol intake and blood pressure. *J. Hypertens.* **1998**, *16*, 175–180. [CrossRef] [PubMed]

124. Rocha, B.S.; Gago, B.; Barbosa, R.M.; Cavaleiro, C.; Rocha, B.S. Ethyl nitrite is produced in the human stomach from dietary nitrate and ethanol, releasing nitric oxide at physiological pH: Potential impact on gastric motility. *Free Radic. Biol. Med.* **2015**, *82*, 160–166. [CrossRef]
125. Álvarez, E.; Rodiño-Janeiro, B.K.; Jerez, M.; Ucieda-Somoza, R.; Núñez, M.J.; González-Juanatey, J.R. Procyanidins from grape pomace are suitable inhibitors of human endothelial NADPH oxidase. *J. Cell. Biochem.* **2012**, *113*, 1386–1396. [CrossRef]
126. Elies, J.; Cuíñas, A.; García-Morales, V.; Orallo, F.; Campos-Toimil, M. Trans-resveratrol simultaneously increases cytoplasmic Ca2+ levels and nitric oxide release in human endothelial cells. *Mol. Nutr. Food Res.* **2011**, *55*, 1237–1248. [CrossRef]
127. Hodge, A.M.; English, D.R.; O'Dea, K.; Giles, G.G. Alcohol intake, consumption pattern and beverage type, and the risk of Type 2 diabetes. *Diabet. Med.* **2006**, *23*, 690–697. [CrossRef]
128. Wannamethee, S.G.; Camargo, C.A.; Manson, J.E.; Willett, W.C.; Rimm, E.B. Alcohol Drinking Patterns and Risk of Type 2 Diabetes Mellitus Among Younger Women. *Arch. Intern. Med.* **2003**, *163*, 1329–1336. [CrossRef]
129. Grønbaek, M. Alcohol, Type of Alcohol, and All-Cause and Coronary Heart Disease Mortality. *Ann. N. Y. Acad. Sci.* **2002**, *957*, 16–20. [CrossRef] [PubMed]
130. Liu, L.; Wang, Y.; Lam, K.S.; Xu, A. Moderate wine consumption in the prevention of metabolic syndrome and its related medical complications. *Endocr. Metab. Immune Disord. Drug Targets* **2008**, *8*, 89–98. [CrossRef] [PubMed]
131. Nova, E.; Martin, I.S.M.; Díaz, L.E.; Marcos, A. Wine and beer within a moderate alcohol intake is associated with higher levels of HDL-c and adiponectin. *Nutr. Res.* **2018**, *63*, 42–50. [CrossRef]
132. Yıldırım, H.K.; Akçay, Y.D.; Güvenc, U.; Sözmen, E.Y. Protection capacity against low-density lipoprotein oxidation and antioxidant potential of some organic and non-organic wines. *Int. J. Food Sci. Nutr.* **2004**, *55*, 351–362. [CrossRef]
133. Muñoz-González, I.; Espinosa-Martos, I.; Rodríguez, J.M.; Jiménez-Girón, A.; Martín-Álvarez, P.J.; Bartolomé, B.; Moreno-Arribas, M.V. Moderate Consumption of Red Wine Can Modulate Human Intestinal Inflammatory Response. *J. Agric. Food Chem.* **2014**, *62*, 10567–10575. [CrossRef]
134. Anand, P.; Kunnumakara, A.B.; Sundaram, C.; Harikumar, K.B.; Tharakan, S.T.; Lai, O.S.; Sung, B.; Aggarwal, B.B. Expert Review Cancer is a Preventable Disease that Requires Major Lifestyle Changes. *Pharm. Res.* **2008**, *25*, 2097–2116. [CrossRef] [PubMed]
135. Caprio, G.G.; Picascia, D.; Dallio, M.; Vitiello, P.P.; Giunta, E.F.; De Falco, V.; Abenavoli, L.; Procopio, A.C.; Famiglietti, V.; Martinelli, E.; et al. Light Alcohol Drinking and the Risk of Cancer Development: A Controversial Relationship. *Rev. Recent Clin. Trials* **2020**, *15*, 164–177. [CrossRef]
136. Iii, G.A.E.; Gamez, N.G.E., Jr.; Calderon, O.; Moreno-Gonzalez, I. Modifiable Risk Factors for Alzheimer's Disease. *Front. Aging Neurosci.* **2019**, *11*, 146. [CrossRef]
137. Barbagallo, M.; Barbagallo, M. Nutritional prevention of cognitive decline and dementia. *Acta Biomed.* **2018**, *89*, 276–290.

Publisher's Note: MDPI stays neutral with regard to jurisdictional claims in published maps and institutional affiliations.

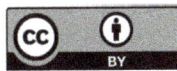

© 2020 by the authors. Licensee MDPI, Basel, Switzerland. This article is an open access article distributed under the terms and conditions of the Creative Commons Attribution (CC BY) license (http://creativecommons.org/licenses/by/4.0/).

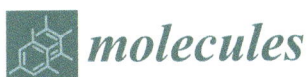

Review

Wine's Phenolic Compounds and Health: A Pythagorean View

Francesco Visioli [1,2,*], Stefan-Alexandru Panaite [1] and Joao Tomé-Carneiro [2]

1. Department of Molecular Medicine, University of Padova, Viale G. Colombo 3, 35121 Padova, Italy; stefan.panaite@outlook.it
2. IMDEA-Food, CEI UAM + CSIC, 28049 Madrid, Spain; joao.estevao@imdea.org
* Correspondence: francesco.visioli@unipd.it

Academic Editors: Paula Silva and Norbert Latruffe
Received: 14 August 2020; Accepted: 5 September 2020; Published: 8 September 2020

Abstract: In support of the J curve that describes the association between wine consumption and all-cause mortality, researchers and the lay press often advocate the health benefits of (poly)phenol consumption via red wine intake and cite the vast amount of in vitro literature that would corroborate the hypothesis. Other researchers dismiss such evidence and call for total abstention. In this review, we take a skeptical, Pythagorean stance and we critically try to move the debate forward by pointing the readers to the many pitfalls of red wine (poly)phenol research, which we arbitrarily treat as if they were pharmacological agents. We conclude that, after 30 years of dedicated research and despite the considerable expenditure, we still lack solid, "pharmacological", human evidence to confirm wine (poly)phenols' biological actions. Future research will eventually clarify their activities and will back the current recommendations of responsibly drinking moderate amounts of wine with meals.

Keywords: wine; polyphenols; flavonoids; diet; clinical trials; metabolites

1. Introduction

The association between alcohol consumption and health follows a J-shaped curve [1]. Moderate alcohol use is associated with better prognosis and lower all-cause death, whereas excessive intake is detrimental to human health [1]. The mechanisms underlying the protective effects of moderate alcohol consumption are under investigation and mostly involve reduced plasminogen levels and lower thrombogenicity observed in moderate drinkers vs. abstainers [1]. Some authors propose the superiority of wine, namely red wine over other alcoholic beverages and attribute such advantage to the (poly)phenolic components of red wine [2]. Even though this notion is not fully proven and is, conversely, often challenged [2], much research is being performed to elucidate the purported biochemical mechanisms through which wine (poly)phenols would afford better health, in particular by lowering cardiovascular risk. The debate on alcohol use and health is becoming heavily polarized: one party underscores a large amount of data in support of the J curve [1,3] whereas the other side dismisses such evidence and calls for total abstention [2,3]. In support of the former, researchers and the lay press often advocate the health benefits of (poly)phenol consumption via red wine intake and cite the vast amount of in vitro literature that would corroborate the hypothesis [4,5].

In this review, we take a skeptical, Pythagorean stance and we critically try to move the debate forward by pointing the readers to the many pitfalls of red wine (poly)phenol research, which we arbitrarily treat as if they were pharmacological agents.

2. Phenolic Compounds and Health

Diet and nutrition are essential to promote and maintain good health throughout life and for many years they have been known to be of crucial importance as risk factors for chronic diseases, making them essential components of prevention activities [6]. The consumption of foods derived from plant products such as wine, fruits, vegetables, nuts, cereals, legumes, spices and others integrated into the Mediterranean or the DASH diets [7], is associated with beneficial health effects and a protective role against the development and progression of diseases, such as cardiovascular disease (CVD) [8]. The ability of some plant-derived foods to reduce disease risk has been associated with the presence of non-nutrient secondary metabolites (phytochemicals) to which a wide variety of biological activities are attributed [9,10]. These metabolites have moderate potency as bioactive compounds and low bioavailability compared to drugs, but when ingested regularly and in significant amounts can have noticeable mid/long term physiological effects. Phytochemicals present in foods associated with a beneficial health effect include glucosinolates, terpenoids and a large group of phenolic compounds (anthocyanins, flavones, flavan-3-ol, stilbenes, etc.) collectively known as (poly)phenols [10,11].

3. Classification and Amounts of Wine Phenolic Compounds

Phenolic compounds have as a common characteristic in their chemical structure the presence of one or more hydroxyl groups attached to one or more aromatic or benzene rings. In general, phenolic compounds that contain more than one phenolic group are called polyphenols to distinguish them from simple phenolics. Typically, these compounds are found in a conjugate form with one or more sugar residues linked by β-glycosidic (O-glycosylated) bonds or by direct linkages of sugar to an aromatic ring carbon atom (C-glycosides) [12]. Phenolic compounds are grouped according to their chemical structure into two main categories, flavonoids and non-flavonoids, each comprising several sub-groups. In wine, sub-groups of flavonoids compounds include flavonols, flavononols (also known as dihydroflavonols), anthocyanins, flavan-3-ols, flavanones and flavones, while non-flavonoids contain hydroxycinnamic and hydroxybenzoic acids, and stilbenes (Table 1). (Poly)phenolic composition varies among different wines according to the type of grape used, vinification process used, type of yeast that participates in the fermentation, and whether grape solids are present in the maceration process [13]. For instance, in grapes, the composition in phenolic compounds is location-dependent, i.e., pulp, skin and seeds have different types and proportions of (poly)phenols; since red wines are exposed to all grape parts during the vinification process they contain more (poly)phenols than white wines, whose contents essentially originate from the pulp. In this sense, the minimum and maximum levels of total phenolic contents reported in a representative set of studies (expressed as the median (Q25–Q75) in mg of gallic acid equivalents (GAE) per liter) were 1531 (983–1898) and 3192 (2700–3624), and 210 (89–282) and 402 (347–434) for red and white wines, respectively (Table 2). The content of polyphenols in rosé wine is intermediate between red and white wines [14,15].

Table 1. Classification of phenolic compounds found in wine.

Group	Subgroup	Main Parent Compounds and Representative Derivatives	
Flavonoids	Flavonols	Kaempferol $R_1 = R_2 = H$ Myricetin $R_1 = R_2 = OH$ Quercetin $R_1 = OH, R_2 = H$	Quercetin-3-O-glucoside
	Flavan-3-ols	(+)-Catechin $R_1 = R_4 = R_5 = OH, R_2 = R_3 = H$ (−)-Epicatechin $R_1 = R_3 = R_5 = OH, R_2 = R_4 = H$	Procyanidin B1

Table 1. Cont.

Group	Subgroup	Main Parent Compounds and Representative Derivatives	
	Anthocyanins	Cyanidin R_1 = OH, R_2 = H Delphinidin R_1 = R_2 = OH Malvidin R_1 = R_2 = OCH$_3$ Peonidin R_1 = OCH$_3$, R_2 = H Petunidin R_1 = OH, R_2 = OCH$_3$	R_3=O-glycoside Malvidin 3-O-glucoside
	Flavanones	Naringenin R_1 = H, R_2 = OH Hesperetin R_1 = OH, R_2 = OCH$_3$	Naringenin 7-O-neohesperidoside
	Flavanolols	Dihydroquercetin R_1 = R_2 = OH Dihydromyricetin R_1 = R_2 = R_3 = OH	Dihydroquercetin 3-rhamnoside
	Flavones	Apigenin R_1 = H Luteolin R_1 = OH	Apigenin-7-glucoside
Non-flavonoids	Hydroxycinnamic acids	Caffeic acid R_1 = R_4 = H, R_2 = R_3 = OH Ferulic acid R_1 = R_4 = H, R_2 = OCH$_3$, R_3 = OH p-Coumaric acid R_1 = R_2 = R_4 = H, R_3 = OH o-Coumaric acid R_1 = OH, R_2 = R_3 = R_4 = H Sinapic acid R_1 = H, R_2 = R_4 = OCH$_3$, R_3 = OH	Caffeoyl tartaric acid
	Hydroxybenzoic acids	2,3-Dihydroxybenzoic acid R_1 = R_2 = H, R_3 = R_4 = OH 2-Hydroxybenzoic acid R_1 = R_2 = R_3 = H, R_4 = OH 4-Hydroxybenzoic acid R_1 = R_3 = R_4 = H, R_2 = OH Gallic acid R_1 = R_2 = R_3 = OH, R_4 = H Gentisic acid R_1 = R_4 = OH, R_3 = R_2 = H Syringic acid R_1 = R_3 = OCH$_3$, R_2 = OH, R_4 = H Protocatechuic acid R_1 = H, R_2 = R_3 = OH, R_4 = H Vanillic acid R_1 = H, R_2 = OH, R_3 = OCH$_3$, R_4 = H	Ethyl gallate
	Stilbenes	Resveratrol R_1 = R_2 = H, R_3 = OH Piceatannol R_1 = H, R_3-R_2 = OH trans-Resveratrol 3-O-glucoside	ε-Viniferin

Table 2. Range of total phenolic content in red and white wines in a representative set of studies.

	Red Wine			White Wine			
	Total Phenolic Content [a]			Total Phenolic Content [a]			
	Range			Range			
	Min.	Max.	n	Min.	Max.	n	Reference
	1615	4177	7	216	854	7	[16]
	1313	2389	16	89	407	17	[17]
	2193	3183	6	292	402	4	[18]
	622	3200	20	-	-	-	[19]
	1724	1936	5	282	434	5	[15]
	2340	3730	23	-	-	-	[20]
	1460	3380	39	210	390	47	[21]
	2082	3184	3	213	277	5	[22]
	1402	3180	24	189	425	11	[14]
	3200	5900	8	-	-	-	[23]
	1788	3070	4	55	370	20	[24]
	1012	3264	11	-	-	-	[25]
	554	2669	2	167	347	3	[26]
	1181	3589	23	-	-	-	[27]
	-	-	-	291	2103	14	[28]
	860	2710	8	-	-	-	[29]
	1602	1968	7	-	-	-	[30]
	1837	3467	6	-	-	-	[31]
	896	6319	38	77	83	2	[32]
Mean ± SD	1538 ± 664	3406 ± 1139		189 ± 85	554 ± 545		
Median (Q25–Q75)	1531 (983–1898)	3192 (2700–3624)		210 (89–282)	402 (347–434)		

[a] Data are expressed as gallic acid equivalents (GAE) in mg/L.

3.1. Flavonoids

Flavonoids have a skeleton with 15 carbon atoms and are represented in a C6-C3-C6 type system, where a benzene ring (designated as B) is joined (in most cases) to the C2 position of a γ-pyran type ring (C) included in a chromane ring (Table 1) [33]. The structure of flavonoids is shaped by different levels of hydroxylation, prenylation, alkalization or glycosylation reactions, which give rise to different sub-groups [34]. In plants, most flavonoids exist as glycosides in combination with monosaccharides such as glucose and rhamnose (most common), followed by galactose, xylose and arabinose [35].

3.2. Flavonols

Flavonols are characterized by a hydroxyl group in C3 (Table 1) and are often named 3-hydroxyflavones. These compounds are known to play a wide range of biological activities and are considered the main active compounds within the flavonoids group [36,37]. Flavonols and their glycosides are present in red and in white wines, influencing their color, taste, and health properties [38]. Flavonols in red wine include aglycons such as myricetin, quercetin, kaempferol, and rutin and their respective glycosides (glucosides, glucuronides, galactosides and diglycosides). Quercetin 3-O-glucoside is the most representative flavonol in wines [39]. Flavonol levels in red wine can reach over 150 mg/L (Table 3).

Table 3. (Poly)phenol contents in red and white wines.

		Red Wine						White Wine					
		Phenol Explorer [a]			USDA [b]			Phenol Explorer [a]			USDA [b]		
	Main representatives	mean	min	max	mean	min	max	mean	min	max	mean	min	max
Flavonoids														
Anthocyanins	Cyanidin [c]	2.9	0.6	11.9	1.9	0.0	45.0	-	-	-	-	-	-
	Delphinidin [c]	16.6	2.4	40.1	20.1	0.2	57.1	-	-	-	-	-	-
	Malvidin [c]	156	12.4	541	138	0.0	536	0.4	0.0	3.5	0.6	0.0	2.4
	Peodinin [c]	18.1	2.5	80.9	12.5	0.2	50.3	-	-	-	-	-	-
	Petunidin [c]	23.6	3.4	61.8	19.8	0.2	56.6	-	-	-	-	-	-
Total		217	21.3	736	193	0.6	745	0.4	0.0	3.5	0.6	0.0	2.4
Dihydroflavonols	Dihydromyricetin 3-O-rhamnoside	44.7	44.7	44.7	-	-	-	3.0	3.0	3.0	-	-	-
Total		54.4	45.8	59.8	-	-	-	5.7	3.7	15.9	-	-	-
Flavanos	(+)-Catechin	68.1	13.8	390	71.4	0.0	390	10.8	0.0	46.0	7.7	0.0	58.0
	(-)-Epicatechin	37.8	0.0	165	37.9	0.0	165	9.5	0.0	60.0	5.5	0.5	60.0
	Proanthocyanidins	355	99.7	560	296	63.1	1354	0.2	0.0	1.5	3.9	0.6	7.3
Total		470	114	1131	407	63.1	1917	20.8	0.0	109	17.1	1.1	125
Flavanones	Naringenin [c]	8.0	7.3	8.8	17.7	10.3	25.1	2.3	1.7	2.9	3.8	0.0	7.7
Total		8.5	7.8	9.4	24.0	13.0	35.0	2.3	1.7	2.9	7.8	3.2	12.5
Flavones	Apigenin	-	-	-	1.3	0.0	4.7	-	-	-	-	-	-
Total		-	-	-	1.7	0.0	8.7	-	-	-	-	-	-
Flavonos	Isorhamnetin [c]	5.9	1.7	11.6	0.2	0.0	1.6	0.0	0.0	0.0	0.0	0.0	0.2
	Kaempferol [c]	10.2	5.7	14.4	0.9	0.0	13.7	0.2	0.0	2.6	0.1	0.0	2.7
	Myricetin [c]	8.3	0.0	17.9	4.2	0.0	17.9	0.0	0.0	0.0	0.1	0.0	1.0
	Quercetin [c]	44.2	12.3	110	10.4	0.0	33.6	4.6	1.3	20.8	0.4	0.0	8.4
Total		68.6	19.7	154	15.7	0.0	66.8	4.8	1.3	23.4	0.5	0.0	9.4

Table 3. Cont.

		Red Wine						White Wine					
		Phenol Explorer [a]			USDA [b]			Phenol Explorer [a]			USDA [b]		
		mean	min	max	mean	min	max	mean	min	max	mean	min	max
Non-flavonoids														
Hydroxybenzoic acids	Gallic	35.9	0.0	126	NA	NA	NA	2.2	0.0	11.0	NA	NA	NA
	Gentisic	4.6	0.0	8.0	NA	NA	NA	18.2	0.0	20.0	NA	NA	NA
	Protocatechuic	1.7	0.0	9.6	NA	NA	NA	3.3	0.1	13.0	NA	NA	NA
	Syringic	2.7	0.0	23.3	NA	NA	NA	0.5	0.0	0.2	NA	NA	NA
	Vanillic	3.2	0.0	7.5	NA	NA	NA	0.4	0.1	1.2	NA	NA	NA
Total		70.1	13.7	221	NA	NA	NA	24.8	0.4	46.8	NA	NA	NA
Hydroxycinnamic acids	Caffeic	18.8	0.0	77.0	NA	NA	NA	2.4	0.0	7.0	NA	NA	NA
	Caftaric	33.5	1.4	179	NA	NA	NA	21.5	21.4	22.0	NA	NA	NA
	Ferulic	0.8	0.0	10.4	NA	NA	NA	0.9	0.3	2.1	NA	NA	NA
	(o- and p-) Coumaric	5.8	0.2	40.4	NA	NA	NA	1.8	0.0	5.6	NA	NA	NA
	Sinapic	0.7	0.0	5.4	NA	NA	NA	0.6	0.0	2.8	NA	NA	NA
Total		100	14.9	378	NA	NA	NA	28.2	21.7	42.4	NA	NA	NA
Stilbenes	Resveratrol [d]	5.8	0.0	61.5	NA	NA	NA	0.9	0.0	3.2	NA	NA	NA
	Resveratrol 3-O-glucoside [d]	12.5	0.0	88.0	NA	NA	NA	5.0	0.4	13.1	NA	NA	NA
	Piceatannol [c]	15.3	6.3	38.8	NA	NA	NA	4.6	1.4	8.0	NA	NA	NA
	Viniferins (δ-, ε-)	7.9	0.1	26.7	NA	NA	NA	0.6	0.0	0.1	NA	NA	NA
	Pallidol	2.0	0.0	2.5	NA	NA	NA	0.7	0.0	0.3	NA	NA	NA
Total		43.5	6.4	218	NA	NA	NA	10.6	1.4	24.7	NA	NA	NA
Other polyphenols	Hydroxybenzaldehydes	7.1	0.0	45.6	NA	NA	NA	4.1	2.4	5.8	NA	NA	NA
	Tyrosols	36.5	6.4	54.3	NA	NA	NA	4.2	2.7	5.7	NA	NA	NA
Total		43.6	6.4	99.9	NA	NA	NA	8.3	5.1	11.5	NA	NA	NA

[a] Data are expressed as milligrams of gallic acid equivalent per litter (mg/GAE/L). [b] Data are expressed as milligrams of gallic acid equivalent per kilogram (mg/GAE/Kg). [c] Plus glucoside derivatives. [d] includes both cis and trans conformations. NA, data not available in the database.

3.3. Flavan-3-Ols

Flavanols or flavan-3-ols are responsible for the astringency, bitterness, and structure of wines, and are found in important concentrations in red wine [40]. They are benzopyrans, having no double bond between C2 and C3, and no C4 carbonyl in Ring C. Furthermore, due to the hydroxylation at C3 flavanols have two chiral centers. (+)-Catechin (*trans* configuration) and (−)-epicatechin (*cis* configuration) are the two main flavan-3-ol isomers found in red wine, with average combined concentration over 100 mg/L (Table 3). Catechins usually occur as aglycones, or esterified with gallic acid, and can form polymers, which are often referred to as proanthocyanidins (or condensed tannins) because an acid-catalyzed cleavage of the polymeric chains produces anthocyanidins. Proanthocyanidins, which present an average concentration over 350 mg/L in red wine, include, for example, procyanidin dimers B1, B2, B3 and B4. Trimers such as procyanidin C1 (three epicatechins) have also been identified.

4. Anthocyanins

Anthocyanic pigments (anthocyanidins and anthocyanins) have a structure based on the flavylium cation (2-phenylbenzopyrylium). In fact, anthocyanins are anthocyanidin glycosides, being the corresponding aglycons (anthocyanidins) obtained by hydrolysis. The great variety of anthocyanins found in nature (more than 500 anthocyanins have been described) is characterized by the different hydroxylated groups, conjugated sugars and acyl moieties they present [41,42]. The main anthocyanidins found in red wine are malvidin (most abundant), petunidin, peonidin, delphinidin and cyanidin. Often anthocyanins are found linked (mainly in position 3) to one or more sugar molecules, usually glucose, and also to acyl substituents bound to sugars, aliphatic acids, and cinnamic acids. Anthocyanins can be present in amounts higher than 700 mg/L in red wine, whereas in white wine they are essentially absent (Table 3).

4.1. Flavanones

Flavanones, also known as dihydroflavones, lack the double bond between carbons 2 and 3 in the C-ring of the flavonoid skeleton. Some flavanones have unique substitution patterns, e.g., prenylated flavanones, furanoflavanones, pyranoflavanones, benzylated flavanones, resulting in a large number of derivatives of this subgroup. One of the main flavonones found in wine is naringenin at levels that can reach 25 mg/kg (Table 3).

4.2. Flavones

Flavones are characterized by absence of a hydroxyl group in the C3 position and a conjugated double bond between C2 and C3 in the flavonoid skeleton. Flavones and their 3-hydroxy derivatives flavonols, including their glycosides, methoxides and other acylated products on all three rings, make this the largest subgroup among all polyphenols. These compounds were found in grape skin and wine in both aglycones and glycosides forms. Apigenin, for example, has been described in red wine only in trace amounts (Table 3).

5. Non-Flavonoids

The non-flavonoid phenolic constituents in wine are divided into hydroxybenzoic acids and hydroxycinnamic acids, stilbenes and other miscellaneous compounds [43]. These phenolic compounds can reach levels that range from 60 to 566 mg/L [44].

6. Hydroxycinnamic Acids

Hydroxycinnamic acids are the foremost group of phenolic compounds in grapes and wine [45]. Caffeic, coumaric, and ferulic acids, essentially conjugated with tartaric acid esters or diesters, are some of the most important compounds in this polyphenol sub-class. For instance, caftaric acid, which is composed of caffeic acid esterified with tartaric acid, is found in the pulp and represents up to 50% of total hydroxycinnamic acids [43,46]. The average amount of hydroxycinnamic acids present in red wine is around 100 and 30 mg/L in red and white wines, respectively (Table 3).

7. Hydroxybenzoic Acids

In comparison with cinnamic acid derivatives, benzoates are present at lower levels in wine (Table 3). Hydroxybenzoic acids are phenolic metabolites with a general C6–C1 structure and occur mainly in their free forms in wine, mainly as p-hydroxybenzoic, gallic, vanillic, gentisic, syringic, salicylic, and protocatechuic acids [43], although ethyl and mehyl esters of these phenolic acids have been also identified [47]. Gallic acid, which is present in important levels in white and, especially, in red wine, is the precursor of all hydrolyzable tannins and is incorporated in condensed tannins [46].

8. Stilbenes

Stilbenes are widely distributed molecules in the Plant Kingdom. However, their presence in the diet is not very significant, being basically restricted to grapes, red wine and, to a lesser extent, peanuts and blueberries [48]. Chemically they are 1,2-diarilethenes and usually have two hydroxyl groups in the meta position of ring A, while ring B is substituted with hydroxyl groups and methoxyl groups in the meta and/or para positions (Table 1). Although its concentration in wine is much lower than other polyphenols, i.e., often traces, resveratrol has received much attention for its biological properties and potential therapeutic effects (see below). The levels of resveratrol aglycone, its piceid glycoside, and its dimeric and trimeric forms (e.g., pallidol, viniferins) combined may range from negligible up to more than 100 mg/L (Table 3) when grapes are exposed to fungi.

9. Effects on Human Health

The Greek philosopher Pythagoras of Samos allegedly used to say "All is number" or "God is number" [49]. He meant that he only believed in what could be measured. This was echoed by William Thomson, 1st Baron Kelvin who, in his *Popular Lectures and Addresses* vol. 1 (1889) 'Electrical Units of Measurement', delivered 3 May 1883 notoriously said "When you can measure what you are speaking about, and express it in numbers, you know something about it, when you cannot express it in numbers, your knowledge is of a meager and unsatisfactory kind; it may be the beginning of knowledge, but you have scarcely, in your thoughts advanced to the stage of science." [50]. What both scientists meant was that we should base our knowledge on hard evidence. More recently, Dr. Archie L. Cochrane set out clearly the vital importance of randomized controlled trials (RCTs) in assessing the effectiveness of treatments [51]. How does this apply to wine (poly)phenols?

We shall start by mentioning that there are thousands of papers published on this topic (a cursory PubMed search ran on August 14th, 2020 retrieved 2954 entries just by entering "wine polyphenols"). The near totality of such studies has been performed in vitro. Needless to say, in vitro studies are indispensable to address mechanisms of action and to propose new avenues of in vivo research. The case of wine (poly)phenols, however, is rather unique and presents us with a paradigmatic opportunity to underscore the current very limits of (poly)phenol research.

In keeping with the above, we would like to discuss the case of resveratrol as an example of molecules for which there exists a strong dyscrasia between the lay public perception of health benefits and hard scientific data.

Resveratrol became popular in 1991, when Drs. Michel de Lorgeril and Serge Renaud appeared in the "60 Minutes" CBS show to talk about the French Paradox and to attribute it to the French habit of drinking red wine, which would theoretically inhibit lipid peroxidation. Note that, back then the "free radical/antioxidant hypothesis" [52] was in full swing and it was commonplace to believe that eating and drinking (poly)phenols would scavenge free radicals and prevent their noxious effects, for example by inhibiting LDL oxidation [53]. This conjecture, now largely proven wrong [54], granted red wine (poly)phenols, namely resveratrol, immediate popularity and trigger the vast amount of well-funded research mentioned above.

Two major issues developed during the nearly three decades that separate the 60 min show from our current knowledge.

The first problem is that we came to realize that (poly)phenols are very weak (if at all effective) in vivo direct antioxidants [55]. For kinetic reasons they do not scavenge free radicals and their bioavailability is generally so low that they contribute very little to the integrated cellular antioxidant machinery, which is mostly composed of enzymes [56–58]. Alas, plenty of investigators still perform research and publish papers on the in vitro antioxidant abilities of individual (poly)phenols or of some raw mixtures of them. Luckily, plenty of researchers correctly use (poly)phenols' metabolites in their in vitro studies [59,60]. The hurdle then becomes the difficulty of synthesizing such metabolites, which are often produced by the organism in different forms. It is worth underscoring that we are making progress in the identification of metabolites, but—until recently—we mainly focused on the liver-derived ones [61]. The relatively recent discovery of microbiota-synthesized metabolites amplifies the list of potential biologically-active molecules produced by the body after the ingestion of (poly)phenol-rich foods [58,62,63].

In consonance with the above, the lay press often overlooks the bioavailability issue. As regards resveratrol, already in 1993 Soleas and Goldberg acted as the harbinger of the subsequent in vivo debacle of the molecule by calling it "a molecule whose time has come and gone" [64]. That conclusive title might have been a bit too harsh, but it's a fact that many years of research and many million dollars invested in it did not yield major results [65,66].

Finally, animal studies often employ very high doses of grape (poly)phenols, e.g., resveratrol and their results cannot be readily transferred to humans, who would need to ingest several grams of extracts to replicate the same effects. Indeed, a discrepancy between animal and human effects has just been underscored [5] and resveratrol's potential toxicity has been recently reviewed [67]. An often overlooked paper reported that resveratrol promoted atherosclerotic development in hypercholesterolemic rabbits, by a mechanism that is independent of observed differences in gross animal health, liver function, plasma cholesterol concentrations, or LDL oxidative status [68].

10. Human Studies of Resveratrol and Red Wine (Poly)Phenols

One of the fields where red wine (poly)phenols are most actively studied is that of weight control, namely obesity and its associated insulin sensitivity [69]. The rationale behind studying red wine (poly)phenols and, particularly, resveratrol is that type II diabetes is rampant in developed countries and that many researchers are looking for fasting mimetics, to approximate the beneficial effects of calorie restriction or intermittent fasting on insulin sensitivity [70]. The results are equivocal, to say the least, as most trials failed to report significant effects, e.g., [71]. The molecular rationale for studying it is the finding that resveratrol and, maybe, other wine (poly)phenols activate SIRT1, a modulator of pathways downstream of calorie restriction that produces beneficial effects on glucose homeostasis and insulin sensitivity [72,73]. This hypothesis is quite controversial for at least two reasons. One is the factual role of sirtuins as longevity promoters [74]. The other one is that several researchers question the reproducibility of those data, e.g., [75]. In summary, the jury is still out [76] and the quixotic search for a substance that would fix the cardiometabolic effects of inordinate diets is not over [77].

Rather than trying to single out individual molecules purportedly responsible for the beneficial effects of moderate wine use (which is a pharmacological approach), an alternative is to test the effects of the whole (poly)phenolic fraction. We retrieved 24 publications of human studies that employed dealcoholized wine (Table S1). Taken together, their results indicate that wine (poly)phenols do exert healthful effects, ranging from anti-inflammatory actions to modulation of the microbiota, which is now gaining traction from an industrial viewpoint [78,79] and might be one of the next applications of these compounds. The extent and precise nature of such activities, however, remains to be fully elucidated. For example, some publications stem from the same study; there are some contradictions between data and their discussion (e.g., LPS and LPB data in [80], fatty acid data in [81], inflammatory markers in [82], etc.); and the true clinical relevance of microbiota modification as related to, e.g., circulating lipids (Table S1) [83–106]. In summary, there is indeed evidence that wine (poly)phenols modulate human physiology, but puffery should be avoided until we can clearly correlate such modifications with undisputable clinical outcomes.

We also searched the literature for acute or short-term human effects of wine (poly)phenols (Table S2) [107–123]. Even though this might be seen as a more classic "pharmacological" approach, even small effects repeated over time might—in the end—affect human physiology and health. Some outcomes fall in the now-outdated "plasma antioxidant capacity" or "oxLDL" areas, i.e., are poor proxies of prognosis. Other data are more physiologically relevant and indicate, e.g., salubrious effects on endothelial function and related flow-mediated dilation. Anti-inflammatory effects have also been reported. Other studies focused on bioavailability, with scant indications of biological effects. It is worth noting that ethical reasons often impede research on alcohol in humans [1].

11. Wine vs. Other Alcoholic Beverages: Does Digestion Make the Difference?

Often miscategorized as direct antioxidants [124] (see above) wine (poly)phenols might act as such during digestion. Several pieces of evidence reveal that, during digestion, lipid peroxides are formed in the stomach at millimolar concentrations [125]. In addition, we eat pre-formed hydroperoxides, whose formation is unavoidable in fat-containing foods. Dr. Kanner called the stomach "a bioreactor" [125] where hydroperoxides are formed and subsequently absorbed. This is particularly noteworthy in the case of red meat (hypothetically because of its iron content [126]), but it is likely to happen with any animal food. Lipid peroxidation during digestion can be decreased by the consumption of (poly)phenol rich foods and beverages such as extra virgin olive oil [127] and—germane to this review—red wine [128,129]. In a wider context, these data experimentally explain the evolutionary-sound habit of eating fruit and vegetables, i.e., (poly)phenols with protein [130]. Further, most cultures have culinary routines that involve drinking (poly)phenols during or after meals, including tea [131], coffee [132,133], red wine [128], etc.

Another place where wine (poly)phenols might act as indirect antioxidants is the liver, where ethanol is metabolized to acetaldehyde by the microsomal ethanol oxidizing system (MEOS), via cyp2E1 [134]. In doing, ROS are generated as by-products. Possibly, (poly)phenols might lessen this untoward effect of ethanol ingestion, through mechanisms that are yet to be elucidated.

12. Conclusions

In this review, we took a pharma-nutritional approach to wine (poly)phenols. Epidemiological evidence describes the association between alcohol use and all-cause mortality as following a J-shaped curve. Many investigators claim the superiority of wine, namely red wine with respect to other alcoholic beverages and call for (poly)phenols to support their hypothesis. The result is that the lay public often believes in this premise, in part because there is plenty of in vitro and some animal data and in part due to wish bias [135]. Indeed, there appears to be a discrepancy between the strength of biochemical data and the scantiness of well-controlled human trials of individual molecules isolated from wine. This is commonplace in nutritional research [136,137] and there is no easy way out of it [138]. In a way, wine (poly)phenols are paradigmatic of the current tension between treating such compounds as non-essential nutritional agents and expecting pharmacological actions from them [139]. In the former case, we must accept the fact that the biological effects of wine (poly)phenols are minimal and very difficult to detect with current technologies and biomarkers [138,139]. The latter scenario involves the unavoidable acceptance of side effects and is not epistemologically applicable to human nutrition. Another limitation of wine (poly)phenol research is that we often use a reductionist approach and look for one single mechanism of action. In the case of wine (poly)phenols and particularly resveratrol, this involves their misclassification as in vivo free radical scavengers and antioxidants, even if their mechanisms of action are manifold and chiefly involve anti-inflammatory actions and, possibly, activation of nrf2 and its downstream pathways via xeno-hormesis [1]. In pharma-nutritional research we should look at a wider picture and acknowledge that phytochemicals contribute to health even though, based on the definition of nutrients, they are not essential. Therefore, these molecules do not fit in the classic and rigorous pharmacological definitions; they can be modified by organisms before they interact with targets, can have different targets depending on their concentration, and do not have a univocal pharmacological mechanism of action.

In conclusion, after 30 years of dedicated research and despite the considerable expenditure, we still lack solid, "pharmacological" human evidence to confirm wine (poly)phenols' biological actions (Figure 1). Future research [138] will eventually clarify their activities and will back the current recommendations of responsibly drinking moderate amounts of wine with meals.

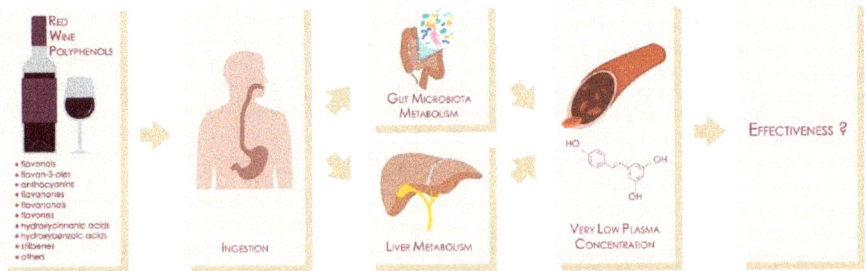

Figure 1. Schematic overview of current pitfalls in wine (poly)phenols research.

Supplementary Materials: The following are available online, Table S1: Human long-term studies with dealcoholized red wine, Table S2: Human acute or short-term studies with dealcoholized red wine.

Author Contributions: This is an Invited Review and all authors (F.V., S.-A.P., and J.T.-C.) contributed to drafting, revising, and finalizing it. All authors have read and agreed to the published version of the manuscript.

Funding: This research received no external funding.

Acknowledgments: This publication was not funded. We thank Paula Silva for inviting us to contribute to this Special Issue. This manuscript forms part of S-A.P. dissertation to obtain his M.D. degree.

Conflicts of Interest: The authors declare no conflict of interest.

References

1. Poli, A.; Marangoni, F.; Avogaro, A.; Barba, G.; Bellentani, S.; Bucci, M.; Cambieri, R.; Catapano, A.L.; Costanzo, S.; Cricelli, C.; et al. Moderate alcohol use and health: A consensus document. *Nutr. Metab. Cardiovasc. Dis.* **2013**, *23*, 487–504. [CrossRef] [PubMed]
2. Holst, C.; Becker, U.; Jorgensen, M.E.; Gronbaek, M.; Tolstrup, J.S. Alcohol drinking patterns and risk of diabetes: A cohort study of 70,551 men and women from the general Danish population. *Diabetologia* **2017**, *60*, 1941–1950. [CrossRef] [PubMed]
3. Costanzo, S.; de Gaetano, G.; Di Castelnuovo, A.; Djousse, L.; Poli, A.; van Velden, D.P. Moderate alcohol consumption and lower total mortality risk: Justified doubts or established facts? *Nutr. Metab. Cardiovasc. Dis.* **2019**, *29*, 1003–1008. [CrossRef] [PubMed]
4. Ditano-Vazquez, P.; Torres-Pena, J.D.; Galeano-Valle, F.; Perez-Caballero, A.I.; Demelo-Rodriguez, P.; Lopez-Miranda, J.; Katsiki, N.; Delgado-Lista, J.; Alvarez-Sala-Walther, L.A. The Fluid Aspect of the Mediterranean Diet in the Prevention and Management of Cardiovascular Disease and Diabetes: The Role of Polyphenol Content in Moderate Consumption of Wine and Olive Oil. *Nutrients* **2019**, *11*, 2833. [CrossRef]
5. Weaver, S.R.; Rendeiro, C.; McGettrick, H.M.; Philp, A.; Lucas, S.J.E. Fine wine or sour grapes? A systematic review and meta-analysis of the impact of red wine polyphenols on vascular health. *Eur. J. Nutr.* **2020**. [CrossRef]
6. WHO. Diet, nutrition and the prevention of chronic diseases. *World Health Organ. Tech. Rep. Ser.* **2003**, *916*, 1–149.

7. Yazdi, F.; Morreale, P.; Reisin, E. First Course DASH, Second Course Mediterranean: Comparing Renal Outcomes for Two "Heart-Healthy" Diets. *Curr. Hypertens Rep.* **2020**, *22*, 54. [CrossRef]
8. Bhupathiraju, S.N.; Tucker, K.L. Coronary heart disease prevention: Nutrients, foods, and dietary patterns. *Clin. Chim. Acta* **2011**, *412*, 1493–1514. [CrossRef]
9. Visioli, F.; Bogani, P.; Grande, S.; Detopoulou, V.; Manios, Y.; Galli, C. Local food and cardioprotection: The role of phytochemicals. *Forum. Nutr.* **2006**, *59*, 116–129. [CrossRef]
10. Holst, B.; Williamson, G. Nutrients and phytochemicals: From bioavailability to bioefficacy beyond antioxidants. *Curr. Opin. Biotechnol.* **2008**, *19*, 73–82. [CrossRef]
11. Barabási, A.; Menichetti, G.; Loscalzo, J. The unmapped chemical complexity of our diet. *Nat. Food* **2019**, *1*, 33–37. [CrossRef]
12. Manach, C.; Scalbert, A.; Morand, C.; Remesy, C.; Jimenez, L. Polyphenols: Food sources and bioavailability. *Am. J. Clin. Nutr.* **2004**, *79*, 727–747. [CrossRef] [PubMed]
13. Baiano, A.; Terracone, C.; Gambacorta, G.; La Notte, E. Phenolic content and antioxidant activity of Primitivo wine: Comparison among winemaking technologies. *J. Food Sci.* **2009**, *74*, C258–C267. [CrossRef] [PubMed]
14. Li, H.; Wang, X.; Li, Y.; Li, P.; Wang, H. Polyphenolic compounds and antioxidant properties of selected China wines. *Food Chem.* **2009**, *112*, 454–460. [CrossRef]
15. Paixão, N.; Perestrelo, R.; Marques, J.C.; Câmara, J.S. Relationship between antioxidant capacity and total phenolic content of red, rosé and white wines. *Food Chem.* **2007**, *105*, 204–214. [CrossRef]
16. Minussi, R.C.; Rossi, M.; Bologna, L.; Cordi, L.v.; Rotilio, D.; Pastore, G.M.; Durán, N. Phenolic compounds and total antioxidant potential of commercial wines. *Food Chem.* **2003**, *82*, 409–416. [CrossRef]
17. Fernández-Pachón, M.S.; Villaño, D.; García-Parrilla, M.C.; Troncoso, A.M. Antioxidant activity of wines and relation with their polyphenolic composition. *Anal. Chim. Acta* **2004**, *513*, 113–118. [CrossRef]
18. Katalinić, V.; Milos, M.; Modun, D.; Musić, I.; Boban, M. Antioxidant effectiveness of selected wines in comparison with (+)-catechin. *Food Chem.* **2004**, *86*, 593–600. [CrossRef]
19. Kallithraka, S.; Tsoutsouras, E.; Tzourou, E.; Lanaridis, P. Principal phenolic compounds in Greek red wines. *Food Chem.* **2006**, *99*, 784–793. [CrossRef]
20. Di Majo, D.; La Guardia, M.; Giammanco, S.; La Neve, L.; Giammanco, M. The antioxidant capacity of red wine in relationship with its polyphenolic constituents. *Food Chem.* **2008**, *111*, 45–49. [CrossRef]
21. Staško, A.; Brezová, V.; Mazúr, M.; Čertík, M.; Kaliňák, M.; Gescheidt, G. A comparative study on the antioxidant properties of Slovakian and Austrian wines. *LWT Food Sci. Technol.* **2008**, *41*, 2126–2135. [CrossRef]
22. Roussis, I.G.; Lambropoulos, I.; Tzimas, P.; Gkoulioti, A.; Marinos, V.; Tsoupeis, D.; Boutaris, I. Antioxidant activities of some Greek wines and wine phenolic extracts. *J. Food Compos. Anal.* **2008**, *21*, 614–621. [CrossRef]
23. Lucena, A.P.S.; Nascimento, R.J.B.; Maciel, J.A.C.; Tavares, J.X.; Barbosa-Filho, J.M.; Oliveira, E.J. Antioxidant activity and phenolics content of selected Brazilian wines. *J. Food Compos. Anal.* **2010**, *23*, 30–36. [CrossRef]
24. Jordão, A.M.; Gonçalves Fj Fau-Correia, A.C.; Correia Ac Fau-Cantão, J.; Cantão J Fau-Rivero-Pérez, M.D.; Rivero-Pérez Md Fau-González Sanjosé, M.L.; González Sanjosé, M.L. Proanthocyanidin content, antioxidant capacity and scavenger activity of Portuguese sparkling wines (Bairrada Appellation of Origin). *J. Sci. Food Agric.* **2010**, *90*, 2144–2152. [CrossRef]
25. Šeruga, M.; Novak, I.; Jakobek, L. Determination of polyphenols content and antioxidant activity of some red wines by differential pulse voltammetry, HPLC and spectrophotometric methods. *Food Chem.* **2011**, *124*, 1208–1216. [CrossRef]
26. Vrček, I.V.; Bojić, M.; Žuntar, I.; Mendaš, G.; Medić-Šarić, M. Phenol content, antioxidant activity and metal composition of Croatian wines deriving from organically and conventionally grown grapes. *Food Chem.* **2011**, *124*, 354–361. [CrossRef]
27. Yoo, Y.J.; Prenzler Pd Fau-Saliba, A.J.; Saliba Aj Fau-Ryan, D.; Ryan, D. Assessment of some Australian red wines for price, phenolic content, antioxidant activity, and vintage in relation to functional food prospects. *J. Food Sci.* **2011**, *76*, C1355–C1364. [CrossRef]
28. Ružić, I.; Škerget, M.; Knez, Ž.; Runje, M. Phenolic content and antioxidant potential of macerated white wines. *Eur. Food Res. Technol.* **2011**, *233*, 465. [CrossRef]
29. Jiang, B.; Zhang, Z.W. Comparison on phenolic compounds and antioxidant properties of cabernet sauvignon and merlot wines from four wine grape-growing regions in China. *Molecules* **2012**, *17*, 8804–8821. [CrossRef]

30. Radovanović, A.N.; Jovančićević Bs Fau-Radovanović, B.C.; Radovanović Bc Fau-Mihajilov-Krstev, T.; Mihajilov-Krstev, T.; Fau-Zvezdanović, J.B.; Zvezdanović, J.B. Antioxidant and antimicrobial potentials of Serbian red wines produced from international Vitis vinifera grape varieties. *J. Sci. Food Agric.* **2012**, *92*, 2154–2161. [CrossRef]
31. Porgalı, E.; Büyüktuncel, E. Determination of phenolic composition and antioxidant capacity of native red wines by high performance liquid chromatography and spectrophotometric methods. *Food Res. Int.* **2012**, *45*, 145–154. [CrossRef]
32. Agatonovic-Kustrin, S.; Hettiarachchi, C.G.; Morton, D.W.; Razic, S. Analysis of phenolics in wine by high performance thin-layer chromatography with gradient elution and high resolution plate imaging. *J. Pharm. Biomed. Anal.* **2015**, *102*, 93–99. [CrossRef] [PubMed]
33. Ferrazzano, G.F.; Amato, I.; Ingenito, A.; Zarrelli, A.; Pinto, G.; Pollio, A. Plant polyphenols and their anti-cariogenic properties: A review. *Molecules* **2011**, *16*, 1486–1507. [CrossRef] [PubMed]
34. Stalikas, C.D. Extraction, separation, and detection methods for phenolic acids and flavonoids. *J. Sep. Sci.* **2007**, *30*, 3268–3295. [CrossRef]
35. Yang, B.; Liu, H.; Yang, J.; Gupta, V.K.; Jiang, Y. New insights on bioactivities and biosynthesis of flavonoid glycosides. *Trends Food Sci. Technol.* **2018**, *79*, 116–124. [CrossRef]
36. Perez-Vizcaino, F.; Duarte, J. Flavonols and cardiovascular disease. *Mol. Aspects Med.* **2010**, *31*, 478–494. [CrossRef]
37. Ku, Y.S.; Ng, M.S.; Cheng, S.S.; Lo, A.W.; Xiao, Z.; Shin, T.S.; Chung, G.; Lam, H.M. Understanding the Composition, Biosynthesis, Accumulation and Transport of Flavonoids in Crops for the Promotion of Crops as Healthy Sources of Flavonoids for Human Consumption. *Nutrients* **2020**, *12*, 1717. [CrossRef]
38. Jeffery, D.W.; Parker, M.; Smith, P.A. Flavonol composition of Australian red and white wines determined by high-performance liquid chromatography. *Aust. J. Grape Wine Res.* **2008**, *14*, 153–161. [CrossRef]
39. Cueva, C.; Gil-Sanchez, I.; Ayuda-Duran, B.; Gonzalez-Manzano, S.; Gonzalez-Paramas, A.M.; Santos-Buelga, C.; Bartolome, B.; Moreno-Arribas, M.V. An Integrated View of the Effects of Wine Polyphenols and Their Relevant Metabolites on Gut and Host Health. *Molecules* **2017**, *22*, 99. [CrossRef]
40. Li, S.Y.; Duan, C.Q. Astringency, bitterness and color changes in dry red wines before and during oak barrel aging: An updated phenolic perspective review. *Crit. Rev. Food Sci. Nutr.* **2019**, *59*, 1840–1867. [CrossRef] [PubMed]
41. Tsao, R. Chemistry and biochemistry of dietary polyphenols. *Nutrients* **2010**, *2*, 1231–1246. [CrossRef] [PubMed]
42. Sanchez-Ilarduya, M.B.; Sanchez-Fernandez, C.; Garmon-Lobato, S.; Abad-Garcia, B.; Berrueta, L.A.; Gallo, B.; Vicente, F. Detection of non-coloured anthocyanin-flavanol derivatives in Rioja aged red wines by liquid chromatography-mass spectrometry. *Talanta* **2014**, *121*, 81–88. [CrossRef]
43. Rentzsch, M.; Wilkens, A.; Winterhalter, P. Non-flavonoid Phenolic Compounds. In *Wine Chemistry and Biochemistry*; Moreno-Arribas, M.V., Polo, M.C., Eds.; Springer: New York, NY, USA, 2009; pp. 509–527. [CrossRef]
44. Castaldo, L.; Narvaez, A.; Izzo, L.; Graziani, G.; Gaspari, A.; Minno, G.D.; Ritieni, A. Red Wine Consumption and Cardiovascular Health. *Molecules* **2019**, *24*, 3626. [CrossRef] [PubMed]
45. Ferreira-Lima, N.; Vallverdu-Queralt, A.; Meudec, E.; Pinasseau, L.; Verbaere, A.; Bordignon-Luiz, M.T.; Le Guerneve, C.; Cheynier, V.; Sommerer, N. Quantification of hydroxycinnamic derivatives in wines by UHPLC-MRM-MS. *Anal. Bioanal. Chem.* **2018**, *410*, 3483–3490. [CrossRef] [PubMed]
46. Garrido, J.; Borges, F. Wine and grape polyphenols—A chemical perspective. *Food Res. Int.* **2013**, *54*, 1844–1858. [CrossRef]
47. Baderschneider, B.; Winterhalter, P. Isolation and characterization of novel benzoates, cinnamates, flavonoids, and lignans from Riesling wine and screening for antioxidant activity. *J. Agric. Food Chem.* **2001**, *49*, 2788–2798. [CrossRef] [PubMed]
48. Neveu, V.; Perez-Jimenez, J.; Vos, F.; Crespy, V.; du Chaffaut, L.; Mennen, L.; Knox, C.; Eisner, R.; Cruz, J.; Wishart, D.; et al. Phenol-Explorer: An online comprehensive database on polyphenol contents in foods. *Database (Oxford)* **2010**, *2010*, bap024. [CrossRef] [PubMed]
49. Kahn, C.H. *Pythagoras and the Pythagoreans: A Brief History*; Hackett Pub Co Inc.: Indianapolis, IN, USA, 2001.
50. Ratcliffe, S. *Oxford Essential Quotation*, 4th ed.; Oxford University Press: Oxford, UK, 2016.

51. Cochrane, A.L. *Effectiveness and Efficiency: Random Reflections on Health Services*; Nuffield Trust: New York, NY, USA, 1972.
52. Koltover, V.K. Free Radical Timer of Aging: From Chemistry of Free Radicals to Systems Theory of Reliability. *Curr. Aging Sci.* **2017**, *10*, 12–17. [CrossRef] [PubMed]
53. Frankel, E.N.; Kanner, J.; German, J.B.; Parks, E.; Kinsella, J.E. Inhibition of oxidation of human low-density lipoprotein by phenolic substances in red wine. *Lancet* **1993**, *341*, 454–457. [CrossRef]
54. Visioli, F.; Keaney, J.F.; Halliwell, B. Antioxidants and cardiovascular disease; panaceas or tonics for tired sheep? *Cardiovasc. Res.* **2000**, *47*, 409. [CrossRef]
55. Forman, H.J.; Davies, K.J.; Ursini, F. How do nutritional antioxidants really work: Nucleophilic tone and para-hormesis versus free radical scavenging in vivo. *Free Radic. Biol. Med.* **2014**, *66*, 24–35. [CrossRef] [PubMed]
56. Lotito, S.B.; Frei, B. Consumption of flavonoid-rich foods and increased plasma antioxidant capacity in humans: Cause, consequence, or epiphenomenon? *Free Radic. Biol. Med.* **2006**, *41*, 1727–1746. [CrossRef]
57. Sies, H. Polyphenols and health: Update and perspectives. *Arch. Biochem. Biophys.* **2010**, *501*, 2–5. [CrossRef] [PubMed]
58. Visioli, F.; De La Lastra, C.A.; Andres-Lacueva, C.; Aviram, M.; Calhau, C.; Cassano, A.; D'Archivio, M.; Faria, A.; Fave, G.; Fogliano, V.; et al. Polyphenols and human health: A prospectus. *Crit. Rev. Food Sci. Nutr.* **2011**, *51*, 524–546. [CrossRef] [PubMed]
59. Rodriguez-Mateos, A.; Vauzour, D.; Krueger, C.G.; Shanmuganayagam, D.; Reed, J.; Calani, L.; Mena, P.; Del Rio, D.; Crozier, A. Bioavailability, bioactivity and impact on health of dietary flavonoids and related compounds: An update. *Arch. Toxicol.* **2014**, *88*, 1803–1853. [CrossRef]
60. Tome-Carneiro, J.; Visioli, F. Polyphenol-based nutraceuticals for the prevention and treatment of cardiovascular disease: Review of human evidence. *Phytomedicine* **2016**, *23*, 1145–1174. [CrossRef]
61. Castellano-Escuder, P.; Gonzalez-Dominguez, R.; Wishart, D.S.; Andres-Lacueva, C.; Sanchez-Pla, A. FOBI: An ontology to represent food intake data and associate it with metabolomic data. *Database (Oxford)* **2020**, *2020*. [CrossRef]
62. Gonzalez-Dominguez, R.; Jauregui, O.; Mena, P.; Hanhineva, K.; Tinahones, F.J.; Angelino, D.; Andres-Lacueva, C. Quantifying the human diet in the crosstalk between nutrition and health by multi-targeted metabolomics of food and microbiota-derived metabolites. *Int. J. Obes. (Lond.)* **2020**. [CrossRef]
63. Scarmozzino, F.; Poli, A.; Visioli, F. Microbiota and cardiovascular disease risk: A scoping review. *Pharmacol. Res.* **2020**, *159*, 104952. [CrossRef]
64. Soleas, G.J.; Diamandis, E.P.; Goldberg, D.M. Resveratrol: A molecule whose time has come? And gone? *Clin. Biochem.* **1997**, *30*, 91–113. [CrossRef]
65. Visioli, F. The resveratrol fiasco. *Pharmacol. Res.* **2014**, *90*, 87. [CrossRef] [PubMed]
66. Tang, P.C.; Ng, Y.F.; Ho, S.; Gyda, M.; Chan, S.W. Resveratrol and cardiovascular health–promising therapeutic or hopeless illusion? *Pharmacol. Res.* **2014**, *90*, 88–115. [CrossRef] [PubMed]
67. Shaito, A.; Posadino, A.M.; Younes, N.; Hasan, H.; Halabi, S.; Alhababi, D.; Al-Mohannadi, A.; Abdel-Rahman, W.M.; Eid, A.H.; Nasrallah, G.K.; et al. Potential Adverse Effects of Resveratrol: A Literature Review. *Int. J. Mol. Sci.* **2020**, *21*, 2084. [CrossRef] [PubMed]
68. Wilson, T.; Knight, T.J.; Beitz, D.C.; Lewis, D.S.; Engen, R.L. Resveratrol promotes atherosclerosis in hypercholesterolemic rabbits. *Life Sci.* **1996**, *59*, PL15–PL21. [CrossRef]
69. Woerdeman, J.; Del Rio, D.; Calani, L.; Eringa, E.C.; Smulders, Y.M.; Serne, E.H. Red wine polyphenols do not improve obesity-associated insulin resistance: A randomized controlled trial. *Diabetes Obes. Metab.* **2018**, *20*, 206–210. [CrossRef]
70. Most, J.; Tosti, V.; Redman, L.M.; Fontana, L. Calorie restriction in humans: An update. *Ageing Res. Rev.* **2017**, *39*, 36–45. [CrossRef]
71. Bo, S.; Ponzo, V.; Ciccone, G.; Evangelista, A.; Saba, F.; Goitre, I.; Procopio, M.; Pagano, G.F.; Cassader, M.; Gambino, R. Six months of resveratrol supplementation has no measurable effect in type 2 diabetic patients. A randomized, double blind, placebo-controlled trial. *Pharmacol. Res.* **2016**, *111*, 896–905. [CrossRef]
72. Milne, J.C.; Lambert, P.D.; Schenk, S.; Carney, D.P.; Smith, J.J.; Gagne, D.J.; Jin, L.; Boss, O.; Perni, R.B.; Vu, C.B.; et al. Small molecule activators of SIRT1 as therapeutics for the treatment of type 2 diabetes. *Nature* **2007**, *450*, 712–716. [CrossRef]

73. Kaeberlein, M.; McDonagh, T.; Heltweg, B.; Hixon, J.; Westman, E.A.; Caldwell, S.D.; Napper, A.; Curtis, R.; DiStefano, P.S.; Fields, S.; et al. Substrate-specific activation of sirtuins by resveratrol. *J. Biol. Chem.* **2005**, *280*, 17038–17045. [CrossRef]
74. Dang, W. The controversial world of sirtuins. *Drug Discov. Today Technol.* **2014**, *12*, e9–e17. [CrossRef]
75. Pacholec, M.; Bleasdale, J.E.; Chrunyk, B.; Cunningham, D.; Flynn, D.; Garofalo, R.S.; Griffith, D.; Griffor, M.; Loulakis, P.; Pabst, B.; et al. SRT1720, SRT2183, SRT1460, and resveratrol are not direct activators of SIRT1. *J. Biol. Chem.* **2010**, *285*, 8340–8351. [CrossRef]
76. Yuan, H.; Marmorstein, R. Biochemistry. Red wine, toast of the town (again). *Science* **2013**, *339*, 1156–1157. [CrossRef] [PubMed]
77. Gliemann, L. Dodging physical activity and healthy diet: Can resveratrol take the edge off the consequences of your lifestyle? *Am. J. Clin. Nutr.* **2020**. [CrossRef] [PubMed]
78. Van de Burgwal, L.H.M.; van der Waal, M.B.; Claassen, E. Accelerating microbiota product development: The Societal Impact Value Cycle as a conceptual model to shape and improve public-private valorization processes. *PharmaNutrition* **2018**, *6*, 157–168. [CrossRef]
79. Flach, J.; dos Ribeiro, C.S.; van der Waal, M.B.; van der Waal, R.X.; Claassen, E.; Van de Burgwal, L.H.M. The Nagoya Protocol on Access to Genetic Resources and Benefit Sharing: Best practices for users of Lactic Acid Bacteria. *PharmaNutrition* **2019**, *9*, 100158. [CrossRef]
80. Clemente-Postigo, M.; Queipo-Ortuno, M.I.; Boto-Ordonez, M.; Coin-Araguez, L.; Roca-Rodriguez, M.M.; Delgado-Lista, J.; Cardona, F.; Andres-Lacueva, C.; Tinahones, F.J. Effect of acute and chronic red wine consumption on lipopolysaccharide concentrations. *Am. J. Clin. Nutr.* **2013**, *97*, 1053–1061. [CrossRef]
81. Banini, A.E.; Boyd, L.C.; Allen, J.C.; Allen, H.G.; Sauls, D.L. Muscadine grape products intake, diet and blood constituents of non-diabetic and type 2 diabetic subjects. *Nutrition* **2006**, *22*, 1137–1145. [CrossRef]
82. Chiva-Blanch, G.; Urpi-Sarda, M.; Llorach, R.; Rotches-Ribalta, M.; Guillen, M.; Casas, R.; Arranz, S.; Valderas-Martinez, P.; Portoles, O.; Corella, D.; et al. Differential effects of polyphenols and alcohol of red wine on the expression of adhesion molecules and inflammatory cytokines related to atherosclerosis: A randomized clinical trial. *Am. J. Clin. Nutr.* **2012**, *95*, 326–334. [CrossRef] [PubMed]
83. Queipo-Ortuno, M.I.; Boto-Ordonez, M.; Murri, M.; Gomez-Zumaquero, J.M.; Clemente-Postigo, M.; Estruch, R.; Cardona Diaz, F.; Andres-Lacueva, C.; Tinahones, F.J. Influence of red wine polyphenols and ethanol on the gut microbiota ecology and biochemical biomarkers. *Am. J. Clin. Nutr.* **2012**, *95*, 1323–1334. [CrossRef]
84. Barden, A.; Shinde, S.; Phillips, M.; Beilin, L.; Mas, E.; Hodgson, J.M.; Puddey, I.; Mori, T.A. The effects of alcohol on plasma lipid mediators of inflammation resolution in patients with Type 2 diabetes mellitus. *Prostaglandins Leukot Essent. Fat. Acids* **2018**, *133*, 29–34. [CrossRef]
85. Barden, A.E.; Chavez, V.; Phillips, M.; Mas, E.; Beilin, L.J.; Croft, K.D.; Mori, T.A.; Puddey, I.B. A Randomized Trial of Effects of Alcohol on Cytochrome P450 Eicosanoids, Mediators of Inflammation Resolution, and Blood Pressure in Men. *Alcohol. Clin. Exp. Res.* **2017**, *41*, 1666–1674. [CrossRef]
86. Mori, T.A.; Burke, V.; Zilkens, R.R.; Hodgson, J.M.; Beilin, L.J.; Puddey, I.B. The effects of alcohol on ambulatory blood pressure and other cardiovascular risk factors in type 2 diabetes: A randomized intervention. *J. Hypertens* **2016**, *34*, 421–428. [CrossRef] [PubMed]
87. Moreno-Indias, I.; Sanchez-Alcoholado, L.; Perez-Martinez, P.; Andres-Lacueva, C.; Cardona, F.; Tinahones, F.; Queipo-Ortuno, M.I. Red wine polyphenols modulate fecal microbiota and reduce markers of the metabolic syndrome in obese patients. *Food Funct.* **2016**, *7*, 1775–1787. [CrossRef]
88. Mori, T.A.; Burke, V.; Beilin, L.J.; Puddey, I.B. Randomized Controlled Intervention of the Effects of Alcohol on Blood Pressure in Premenopausal Women. *Hypertension* **2015**, *66*, 517–523. [CrossRef]
89. Boto-Ordonez, M.; Urpi-Sarda, M.; Queipo-Ortuno, M.I.; Tulipani, S.; Tinahones, F.J.; Andres-Lacueva, C. High levels of Bifidobacteria are associated with increased levels of anthocyanin microbial metabolites: A randomized clinical trial. *Food Funct.* **2014**, *5*, 1932–1938. [CrossRef] [PubMed]
90. Jimenez-Giron, A.; Queipo-Ortuno, M.I.; Boto-Ordonez, M.; Munoz-Gonzalez, I.; Sanchez-Patan, F.; Monagas, M.; Martin-Alvarez, P.J.; Murri, M.; Tinahones, F.J.; Andres-Lacueva, C.; et al. Comparative study of microbial-derived phenolic metabolites in human feces after intake of gin, red wine, and dealcoholized red wine. *J. Agric. Food Chem.* **2013**, *61*, 3909–3915. [CrossRef] [PubMed]

91. Chiva-Blanch, G.; Urpi-Sarda, M.; Ros, E.; Valderas-Martinez, P.; Casas, R.; Arranz, S.; Guillen, M.; Lamuela-Raventos, R.M.; Llorach, R.; Andres-Lacueva, C.; et al. Effects of red wine polyphenols and alcohol on glucose metabolism and the lipid profile: A randomized clinical trial. *Clin. Nutr.* **2013**, *32*, 200–206. [CrossRef] [PubMed]
92. Chiva-Blanch, G.; Urpi-Sarda, M.; Ros, E.; Arranz, S.; Valderas-Martinez, P.; Casas, R.; Sacanella, E.; Llorach, R.; Lamuela-Raventos, R.M.; Andres-Lacueva, C.; et al. Dealcoholized red wine decreases systolic and diastolic blood pressure and increases plasma nitric oxide: Short communication. *Circ. Res.* **2012**, *111*, 1065–1068. [CrossRef]
93. Vazquez-Fresno, R.; Llorach, R.; Alcaro, F.; Rodriguez, M.A.; Vinaixa, M.; Chiva-Blanch, G.; Estruch, R.; Correig, X.; Andres-Lacueva, C. (1)H-NMR-based metabolomic analysis of the effect of moderate wine consumption on subjects with cardiovascular risk factors. *Electrophoresis* **2012**, *33*, 2345–2354. [CrossRef]
94. Schrieks, I.C.; van den Berg, R.; Sierksma, A.; Beulens, J.W.; Vaes, W.H.; Hendriks, H.F. Effect of red wine consumption on biomarkers of oxidative stress. *Alcohol. Alcohol.* **2013**, *48*, 153–159. [CrossRef]
95. Noguer, M.A.; Cerezo, A.B.; Donoso Navarro, E.; Garcia-Parrilla, M.C. Intake of alcohol-free red wine modulates antioxidant enzyme activities in a human intervention study. *Pharmacol. Res.* **2012**, *65*, 609–614. [CrossRef] [PubMed]
96. Imhof, A.; Plamper, I.; Maier, S.; Trischler, G.; Koenig, W. Effect of drinking on adiponectin in healthy men and women: A randomized intervention study of water, ethanol, red wine, and beer with or without alcohol. *Diabetes Care* **2009**, *32*, 1101–1103. [CrossRef] [PubMed]
97. Ellinger, S.; Arendt, B.M.; Fimmers, R.; Stehle, P.; Spengler, U.; Goerlich, R. Bolus ingestion but not regular consumption of native or dealcoholized red wine modulates selected immunological functions of leukocytes in healthy volunteers. *Ann. Nutr. Metab.* **2008**, *52*, 288–295. [CrossRef] [PubMed]
98. Beulens, J.W.; van Beers, R.M.; Stolk, R.P.; Schaafsma, G.; Hendriks, H.F. The effect of moderate alcohol consumption on fat distribution and adipocytokines. *Obes. (Silver Spring)* **2006**, *14*, 60–66. [CrossRef]
99. Arendt, B.M.; Ellinger, S.; Kekic, K.; Geus, L.; Fimmers, R.; Spengler, U.; Muller, W.U.; Goerlich, R. Single and repeated moderate consumption of native or dealcoholized red wine show different effects on antioxidant parameters in blood and DNA strand breaks in peripheral leukocytes in healthy volunteers: A randomized controlled trial (ISRCTN68505294). *Nutr. J.* **2005**, *4*, 33. [CrossRef]
100. Zilkens, R.R.; Burke, V.; Hodgson, J.M.; Barden, A.; Beilin, L.J.; Puddey, I.B. Red wine and beer elevate blood pressure in normotensive men. *Hypertension* **2005**, *45*, 874–879. [CrossRef]
101. Watzl, B.; Bub, A.; Pretzer, G.; Roser, S.; Barth, S.W.; Rechkemmer, G. Daily moderate amounts of red wine or alcohol have no effect on the immune system of healthy men. *Eur. J. Clin. Nutr.* **2004**, *58*, 40–45. [CrossRef]
102. Abu-Amsha Caccetta, R.; Burke, V.; Mori, T.A.; Beilin, L.J.; Puddey, I.B.; Croft, K.D. Red wine polyphenols, in the absence of alcohol, reduce lipid peroxidative stress in smoking subjects. *Free Radic. Biol. Med.* **2001**, *30*, 636–642. [CrossRef]
103. McDonald, J.T.; Margen, S. Wine versus ethanol in human nutrition. IV. Zinc balance. *Am. J. Clin. Nutr.* **1980**, *33*, 1096–1102. [CrossRef]
104. McDonald, J.T.; Margen, S. Wine versus ethanol in human nutrition. III. Calcium, phosphorous, and magnesium balance. *Am. J. Clin. Nutr.* **1979**, *32*, 823–833. [CrossRef]
105. McDonald, J.T.; Margen, S. Wine versus ethanol in human nutrition. II. Fluid, sodium, and potassium balance. *Am. J. Clin. Nutr.* **1979**, *32*, 817–822. [CrossRef]
106. McDonald, J.T.; Margen, S. Wine versus ethanol in human nutrition. I. Nitrogen and calorie balance. *Am. J. Clin. Nutr.* **1976**, *29*, 1093–1103. [CrossRef] [PubMed]
107. Perez-Mana, C.; Farre, M.; Rodriguez-Morato, J.; Papaseit, E.; Pujadas, M.; Fito, M.; Robledo, P.; Covas, M.I.; Cheynier, V.; Meudec, E.; et al. Moderate consumption of wine, through both its phenolic compounds and alcohol content, promotes hydroxytyrosol endogenous generation in humans. A randomized controlled trial. *Mol. Nutr. Food Res.* **2015**, *59*, 1213–1216. [CrossRef] [PubMed]
108. Barden, A.E.; Croft, K.D.; Beilin, L.J.; Phillips, M.; Ledowski, T.; Puddey, I.B. Acute effects of red wine on cytochrome P450 eicosanoids and blood pressure in men. *J. Hypertens* **2013**, *31*, 2195–2202. [CrossRef] [PubMed]
109. Kiviniemi, T.O.; Saraste, A.; Lehtimaki, T.; Toikka, J.O.; Saraste, M.; Raitakari, O.T.; Hartiala, J.J.; Viikari, J.; Koskenvuo, J.W. Decreased endothelin-1 levels after acute consumption of red wine and de-alcoholized red wine. *Atherosclerosis* **2010**, *211*, 283–286. [CrossRef]

110. Kiviniemi, T.O.; Saraste, A.; Lehtimaki, T.; Toikka, J.O.; Saraste, M.; Raitakari, O.T.; Parkka, J.P.; Hartiala, J.J.; Viikari, J.; Koskenvuo, J.W. High dose of red wine elicits enhanced inhibition of fibrinolysis. *Eur J Cardiovasc. Prev. Rehabil.* **2009**, *16*, 161–163. [CrossRef]
111. Kiviniemi, T.O.; Saraste, A.; Toikka, J.O.; Saraste, M.; Raitakari, O.T.; Parkka, J.P.; Lehtimaki, T.; Hartiala, J.J.; Viikari, J.; Koskenvuo, J.W. A moderate dose of red wine, but not de-alcoholized red wine increases coronary flow reserve. *Atherosclerosis* **2007**, *195*, e176–e181. [CrossRef]
112. Modun, D.; Music, I.; Vukovic, J.; Brizic, I.; Katalinic, V.; Obad, A.; Palada, I.; Dujic, Z.; Boban, M. The increase in human plasma antioxidant capacity after red wine consumption is due to both plasma urate and wine polyphenols. *Atherosclerosis* **2008**, *197*, 250–256. [CrossRef]
113. Karatzi, K.; Papamichael, C.; Karatzis, E.; Papaioannou, T.G.; Voidonikola, P.T.; Lekakis, J.; Zampelas, A. Acute smoking induces endothelial dysfunction in healthy smokers. Is this reversible by red wine's antioxidant constituents? *J. Am. Coll. Nutr.* **2007**, *26*, 10–15. [CrossRef]
114. Boban, M.; Modun, D.; Music, I.; Vukovic, J.; Brizic, I.; Salamunic, I.; Obad, A.; Palada, I.; Dujic, Z. Red wine induced modulation of vascular function: Separating the role of polyphenols, ethanol, and urates. *J. Cardiovasc. Pharmacol.* **2006**, *47*, 695–701. [CrossRef]
115. Karatzi, K.N.; Papamichael, C.M.; Karatzis, E.N.; Papaioannou, T.G.; Aznaouridis, K.A.; Katsichti, P.P.; Stamatelopoulos, K.S.; Zampelas, A.; Lekakis, J.P.; Mavrikakis, M.E. Red wine acutely induces favorable effects on wave reflections and central pressures in coronary artery disease patients. *Am. J. Hypertens* **2005**, *18*, 1161–1167. [CrossRef]
116. Pal, S.; Naissides, M.; Mamo, J. Polyphenolics and fat absorption. *Int. J. Obes. Relat. Metab. Disord.* **2004**, *28*, 324–326. [CrossRef] [PubMed]
117. Papamichael, C.; Karatzis, E.; Karatzi, K.; Aznaouridis, K.; Papaioannou, T.; Protogerou, A.; Stamatelopoulos, K.; Zampelas, A.; Lekakis, J.; Mavrikakis, M. Red wine's antioxidants counteract acute endothelial dysfunction caused by cigarette smoking in healthy nonsmokers. *Am. Heart J.* **2004**, *147*, E5. [CrossRef]
118. Watzl, B.; Bub, A.; Briviba, K.; Rechkemmer, G. Acute intake of moderate amounts of red wine or alcohol has no effect on the immune system of healthy men. *Eur. J. Nutr.* **2002**, *41*, 264–270. [CrossRef] [PubMed]
119. Bub, A.; Watzl, B.; Heeb, D.; Rechkemmer, G.; Briviba, K. Malvidin-3-glucoside bioavailability in humans after ingestion of red wine, dealcoholized red wine and red grape juice. *Eur. J. Nutr.* **2001**, *40*, 113–120. [CrossRef] [PubMed]
120. Bell, J.R.; Donovan, J.L.; Wong, R.; Waterhouse, A.L.; German, J.B.; Walzem, R.L.; Kasim-Karakas, S.E. (+)-Catechin in human plasma after ingestion of a single serving of reconstituted red wine. *Am. J. Clin. Nutr.* **2000**, *71*, 103–108. [CrossRef] [PubMed]
121. Caccetta, R.A.; Croft, K.D.; Beilin, L.J.; Puddey, I.B. Ingestion of red wine significantly increases plasma phenolic acid concentrations but does not acutely affect ex vivo lipoprotein oxidizability. *Am. J. Clin. Nutr.* **2000**, *71*, 67–74. [CrossRef]
122. Agewall, S.; Wright, S.; Doughty, R.N.; Whalley, G.A.; Duxbury, M.; Sharpe, N. Does a glass of red wine improve endothelial function? *Eur. Heart J.* **2000**, *21*, 74–78. [CrossRef]
123. Donovan, J.L.; Bell, J.R.; Kasim-Karakas, S.; German, J.B.; Walzem, R.L.; Hansen, R.J.; Waterhouse, A.L. Catechin is present as metabolites in human plasma after consumption of red wine. *J. Nutr.* **1999**, *129*, 1662–1668. [CrossRef]
124. Yang, C.S.; Ho, C.T.; Zhang, J.; Wan, X.; Zhang, K.; Lim, J. Antioxidants: Differing Meanings in Food Science and Health Science. *J. Agric. Food Chem.* **2018**, *66*, 3063–3068. [CrossRef]
125. Gorelik, S.; Ligumsky, M.; Kohen, R.; Kanner, J. The stomach as a "bioreactor": When red meat meets red wine. *J. Agric. Food Chem.* **2008**, *56*, 5002–5007. [CrossRef] [PubMed]
126. Timmers, P.; Wilson, J.F.; Joshi, P.K.; Deelen, J. Multivariate genomic scan implicates novel loci and haem metabolism in human ageing. *Nat. Commun.* **2020**, *11*, 3570. [CrossRef] [PubMed]
127. Tirosh, O.; Shpaizer, A.; Kanner, J. Lipid Peroxidation in a Stomach Medium Is Affected by Dietary Oils (Olive/Fish) and Antioxidants: The Mediterranean versus Western Diet. *J. Agric. Food Chem.* **2015**, *63*, 7016–7023. [CrossRef] [PubMed]
128. Natella, F.; Ghiselli, A.; Guidi, A.; Ursini, F.; Scaccini, C. Red wine mitigates the postprandial increase of LDL susceptibility to oxidation. *Free Radic. Biol. Med.* **2001**, *30*, 1036–1044. [CrossRef]

129. Kanner, J.; Gorelik, S.; Roman, S.; Kohen, R. Protection by polyphenols of postprandial human plasma and low-density lipoprotein modification: The stomach as a bioreactor. *J. Agric. Food Chem.* **2012**, *60*, 8790–8796. [CrossRef]
130. Kanner, J.; Selhub, J.; Shpaizer, A.; Rabkin, B.; Shacham, I.; Tirosh, O. Redox homeostasis in stomach medium by foods: The Postprandial Oxidative Stress Index (POSI) for balancing nutrition and human health. *Redox. Biol.* **2017**, *12*, 929–936. [CrossRef]
131. Ellinger, S.; Muller, N.; Stehle, P.; Ulrich-Merzenich, G. Consumption of green tea or green tea products: Is there an evidence for antioxidant effects from controlled interventional studies? *Phytomedicine* **2011**, *18*, 903–915. [CrossRef]
132. Higdon, J.V.; Frei, B. Coffee and health: A review of recent human research. *Crit. Rev. Food Sci. Nutr.* **2006**, *46*, 101–123. [CrossRef]
133. van Dam, R.M.; Hu, F.B.; Willett, W.C. Coffee, Caffeine, and Health. *N. Engl. J. Med.* **2020**, *383*, 369–378. [CrossRef]
134. Comporti, M.; Signorini, C.; Leoncini, S.; Gardi, C.; Ciccoli, L.; Giardini, A.; Vecchio, D.; Arezzini, B. Ethanol-induced oxidative stress: Basic knowledge. *Genes Nutr.* **2010**, *5*, 101–109. [CrossRef]
135. Wynder, E.L.; Higgins, I.T.; Harris, R.E. The wish bias. *J. Clin. Epidemiol.* **1990**, *43*, 619–621. [CrossRef]
136. Ioannidis, J.P. We need more randomized trials in nutrition-preferably large, long-term, and with negative results. *Am. J. Clin. Nutr.* **2016**, *103*, 1385–1386. [CrossRef] [PubMed]
137. Trepanowski, J.F.; Ioannidis, J.P.A. Perspective: Limiting Dependence on Nonrandomized Studies and Improving Randomized Trials in Human Nutrition Research: Why and How. *Adv. Nutr.* **2018**, *9*, 367–377. [CrossRef] [PubMed]
138. Laville, M.; Segrestin, B.; Alligier, M.; Ruano-Rodriguez, C.; Serra-Majem, L.; Hiesmayr, M.; Schols, A.; La Vecchia, C.; Boirie, Y.; Rath, A.; et al. Evidence-based practice within nutrition: What are the barriers for improving the evidence and how can they be dealt with? *Trials* **2017**, *18*, 425. [CrossRef] [PubMed]
139. Visioli, F. Can experimental pharmacology be always applied to human nutrition? *Int. J. Food Sci. Nutr.* **2012**, *63* (Suppl. 1), 10–13. [CrossRef]

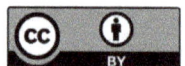

© 2020 by the authors. Licensee MDPI, Basel, Switzerland. This article is an open access article distributed under the terms and conditions of the Creative Commons Attribution (CC BY) license (http://creativecommons.org/licenses/by/4.0/).

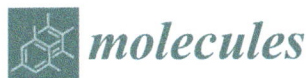

Review

Wine Consumption and Oral Cavity Cancer: Friend or Foe, Two Faces of Janus

Paula Silva [1,*], Norbert Latruffe [2] and Giovanni de Gaetano [3]

1. Laboratory of Histology and Embryology, Institute of Biomedical Sciences Abel Salazar (ICBAS), University of Porto, Rua de Jorge Viterbo Ferreira n°228, 4050-313 Porto, Portugal
2. BioPeroxIL laboratory, Université de Bourgogne, 6, Boulevard Gabriel, 21000 Dijon, France; Norbert.Latruffe@u-bourgogne.fr
3. Department of Epidemiology and Prevention, IRCCS Istituto Neurologico Mediterraneo Neuromed, 86077 Pozzilli, Italy; giovanni.degaetano@moli-sani.org or giovanni.degaetano@neuromed.it
* Correspondence: psilva@icbas.up.pt

Academic Editors: Paula Silva and Norbert Latruffe
Received: 19 March 2020; Accepted: 28 May 2020; Published: 31 May 2020

Abstract: The health benefits of moderate wine consumption have been extensively studied during the last few decades. Some studies have demonstrated protective associations between moderate drinking and several diseases including oral cavity cancer (OCC). However, due to the various adverse effects related to ethanol content, the recommendation of moderate wine consumption has been controversial. The polyphenolic components of wine contribute to its beneficial effects with different biological pathways, including antioxidant, lipid regulating and anti-inflammatory effects. On the other hand, in the oral cavity, ethanol is oxidized to form acetaldehyde, a metabolite with genotoxic properties. This review is a critical compilation of both the beneficial and the detrimental effects of wine consumption on OCC.

Keywords: wine; ethanol; acetaldehyde; oral cavity cancer; carcinogenesis; resveratrol

---

1. Introduction

Oral cavity cancer (OCC) is a neoplastic condition characterized by the malignant transformation of the lips, oral cavity or oropharynx cells. In 2018, the worldwide estimate was 177,384 deaths and 354,864 new cases of OCC, which is the fourth most common cancer and the sixth most common cause of cancer deaths in low- and middle-income countries [1]. The consumption of alcoholic beverages has been pointed out as one key risk factor for OCC. The population-attributable risk of OCC for alcohol consumption alone is lower than 18% [2]. Epidemiological studies indicate that the risk associated with OCC increases when it is treated as an independent effect in people who consume ≥30 grams of ethanol per day [3–12]. The relative risk of cancers of the oral cavity and pharynx, esophagus and larynx are around five for an amount of around 50 g/day of ethanol [13]. These values are higher than the ones that define moderate consumption (up to one drink—equivalent to about 12 g of ethanol—per day in women and up to two in men, of all types of alcoholic beverages combined) [13]. Higher consumption, of more than three drinks per day, over a short period (a few years) has a higher risk of oral cancer than a lower intake over a longer period (many years) [14].

Wine is known for its large quantities of polyphenols, which have antioxidant properties that may counteract the potential pro-oxidant effect of ethanol. Numerous studies of animals and humans have shown that the bioavailability of phenolic compounds is low [15]. However, oral cavity tissues are in direct contact with wine and its compounds. The levels of salivary polyphenols peaked soon after red wine intake in healthy volunteers [16,17]. The effects of phenolic compounds in the oral cavity derive mainly from a reservoir adhering to oral mucosa rather than from systemic absorption. Therefore, it seems that the intra-oral actions of both ethanol and the phenolic portion of the wine overlap with the systemic ones, which makes OCC a peculiar type of disease to study.

In this review, we analyze the molecular mechanisms of ethanol-related carcinogenesis and phenolic-related preventive-carcinogenesis in the oral cavity and explore the possibility of a dual contrasting effect of these wine components in the development of OCC.

2. Wine as Oral Cavity Cancer-Enhancer

2.1. Formation and Accumulation of Acetaldehyde in Oral Cavity after Wine Ingestion

Wine contains ethanol, which by itself is not a carcinogen; however, acetaldehyde, which is associated with wine consumption, is classified as "carcinogenic to humans" by the International Agency for Research on Cancer (IARC), based, in large part, on the elevated risk of oral and esophageal cancers in alcohol abusers [18,19]. The concentration of acetaldehyde varies among wine types (e.g., white, red, sparkling and fortified wines) as a result of the different winemaking conditions, particularly with the quantity of SO_2 added to the medium. Therefore, different values appear in the literature. Acetaldehyde has been detected at concentration levels of 80 mg/L for white wines, 30 mg/L for red wines and 300 mg/L for sherries [20]. Jackowetz and Orduña [21] reported a final wine concentration of acetaldehyde of 25 mg/L in reds and 40 mg/L in white wines. Different values were found in another study, where acetaldehyde content was measured in a large collection of different alcoholic beverages (over 1500 samples), in which the amount found was 34 mg/L and 118 ± 120 mg/L in wine and in fortified wines, respectively [22]. In a study carried out to measure the acetaldehyde concentration in different beverages consumed in Italy, acetaldehyde concentrations of 55.8 mg/L in red, 67 mg/L in white, 81.7 mg/L in rosé and 123 mg/L in sparkling wine and champagne were found [23]. Linderborg et al. [24] found a lower concentration of acetaldehyde in wine samples (12.1 mg/L ± 10.4 mg/L). Recently, acetaldehyde levels ranging from 2.49 ± 0.34 to 29.27 ± 4.69 mg/L were found in Cabernet Sauvignon wines and this declined by close to 40% during aging under screw cap closures which admitted very little oxygen [25]. Despite the differences found among studies, wine contains acetaldehyde levels above the mutagenic limit (4.4 mg/L). Moreover, the IARC classification includes both acetaldehyde present in wine and acetaldehyde formed from ethanol via endogenous metabolism [22,24,26–28]. In fact, one of the key mechanisms in the oral formation of acetaldehyde is the metabolism of ethanol by the microbial flora of the oral mucosa [18,29,30]. Ethanol is oxidized by mucosal and microbial cells to form acetaldehyde by alcohol dehydrogenase (ADH), mainly alcohol dehydrogenase-1B (ADH1B) (Figure 1). Acetaldehyde is further metabolized by aldehyde dehydrogenase (ALDH, mostly by aldehyde dehydrogenase-2 (ALDH2)), yielding acetate, which is a less toxic and less harmful compound (Figure 1). Despite this process primarily occurring in the liver, the required enzymes are also expressed in the oral mucosa and gingiva. Oral microflora appears to be the main origin of acetaldehyde concentration in saliva. Some *Streptococcus* species have produced high quantities of acetaldehyde and showed significant ADH activity, suggesting that they may participate in metabolizing ethanol to form carcinogenic acetaldehyde in the oral cavity (Figure 1) [31]. As revealed by an in vitro characterization of the oral microbiome, both the *Neisseria* and *Candida* species are among the most potent microbial producers of acetaldehyde [32–35].

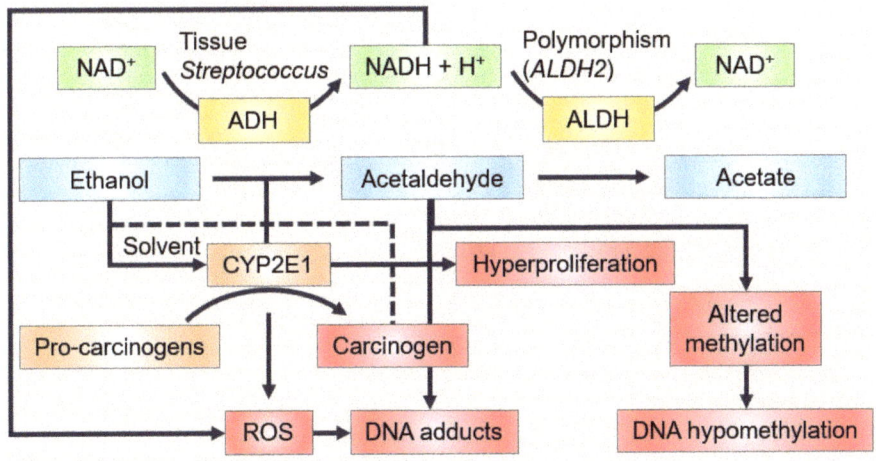

Figure 1. Scheme of the mechanisms by which ethanol may affect oral carcinogenesis. Ethanol is metabolized to form acetaldehyde by alcohol dehydrogenase (ADH) and cytochrome P450 2E1 (CYP2E1) in the oral cavity and is further oxidized to form acetate by acetaldehyde dehydrogenase (ALDH). ADH-mediated ethanol metabolism results in the generation of reducing equivalents in the form of reduced nicotinamide adenine dinucleotide (NADH) and acetaldehyde, whereas ethanol oxidation by CYP2E1 leads to the production of acetaldehyde but also to the generation of reactive oxygen species (ROS). Single nucleotide polymorphisms of ALDH2 cause the production and/or oxidation of acetaldehyde to vary between individuals. Increased CYP2E1 activity not only leads to an increased generation of ROS but also leads to an increased activation of various environmental agents such as the pro-carcinogens present in tobacco smoke. Ethanol may also act as a solvent for these carcinogens to enter the cell. Acetaldehyde can bind to DNA, forming stable adducts, and ROS results in lipid peroxidation products, such as 4-hydroxynonenal (4-HNE), which bind to DNA to form mutagenic adducts. During cancer promotion, ethanol and acetaldehyde alter methyl transfer, leading to DNA hypomethylation that could change the expression of oncogenes and tumor-suppressor genes. Finally, ethanol-associated immune suppression may facilitate tumor cell spreading.

From that which has been reported above, it is clear that in order to evaluate the OCC risk of wine, it is important to measure the acetaldehyde content in saliva after wine ingestion. In vivo findings in humans have shown that acetaldehyde concentrations in saliva range between 0.793 mg/L and 4.41 mg/L after a dose of alcohol containing 0.5 g ethanol/kg body weight [17,36,37]. A study that was carried out to clarify the effects of alcohol beverage type on salivary and blood acetaldehyde and ethanol levels, after a moderate dose of alcoholic beverages in healthy Japanese volunteers, showed that the type of alcoholic beverage (13% ethanol Calvados, 13% ethanol shochu, 13% ethanol red wine and 5% ethanol beer) had no effect on the salivary acetaldehyde levels that were measured 30 min or more after the completion of drinking. However, the salivary acetaldehyde concentration after drinking red wine was significantly lower than that after drinking any of the other beverages [36].

Ethanol may also be metabolized to form acetaldehyde by the cytochrome P450 2E1 (CYP2E1) present in the keratinocytes of buccal mucosa (Figure 1) [38]. The increase in CYP2E1 activity is due to ethanol consumption and, consequently, the generation of reactive oxygen and reactive nitrogen species (ROS, RNS). Some studies suggest that the initiation of OCC results from DNA damage by ROS/RNS via the activation of proto-oncogenes and the inactivation of tumor suppressor genes. An accumulation of 8-nitroguanine, which is a potentially mutagenic DNA lesion, and 8-hydroxy-deoxyguanosine, one of the most frequent DNA base modifications associated with oxidative damage, has been found in the tissue of patients with oral lichen planus (OLP) [38,39], oral squamous cell carcinoma (OSCC) [38] and leucoplakia [40], though no immune-reactivity was observed in normal oral mucosa [38]. The formation of 8-nitroguanine and 8-oxodG may contribute to the development of oral cancer from OLP and leucoplakia [41]. It was also observed that inducible nitric oxide synthase dependent DNA damage may stimulate tumor protein p53 accumulation in OLP, leukoplakia and OSCC [41]. Increased levels of 4-hydroxy-2-nonenal and malondialdehyde, which result from the lipid peroxidation of cell membranes by ROS, have been reported in oral cancer and pre-cancer patients [42–45].

Ethanol may directly affect the oral mucosa since it can act as a solvent, removing some of mucosa lipid content, thereby making it considerably more permeable, which also facilitates the development of tumors on such exposed locations by the increased absorption of other carcinogenic substances [46–48].

2.2. Ethanol/Acetaldehyde Genotoxicity

Acetaldehyde's genotoxicity is linked to its reactivity, forming DNA adducts and interfering with DNA synthesis and repair as well as binding to proteins, altering their structure and function. Mutagenic DNA adducts can be formed when acetaldehyde is present in concentrations equal to or higher than 6.30 mg/L [49,50]. The major acetaldehyde-derived DNA adduct in the human body is a Schiff base, N2-ethylidene-2′-deoxyguanosine (N2-ethylidene-dG) [51]. Since the N2-ethylidene-dG adduct is unstable in the single 2′-deoxynucleoside form, with a half-life of just 5 min, an analytical approach was developed for quantifying N2-ethyl-2′-deoxyguanosine (N2-ethyl-dG): this is a compound which is more stable and easier to detect than results from the reduction of N2-ethylidene-dG by sodium cyanoborohydride ($NaBH_3CN$) (Figure 2) [52]. Therefore, for assessing the effects of alcohol consumption on DNA in studies of alcohol-related carcinogenicity, N2-ethyl-dG has been used as a biomarker (Figure 2). The detection of N2-ethyl-dG supported epidemiological studies showing a higher risk of oral and esophageal cancer in ALDH2-deficient individuals who drink chronically [53]. Balbo et al. [54] used N2-ethyl-dG to investigate, for the first time, the effects of alcohol consumption on the time course of DNA adduct production in the oral cavities of healthy volunteers. A clear dose–response relationship between the levels of N2-ethyl-dG produced and the amount of alcohol consumed was observed. The most interesting result of this bio-kinetic study was that the adduct levels returned to baseline values after 24 h. Since the half-life of N2-ethylidene-dG in DNA is 24 h at 37 °C, the elimination of adducts can be explained by either DNA repair or cell turnover [54,55]. It is possible that the nucleotide excision repair mechanism could remove the lesion, since neither base deletion repair nor direct repair have been shown to be able to remove N2-ethyl-dG (used as a substitute for N2-ethylidene-dG). The other possibility is that the return of the adduct levels to baseline values reflects changes in the cell population that is being sampled. Cells in the basal layer of the epithelium appropriately undergo mitosis to provide cell renewal. As these cells differentiate, they are pushed toward the surface by new cells in the basal layer. Therefore, the cells sampled at the 24 h time point would have been in a different epithelial layer relative to the surface during the alcohol drinking and immediately afterwards, when salivary acetaldehyde levels would be at their highest [54,55]. The condensation of two molecules of acetaldehyde may also produce a reactive electrophile, croton-aldehyde, which can also form a Schiff base on the same amino group of deoxyguanosine (dG), which results in the formation of other adducts the croton-aldehyde-derived propano-dG ones. Under the in vitro conditions that were investigated, these adducts proved to be very unstable. Further investigation is needed to clarify the biological significance of these adducts [56].

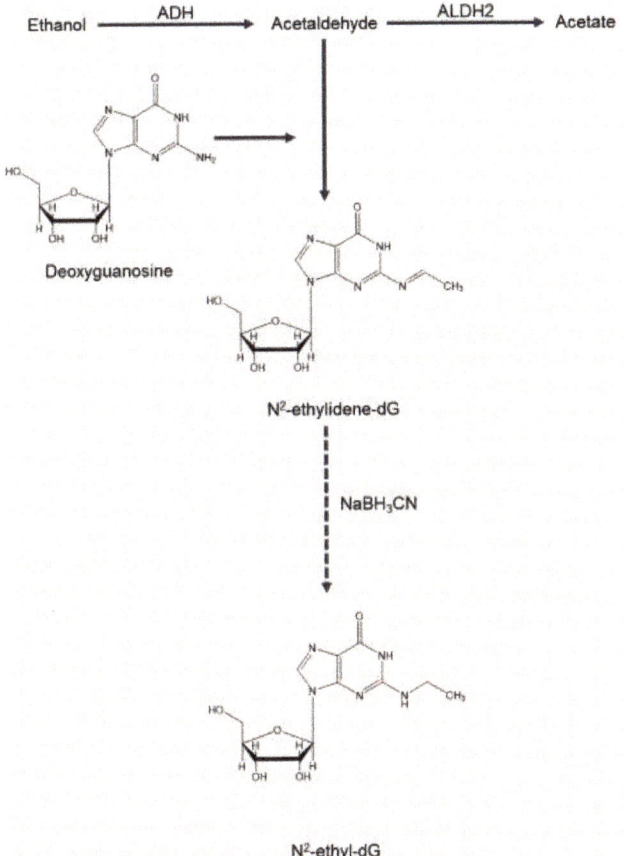

Figure 2. Formation of the N2-ethylidene-dG adduct and the N2-ethyl-dG adduct due to acetaldehyde production from ethanol. Acetaldehyde can interact with deoxyguanosine (dG) to form a Schiff base N2-ethylidene-dG. During the reduction step, the unstable N2-ethylidene-dG is expected to be converted to the stable N2-ethyl-dG.

2.3. Ethanol/Acetaldehyde and Pre-Cancerous Lesions

Acetaldehyde also damages oral mucosa, which promotes the stimulation of cell regeneration. DNA mutation may result from the spreading out of the proliferative cell compartment and hyper-regeneration. The various alterations in DNA can progress from a normal oral epithelial cell to a pre-malignant or a potentially malignant oral epithelial cell that is characterized by the ability to proliferate in a non-controlled mode. Genetic alterations may then cause the development of pre-cancerous lesions, which develop in the form of benign or malignant tumors. Pre-cancerous lesions can be in the form of leukoplakia, erythroplakia, erythroleukoplakia (Figure 3) or oral sub-mucous fibrosis, and all these can potentially give rise to a primary tumor in the oral cavity [56–60]. OCC involves changes in the mucosal layers that most probably occur in the entire epithelial surface of the oral cavity and are followed by the invasion of tumor cells [61]. Changes in over approximately 100 genes have been involved in OCC, the overexpression of oncogenes and/or the silencing of tumor suppressor genes being the focus of the scientific community [62].

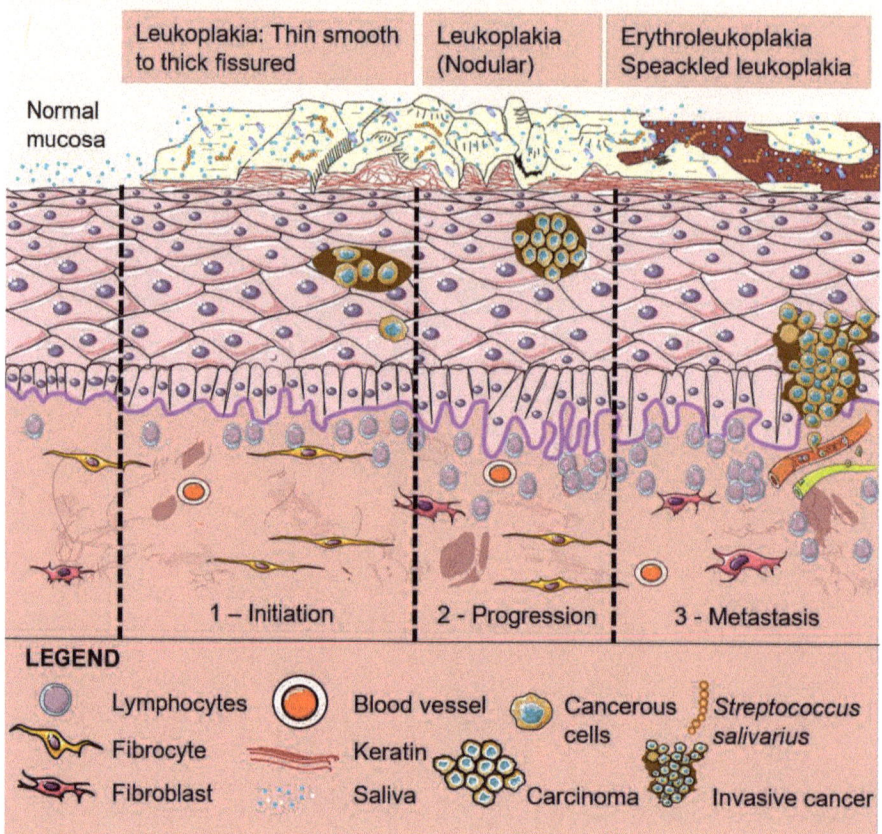

Figure 3. The various clinical appearances of leukoplakia with expected underlying microscopic changes are shown. Leukoplakia is a pre-malignant, pre-cancerous or potentially malignant lesion or condition, which means that there is an increased risk of future malignant transformation into a squamous cell carcinoma either at the site of the leukoplakia or elsewhere in the oral cavity. Lesions become progressively more "severe" toward the right, culminating in erythroleukoplakia, which most frequently demonstrates severe epithelial dysplasia and carcinoma in situ when studied histologically. It should be emphasized that the scheme does not necessarily represent a chronological change, but rather it shows the potential presentations of leukoplakia. Homogeneous leukoplakia is a uniform, flat, thin and white plaque, with or without fissuring and with a gradual increase of hyperkeratosis and acanthosis. Leukoplakia can also be non-homogeneous, being nodular or flat with a mixed white and red discoloration ("erythroleukoplakia"). The histopathologic features of leukoplakia may vary from hyperkeratosis with or without epithelial dysplasia to various degrees of epithelial dysplasia, carcinoma in situ and even invasive squamous cell carcinoma.

A case–control study in Kenya revealed a weak to moderate association between wine intake and oral leukoplakia [63]. No relationship was found in a case–control study investigating the role of alcohol consumption in the development of oral leukoplakia in Southern Taiwan. Subjects who had drunk a bottle or more of an alcoholic beverage per month for at least one year did not develop oral leukoplakia [64]. According to Petti et al. [65], regular intake of a moderate quantity of wine could reduce the risk of oral leukoplakia. Consumption of beer and hard liquor, but not wine, is more strongly associated with oral cancer than oral epithelial dysplasia [66]. Jaber et al. [67] carried out a study that aimed to provide an assessment of the importance of tobacco and alcohol consumption in the development of oral epithelial dysplasia in a large group of European patients. These authors found no relationship between the degree of wine consumption and risk of oral epithelial dysplasia. However, increased risk of oral epithelial dysplasia was associated with the consumption of fortified wines [67]. A retrospective case–control study showed no overall increased risk from wine and other alcoholic beverages of oral dysplasia. However, the proportion of subjects who drank spirits was significantly higher among cases than controls [68]. Morse et al. [69] found a two-fold increase in the risk of oral epithelial dysplasia associated with drinking seven or more drinks of beer and hard liquor per week but no excess risk with drinking an equivalent amount of wine. A study in Puerto Rico also suggests that any type of alcoholic beverage consumption, including wine, is positively associated with an increased risk of potentially malignant oral disorders [70]. Conflicting evidence exists to support alcohol's role in the development of pre-cancerous lesions but apparently wine has little to no effect on their development. In general, these results corroborate the ones obtained by Purdue et al. [71], who found that among wine-only drinkers, the odds ratio for moderate levels of consumption frequency approached null. According to their study, only individuals with higher wine consumption levels were comparable to drinkers of other beverage types.

In summary, it seems that ethanol may act as an OCC promoter by multiple pathways. However, important questions remain to be answered about the mechanistic and dynamic bases of this relationship.

3. Wine as Oral Cavity Cancer-Preventer

Grapes contain phenolic compounds: these are highly specific metabolites that are important in plant regulatory mechanisms and play an important role in the response and resistance of plants to infection by pathogenic microorganisms. Phenolic compounds also directly contribute to the sensory properties, such as color, astringency, bitterness and roughness, of wine. They are involved in redox reactions, protein interactions and wine-aging processes [72]. The primary constituents of the phenolic compounds are flavonoids and non-flavonoids. Flavonoids make up approximately 85% of the total phenolic content of red wine but less than 20% of that of white wine [73]. Phenolic compounds have important effects on human physiology and are considered to have beneficial effects in relation to cancer and diabetes, microbial, inflammatory, neurodegenerative and kidney diseases and aging [74]. Herein, we will review the literature related to the chemoprevention potential of wine polyphenols, i.e., their potential for controlling the transformation of pre-malignant or potentially malignant lesions into invasive OCC.

3.1. In Vitro Studies

Wine contains the same flavanol derivatives as green tea, namely catechins; the latter have been extensively studied for their chemo-preventive potential, showing efficacy against multiple cancers including OCC [75,76]. Therefore, it is reasonable to suppose that wine flavanols could have similar OCC protective effects. Oral and head and neck cancer cells exposed to green tea and epigallocatechin-3-gallate (EGCG), respectively, lead to a decrease in the expression of the phosphorylated epidermal growth factor receptor (EGFR), suggesting that catechins are potential cancer chemo-therapeutic or chemo-preventive agents [77,78]. In vitro, tea catechins promote a decrease in the proliferation of different human head and neck squamous cell carcinoma (HNSCC) cell lines [77–82]. Li et al. [82] found that EGCG affects the proliferation, apoptosis, migration and invasion of tongue squamous cell carcinoma cells through the Hippo-TAZ signaling pathway. Polyphenols extracted from green tea have a synergistic beneficial effect with lactoferrin on oral carcinoma cells' cytotoxicity and apoptosis. Moreover, polyphenols alone induce G0/G1 cell-cycle arrest and apoptosis [83]. EGCG also induces the G1 phase arrest of human OSCC cells [81]. Activation of the p53 tumor suppressor gene by green tea polyphenols could explain the induction of cell cycle arrest and apoptosis [84]. Treatment with EGCG increases caspase-3 and -7 activities and the percentage of apoptotic cells [81]. In addition, it was observed that EGCG induces cell apoptosis and autophagy and inhibits multi-drug resistance gene (MDR1) expression in oral cancer cells [85]. The in vitro effects of EGCG on oral cancer cells include three main phases: (i) inhibition of cell proliferation via apoptosis induction and cell cycle arrest; (ii) modulation of transcription factors, namely nuclear factor kappa-light-chain-enhancer (NF-κB) and activator protein; and (iii) reduction of cell migration and invasion by decreasing the production of matrix metallo-proteinases (MMPs) [86,87].

Quercetin is an efficient anti-cancer agent as evidenced by an EGFR decrease in EGFR-overexpressing HNSCC [88]. An in vitro study with human OSCC cells suggested that quercetin chemo-preventive mechanisms start by inducing a stress response, resulting in cell necrosis. Then, the surviving cells die by apoptosis after prolonged exposure to quercetin, presumably mediated by the inhibition of thymidylate synthase protein, a key S-phase enzyme [89].

The combination of quercetin with chemo-therapeutic drugs not only induces apoptosis but also decreases the cells' resistance to the chemo-therapeutic medication [90,91]. The bio-pharmacological effects of quercetin on cell growth and invasion/migration inhibition involve cellular and molecular mechanisms, mainly via cell cycle arrest accompanied by mitochondria-mediated apoptosis. The caspase-3-dependent apoptosis of OSCC cells is one of the mechanisms that has been proposed to explain the anti-OCC properties of quercetin [92].

Quercetin efficiently inhibits the cellular migration and invasion of the HNSCC cell lines, HSC-3 and FaDu, and human oral cancer cells (SAS) via suppression of the MMP-2 and MMP-9 activation [88,93]. MMPs inhibition occurs via the down-regulation of protein kinase C and the blocking of mitogen activated protein kinases (MAPK) and phosphatidylinositide-3 kinases (PI3K) signaling pathways and both cyclo-oxygenase-2 (COX-2) and NF-κB [93]. Moreover, quercetin affects the ratio of anti-/pro-apoptotic proteins in SAS cell lines, which may lead to the dysfunction of mitochondria followed by the release of cytochrome c (cyto c), apoptosis-inducing factors and endonuclease G from mitochondria, inducing cell-destruction by triggering apoptosis [94].

Quercetin treatment enhances microRNA-16 (miR-16) expression and inhibits homeobox A10 (HOXA10) levels. The overexpression of miR-16 blocks cell viability, migration and invasion by targeting HOXA10, and its knockdown reverses the quercetin-mediated progression of oral cancer cells [95].

Several lines of evidence both in vitro and in vivo support the notion that quercetin is a potential therapeutic agent for a subset of human OSCC involving the activation of fork-head box O (FOXO1). In fact, quercetin suppresses cancer cell growth and promotes phase G2 cell cycle arrest and apoptosis in EGFR-overexpressing HSC-3 and TW206 cells, thus inducing the activation of FOXO1, the knockdown of which attenuates the quercetin induction of p21 and Fas ligand (FasL) expression [96]. From the above, it can be concluded that quercetin exerts chemo-preventive effects on the oral keratinocytes, and after a tumor has formed, quercetin could continue to have beneficial anti-tumor effects at higher doses by exerting cytotoxic effects.

Anthocyanins are flavonoids found mainly in grape skin and are responsible for the bluish-red color of the skin of red grapes and, therefore, for the color of red wine. Grape seed proanthocyanidins (GSPs) reduce cell viability and induce cell death in a dose- and time-dependent manner in human HNSCC cell lines from different sub-sites such as the oral cavity (SCC1), larynx (SCC5), tongue (OSC19) and pharynx (FaDu). GSPs reduce the expression of EGFR in those cell lines. Moreover, these anthocyanins increase the apoptosis of SCC1 and OSC19 cells with the induction of Bax (Bcl-2-associated X protein), reduction of the expression of Bcl-2 and the activation of caspase-3 [97]. GSPs inhibit the proliferation, migration and invasion of tongue squamous cell carcinoma cells (Tca8113) through suppression of the Akt/NF-κB signaling pathway [98].

Blueberries, a rich source of anthocyanins, and malvidin inhibit STAT-3 (signal transducers and activators of transcription-3), which prevents the proliferation and induces the apoptosis of oral cancer cells in vitro, a result further confirmed in vivo. Blueberry and malvidin suppress STAT-3 phosphorylation, block the nuclear translocation of the active dimer and prevent the transactivation of the STAT3 target genes that play crucial roles in cell proliferation and apoptosis [99]. Anthocyanins from the wild blueberries of Inner Mongolia suppress the growth of the oral cancer cell line KB in a dose-dependent manner as well as induce G2/M cell cycle arrest and apoptosis of the cells. Anthocyanin treatment increases the expression of caspase-9 and cyto c. Anthocyanins can also down-regulate the methylation of tumor protein p53 [100]. In a different study, it was observed that besides blueberry, cranberry, blackberry, black raspberry, red raspberry and strawberry extracts also inhibit the proliferation of human oral cancer cell lines [101,102]. The result for black raspberry was observed in another study in which extracts of this fruit inhibited the growth of oral pre-malignant and malignant cells by targeting cell cycle regulatory proteins [103]. Isolated cell lines from human OSCC tumors were used to investigate the effects of a freeze-dried black raspberry ethanol extract on cellular growth [104]. As in the other studies, black raspberry extracts suppressed cell proliferation without perturbing viability, inhibited the translation of the complete angiogenic cytokine vascular endothelial growth factor (VEGF), suppressed nitric oxide synthase activity and induced both apoptosis and terminal differentiation [104].

Crude extracts of strawberry and pure anthocyanins, namely cyanidin-3-O-glucoside, pelargonidin and pelargonidin-3-O-rutinoside, inhibit the proliferation of KB and CAL27 human oral cancer cells, which has been associated with an antioxidant mechanism of action [105]. In human oral CAL 27 cells, it has also been observed that anthocyanins from a species of black rice could decrease cells' metastasis by the reduction of MMP-2, MMP-9 and NF-κB p65 expression through the suppression of the PI3K/Akt pathway and the inhibition of NF-κB levels [106]. Recently, it was shown that anthocyanin promotes the death of OSCC cells through the activation of pyroptosis [107].

The mechanism of action of anthocyanins seems to involve their ability to modulate epithelial cell growth and quench ROS, which is achieved because anthocyanins affect intracellular signaling and gene expression [108]. In fact, the anti-mutagenic and anti-carcinogenic activities of anthocyanins are generally ascribed to their antioxidant properties as conveyed by their phenolic structure. They may play an important role in the anti-cancer effects in OCC and are worthy of further investigation.

Resveratrol is a stilbene and the major non-flavonoid found in red wines, and it can modulate the signal transduction pathways that control cell division and growth, apoptosis, inflammation, angiogenesis and metastasis [109,110]. Its anti-cancer properties have been shown on various types of cancer cells including those of HNSCC origin [110,111]. Resveratrol's anti-cancer effects are related to the inhibition of the proliferation of different oral cancer cells through the induction of apoptosis [112,113]. Moreover, resveratrol has considerable efficacy against the growth and proliferation of HNSCC through its selective induction of DNA damage and apoptosis, independently of Smad4 status, the mutation/absence of which is one of the primary causes of failed cellular DNA repair machinery in HNSCC [114].

Another study aimed to find potential compounds for the treatment of OCC, based on a large scale of reliable compound- and bioactivity-databases which showed that resveratrol is a natural product with a high potential to treat OCC. Resveratrol inhibits matrix MMP-9 expression and metastasis in oral cancer cells by down-regulating the signaling pathways of c-Jun N-terminal kinase1/2 and extra-cellular signal-regulated kinase1/2 signals, thus exerting beneficial effects in chemo-prevention [115]. Concentrations of 100 µM resveratrol decrease the adhesion, migration and invasion of OSCC cells (KB) [116] and of human oral cancer cell lines (SCC-9) [115]. Cell migration induced by 12-O-tetradecanoylphorbol-13-acetate (TPA) is also inhibited by resveratrol, which reduces the expression of MMP-9 and blocks the extra-cellular signal-regulated kinase (ERK) and JNK-MAPK (c-Jun N-terminal protein kinase family of mitogen-activated protein kinases) pathways. The reduction of MMP-9 activity by resveratrol is related to the suppression of the phosphorylation of ERK and JNK induced by TPA [115]. Using the oral cancer cell line SAS, it was observed that resveratrol induces apoptosis through nuclear factor-erythroid 2-related factor 2, heme oxygenase 1, tumor protein p53 and Bax signaling pathways [117].

The exposition of an OSCC cell line to a combination of resveratrol and doxorubicin loaded in liposomal nanoparticles exerts apoptosis-inducing effects by controlling the cell cycle and downstream apoptosis-inducing proteins such as caspase-3 and ribose polymerase-1 [118]. Their data indicate that the drug-loaded nanoparticle exerted apoptosis-inducing effects by controlling the cell cycle and downstream apoptosis by inducing proteins such as caspase-3 and poly (ADP-ribose) polymerase 1.

Nano-diamino-tetrac (NDAT) inhibits programmed death-ligand 1 (PD-L1) expression which is essential for proliferation in oral cancer cells. Recently, it was shown that a combined treatment of resveratrol and NDAT is more effective in reducing programmed death-ligand 1 expression and anti-proliferation as compared with resveratrol treatment alone in two oral cancer cell lines [119]. Thyroxine is an enhancer of the proliferation and progression of oral cancer cells by the down-regulation of apoptotic factor BAD (B-cell lymphoma 2 (Bcl-2)-associated agonist of cell death) and up-regulation of PD-L1. Resveratrol inhibits the function of thyroxine so that resveratrol supplementation enhances the expression of BAD and inhibits PD-1 to suppress oral cancer cells [120]. Chen et al [121] found that blocking expressions of inflammatory genes in oral cancer cells makes resveratrol an attractive agent that could possibly be employed in combination with other anti-STAT3 drugs.

Hayashi et al. [122] found that the overexpression of tripartite motif family-like 2 (TRIML2) contributes to tumor growth at the G1 phase as seen by cell cycle analysis, which results in insufficient control by the down-regulation of $p21^{Cip1}$ expression. The authors also observed that resveratrol caused the up-regulation of $p21^{Cip1}$ through the TRIML2 expression. Therefore, the authors concluded that the expression status of TRIML2 might be an indicator of OSCC progression and resveratrol may be a potential new therapeutic drug for oral cancer therapy via TRIML2 [122].

The combination of 50 µM resveratrol with 10, 25 and 50 µM of quercetin resulted in a significant inhibitory effect on cell growth and DNA synthesis [123]. Resveratrol is the major compound of *Polygonum cuspidatum* (PCE), which reduces human oral cancer cells' viability in a concentration- and time-dependent mode PCE treatment induced autophagic and apoptotic cell death. PCE also stimulated caspase-9 and -3. These findings also suggest that resveratrol may be potentially efficacious for the treatment of cisplatin-resistant human oral cancer [124]. Pinostilbene hydrate, a methylated derivative of resveratrol, inhibits the migration and invasion ability, reducing the protein activity and expression of matrix MMP-2 in three oral cancer cell lines (SCC-9, SAS and HSC) by down-regulating the p38/ERK1/2 pathway, and it might be a promising agent for preventing OSCC cell metastasis [125].

3.2. In Vivo Studies

The chemo-preventive activity of grape skin extracts in oral carcinogenesis was evaluated in 4-nitroquinoline 1-oxide (4-NQO)-induced rats. After 12 weeks of treatment, a significant reduction in epithelial dysplasia was observed. Moreover, 8-hydroxy-2′–deoxyguanosine and ki-67 immuno-expression was reduced in animals treated with grape skin extracts. A Western blot analysis showed a significant decrease in p-NFκBp50 and myeloid differentiation primary response 88 protein expression in the groups treated with grape skin extracts. The authors concluded that grape skin extracts displayed chemo-preventive activity in oral carcinogenesis assays, as depicted by its antioxidant, anti-proliferative and anti-inflammatory properties [126].

Green tea polyphenols are also able to mitigate OCC in vivo. In 4-NQO-induced rats, green tea polyphenols decreased the levels of glutathione reductase and total thiols while increasing the levels of glutathione oxidase and conjugated dienes and increasing γ-glutamyl transferase activity. Supplementation with green tea polyphenols also reduced the activity of γ-glutamyl transferase, a tumor growth marker [127]. In a xenograft experiment on mice, EGCG treatment resulted in a 45.2% reduction in tumor size without a loss of body weight [81].

The chemo-prevention potential of quercetin has also been tested in vivo. Quercetin reduced tumor incidence and induced apoptosis through the modulation of NF-kB signaling and its target genes Bcl-2 and Bax in the DMBA (7,12-dimethylbenz(a)anthracene)-induced carcinogenesis hamster model [128].

In DMBA-induced hamster cheek pouch tumors, the dietary administration of freeze-dried black raspberries at a concentration of 5% of the diet inhibited the incidence, total number, multiplicity and size of tumors [129]. The environmental pollutant and tobacco smoke constituent dibenzo[def,p]chrysene (DBP) was used to induce OSCC in mice and to explore the effects of 5% dietary black raspberry. A reduction in the levels of DBP-DNA adducts in the mouse oral cavity with a comparable effect to those of its constituents was observed [130].

The effect of dietary GSPs was assessed on the in vivo tumor xenograft growth of SCC1 cells using athymic nude mice; these anthocyanins showed identical chemo-therapeutic efficacy to that which was observed in vitro in the same study, as mentioned above. This efficiency was found to be associated with the: (i) control of cell cycle regulation and (ii) induction of the apoptotic cell death of tumor cells, as indicated by the analysis of the proteins of the Bcl-2 family, TUNEL-positive and activated caspase-3-positive cells [97].

Resveratrol locally applied and complexed with 2-Hydroxypropyl-beta-cyclodextrin (HPβCD) (cream and mouthwash) in DMBA-induced OSCC in Syrian hamster cheek pouches prevents oral pre-neoplastic lesions and OSCC appearance and growth. HPβCD-formulations (mainly mouthwash) show the best chemo-preventive effects in terms of lesions' prevalence, multiplicity, dimension and histological signs of malignancy [131]. Recently, an in vivo study was carried out using loaded GE11-conjugated liposomes (RSV-GL) and it was found that RSV-GL exhibited a two-fold decrease in tumor volume compared with the free resveratrol and a three-fold decrease in volume compared with the control [132].

3.3. Human Studies

There are few human studies, most of which have been conducted with green tea polyphenols. In a phase II clinical trial, patients with high-risk oral pre-malignant lesions receiving 500–1000 mg/m^2 of green tea extract for 12 weeks exhibited reduced VEGF levels, which are angiogenic stimuli for tumors [133]. A double-blind intervention trial in patients with pre-cancerous lesions of the oral mucosa (leukoplakia) found that a treatment regimen of green and black tea polyphenols (3 g/day orally and a 10% ointment applied to lesions three times daily) resulted in lower numbers of micronucleated cells from oral lesions, normal oral mucosa and peripheral blood lymphocytes, thus providing some direct evidence for the protective effects of tea on OCC [134]. In patients with oral field cancerization, at a high risk for developing recurrent oral pre-cancerous and cancer lesions, EGCG was administered in a form of mouthwash for seven days and a decrease was found in the expression levels of some oral carcinogenesis biomarkers [135].

A clinical study was conducted to assess the effects of topical application of 10% freeze-dried black raspberry gel on oral intraepithelial neoplasia. The results showed histologic regression in a subset of patients and a reduction in the loss of heterozygosity at tumor suppressor gene-associated loci [136]. The berry gel application uniformly suppressed genes associated with RNA processing, growth factor recycling and the inhibition of apoptosis and suppression of epithelial COX-2 levels [137]. OSCC patients who were treated with black raspberries showed an enhanced expression of pro4-survival genes, such as EGFR, and a reduction in other pro-inflammatory genes, such as NF-kB1 and prostaglandin-endoperoxide synthase 2 [138].

Moreover, adherence to a Mediterranean diet based on ingredients of polyunsaturated fatty acid, polyphenols from olive oil and polyphenols from grapes, including the ones present in wine, decreased the risk of developing head and neck cancer [139].

4. Conclusions

At the experimental level, some studies were carried out to explore ethanol's carcinogenic mechanisms whereas others analyzed the phenolic protective mechanisms. In the former group, the in vivo bio-kinetic studies were mainly focused on the analysis of salivary acetaldehyde. In contrast, the chemo-preventive/therapeutic properties of phenolic compounds against oral carcinogenesis were mainly studied using in vitro and in vivo test systems. Acetaldehyde resulting from wine intake damages oral mucosa, which promotes the stimulation of cell regeneration. The various alterations in DNA can result in the development of a pre-malignant or a potentially malignant oral epithelial cell characterized by the ability to proliferate in a non-controlled mode. In fact, acetaldehyde leads to the overexpression of oncogenes and/or the silencing of tumor suppressor genes. On other hand, several studies showed that polyphenols activate the p53 tumor suppressor gene. This could explain the induction of cell cycle arrest and apoptosis by polyphenols that was reported in some studies. Acetaldehyde's genotoxicity also results in the formation of DNA adducts, which can also be reduced by polyphenols, as observed with black raspberry administration in vivo. On the other hand, polyphenols are potent antioxidants and, therefore, they counteract ROS/RNS generation due to an increase in CYP2E1 activity as promoted by ethanol consumption. Likely, the phenolic compounds from wine mitigate the deleterious effects of ethanol, decreasing the risk of OCC. Although all these studies have yielded important data for understanding the mechanisms of action of either ethanol or phenolic compounds on either normal or tumor keratinocyte cells from the oral cavity, much remains to be studied. More adequately powered, randomized, placebo-controlled human studies, as well as experimental animal models, are required for a better understanding of the effect(s) of wine, particularly when consumed regularly in moderate doses, on oral cells.

In conclusion, this area warrants further investigation as a new way of thinking, which is to assess the wine-specific intake risk while considering the additive/synergistic or contrasting effects of its different compounds.

Author Contributions: Conceptualization—P.S., N.L. and G.d.G. Writing, editing and reviewing—P.S., N.L. and G.d.G. All three authors have read and agreed to the published version of the manuscript.

Funding: This research received no external funding.

Conflicts of Interest: Paula Silva and Norbert Latruffe declare no conflict of interest. Giovanni de Gaetano is a member of the International Scientific Forum on Alcohol Research, an independent organization of scientists that prepares critiques of emerging research reports on alcohol and health. The members of the Forum donate their time and effort in the review of papers and receive no financial support. The Forum itself receives no support from any organization or company in the alcoholic beverage industry. Giovanni de Gaetano was also a consultant to the Web Newsletter of Assobirra, the Italian Association of the Beer and Malt Industries and is a corresponding member of the non-profit Accademia Italiana della Vite e del Vino. He reports personal fees for given lectures at the 8th European Beer and Health Symposium (2017), Beer and Health Initiative (The Dutch Beer Institute foundation—The Brewers of Europe), outside the submitted work.

References

1. Ferlay, J.; Ervik, M.; Lam, F.; Colombet, M.; Mery, L.; Piñeros, M.; Znaor, A.; Soerjomataram, I.; Bray, F. Global cancer observatory: Cancer today. *Lyon Fr. Int. Agency Res. Cancer* **2018**, *144*, 1941–1953.
2. Radoi, L.; Luce, D. A review of risk factors for oral cavity cancer: The importance of a standardized case definition. *Community Dent. Oral Epidemiol.* **2013**, *41*, 97–109. [CrossRef] [PubMed]
3. Lewin, F.; Norell, S.E.; Johansson, H.; Gustavsson, P.; Wennerberg, J.; Biorklund, A.; Rutqvist, L.E. Smoking tobacco, oral snuff, and alcohol in the etiology of squamous cell carcinoma of the head and neck: A population-based case-referent study in Sweden. *Cancer* **1998**, *82*, 1367–1375. [CrossRef]
4. Moreno-Lopez, L.A.; Esparza-Gomez, G.C.; Gonzalez-Navarro, A.; Cerero-Lapiedra, R.; Gonzalez-Hernandez, M.J.; Dominguez-Rojas, V. Risk of oral cancer associated with tobacco smoking, alcohol consumption and oral hygiene: A case-control study in Madrid, Spain. *Oral Oncol.* **2000**, *36*, 170–174. [CrossRef]
5. Radoi, L.; Paget-Bailly, S.; Cyr, D.; Papadopoulos, A.; Guida, F.; Schmaus, A.; Cenee, S.; Menvielle, G.; Carton, M.; Lapotre-Ledoux, B.; et al. Tobacco smoking, alcohol drinking and risk of oral cavity cancer by subsite: Results of a French population-based case-control study, the ICARE study. *Eur. J. Cancer Prev.* **2013**, *22*, 268–276. [CrossRef] [PubMed]
6. Andre, K.; Schraub, S.; Mercier, M.; Bontemps, P. Role of alcohol and tobacco in the aetiology of head and neck cancer: A case-control study in the Doubs region of France. *Eur. J. Cancer B Oral Oncol.* **1995**, *31*, 301–309. [CrossRef]

7. Brugere, J.; Guenel, P.; Leclerc, A.; Rodriguez, J. Differential effects of tobacco and alcohol in cancer of the larynx, pharynx, and mouth. *Cancer* **1986**, *57*, 391–395. [CrossRef]
8. Franceschi, S.; Talamini, R.; Barra, S.; Baron, A.E.; Negri, E.; Bidoli, E.; Serraino, D.; La Vecchia, C. Smoking and drinking in relation to cancers of the oral cavity, pharynx, larynx, and esophagus in northern Italy. *Cancer Res.* **1990**, *50*, 6502–6507.
9. Mashberg, A.; Boffetta, P.; Winkelman, R.; Garfinkel, L. Tobacco smoking, alcohol drinking, and cancer of the oral cavity and oropharynx among U.S. veterans. *Cancer* **1993**, *72*, 1369–1375. [CrossRef]
10. Merletti, F.; Boffetta, P.; Ciccone, G.; Mashberg, A.; Terracini, B. Role of tobacco and alcoholic beverages in the etiology of cancer of the oral cavity/oropharynx in Torino, Italy. *Cancer Res.* **1989**, *49*, 4919–4924.
11. Tuyns, A.J.; Esteve, J.; Raymond, L.; Berrino, F.; Benhamou, E.; Blanchet, F.; Boffetta, P.; Crosignani, P.; Del Moral, A.; Lehmann, W.; et al. Cancer of the larynx/hypopharynx, tobacco and alcohol: IARC international case-control study in Turin and Varese (Italy), Zaragoza and Navarra (Spain), Geneva (Switzerland) and Calvados (France). *Int. J. Cancer* **1988**, *41*, 483–491. [CrossRef] [PubMed]
12. Maasland, D.H.; Brandt, P.A.V.D.; Kremer, B.; Goldbohm, R.A.; Schouten, L.J. Alcohol consumption, cigarette smoking and the risk of subtypes of head-neck cancer: Results from the Netherlands Cohort Study. *BMC Cancer* **2014**, *14*, 187. [CrossRef] [PubMed]
13. De Gaetano, G.; Costanzo, S.; Di Castelnuovo, A.; Badimon, L.; Bejko, D.; Alkerwi, A.; Chiva-Blanch, G.; Estruch, R.; La Vecchia, C.; Panico, S.; et al. Effects of moderate beer consumption on health and disease: A consensus document. *Nutr. Metab. Cardiovasc. Dis.* **2016**, *26*, 443–467. [CrossRef] [PubMed]
14. Conway, D.I.; Purkayastha, M.; Chestnutt, I.G. The changing epidemiology of oral cancer: Definitions, trends, and risk factors. *Br. Dent. J.* **2018**, *225*, 867–873. [CrossRef] [PubMed]
15. Meng, X.; Maliakal, P.; Lu, H.; Lee, M.-J.; Yang, C.S. Urinary and Plasma Levels of Resveratrol and Quercetin in Humans, Mice, and Rats after Ingestion of Pure Compounds and Grape Juice. *J. Agric. Food Chem.* **2004**, *52*, 935–942. [CrossRef] [PubMed]
16. Rotches-Ribalta, M.; Andres-Lacueva, C.; Estruch, R.; Escribano-Ferrer, E.; Urpi, M. Pharmacokinetics of resveratrol metabolic profile in healthy humans after moderate consumption of red wine and grape extract tablets. *Pharm. Res.* **2012**, *66*, 375–382. [CrossRef]
17. Lachenmeier, D.W.; Monakhova, Y.B. Short-term salivary acetaldehyde increase due to direct exposure to alcoholic beverages as an additional cancer risk factor beyond ethanol metabolism. *J. Exp. Clin. Cancer Res.* **2011**, *30*, 3. [CrossRef]
18. Seitz, H.K.; Stickel, F. Molecular mechanisms of alcohol-mediated carcinogenesis. *Nat. Rev. Cancer* **2007**, *7*, 599–612. [CrossRef]
19. Lauby-Secretan, B.; Straif, K.; Baan, R.; Grosse, Y.; El Ghissassi, F.; Bouvard, V.; Benbrahim-Tallaa, L.; Guha, N.; Freeman, C.; Galichet, L.; et al. A review of human carcinogens—Part E: Tobacco, areca nut, alcohol, coal smoke, and salted fish. *Lancet Oncol.* **2009**, *10*, 1033–1034. [CrossRef]
20. Mccloskey, L.P.; Mahaney, P. An Enzymatic Assay for Acetaldehyde in Grape Juice and Wine. *Am. J. Enol. Vitic.* **1981**, *32*, 159–162.
21. Jackowetz, J.; De Orduña, R.M. Survey of SO_2 binding carbonyls in 237 red and white table wines. *Food Control.* **2013**, *32*, 687–692. [CrossRef]
22. Lachenmeier, D.W.; Sohnius, E.M. The role of acetaldehyde outside ethanol metabolism in the carcinogenicity of alcoholic beverages: Evidence from a large chemical survey. *Food Chem. Toxicol.* **2008**, *46*, 2903–2911. [CrossRef] [PubMed]
23. Paiano, V.; Bianchi, G.; Davoli, E.; Negri, E.; Fanelli, R.; Fattore, E. Risk assessment for the Italian population of acetaldehyde in alcoholic and non-alcoholic beverages. *Food Chem.* **2014**, *154*, 26–31. [CrossRef] [PubMed]
24. Linderborg, K.; Joly, J.P.; Visapää, J.-P.; Salaspuro, M. Potential mechanism for Calvados-related oesophageal cancer. *Food Chem. Toxicol.* **2008**, *46*, 476–479. [CrossRef]
25. Han, G.; Webb, M.R.; Waterhouse, A.L. Acetaldehyde reactions during wine bottle storage. *Food Chem.* **2019**, *290*, 208–215. [CrossRef] [PubMed]
26. Kanteres, F.; Lachenmeier, D.W.; Rehm, J. Alcohol in Mayan Guatemala: Consumption, distribution, production and composition of cuxa. *Addiction* **2009**, *104*, 752–759. [CrossRef]
27. Lachenmeier, D.W.; Sohnius, E.M.; Attig, R.; Lopez, M.G. Quantification of selected volatile constituents and anions in Mexican Agave spirits (Tequila, Mezcal, Sotol, Bacanora). *J. Agric. Food Chem.* **2006**, *54*, 3911–3915. [CrossRef]

28. Oliveira, V.A.; Vicente, M.A.; Fietto, L.G.; Castro, I.M.D.; Coutrim, M.X.; Schüller, D.; Alves, H.; Casal, M.; Santos, J.D.O.; Araújo, L.D.; et al. Biochemical and Molecular Characterization of Saccharomyces cerevisiae Strains Obtained from Sugar-Cane Juice Fermentations and Their Impact in Cachaça Production. *Appl. Environ. Microbiol.* **2008**, *74*, 693–701. [CrossRef]
29. Salaspuro, M. Acetaldehyde as a common denominator and cumulative carcinogen in digestive tract cancers. *Scand. J. Gastroenterol.* **2009**, *44*, 912–925. [CrossRef]
30. Salaspuro, M. Acetaldehyde and gastric cancer. *J. Dig. Dis.* **2011**, *12*, 51–59. [CrossRef]
31. Gaonkar, P.P.; Patankar, S.R.; Tripathi, N.; Sridharan, G. Oral bacterial flora and oral cancer: The possible link. *J. Oral Maxillofac. Pathol.* **2018**, *22*, 234–238. [CrossRef] [PubMed]
32. Cirauqui, M.L.G.; Nieminen, M.; Novak-Frazer, L.; Aguirre-Urizar, J.M.; Moragues, M.-D.; Rautemaa, R. Production of carcinogenic acetaldehyde byCandida albicansfrom patients with potentially malignant oral mucosal disorders. *J. Oral Pathol. Med.* **2012**, *42*, 243–249. [CrossRef] [PubMed]
33. Alnuaimi, A.D.; Ramdzan, A.N.; Wiesenfeld, D.; Kolev, S.D.; O'Brien-Simpson, N.M.; Reynolds, E.C.; McCullough, M. Candida virulence and ethanol-derived acetaldehyde production in oral cancer and non-cancer subjects. *Oral Dis.* **2016**, *22*, 805–814. [CrossRef] [PubMed]
34. Muto, M.; Hitomi, Y.; Ohtsu, A.; Shimada, H.; Kashiwase, Y.; Sasaki, H.; Yoshida, S.; Esumi, H. Acetaldehyde production by non-pathogenic Neisseria in human oral microflora: Implications for carcinogenesis in upper aerodigestive tract. *Int. J. Cancer* **2000**, *88*, 342–350. [CrossRef]
35. Moritani, K.; Takeshita, T.; Shibata, Y.; Ninomiya, T.; Kiyohara, Y.; Yamashita, Y. Acetaldehyde production by major oral microbes. *Oral Dis.* **2015**, *21*, 748–754. [CrossRef] [PubMed]
36. Yokoyama, A.; Tsutsumi, E.; Imazeki, H.; Suwa, Y.; Nakamura, C.; Mizukami, T.; Yokoyama, T. Salivary Acetaldehyde Concentration According to Alcoholic Beverage Consumed and Aldehyde Dehydrogenase-2 Genotype. *Alcohol. Clin. Exp. Res.* **2008**, *32*, 1607–1614. [CrossRef]
37. Homann, N.; Jousimies-Somer, H.; Jokelainen, K.; Heine, R.; Salaspuro, M. High acetaldehyde levels in saliva after ethanol consumption: Methodological aspects and pathogenetic implications. *Carcinogenesis* **1997**, *18*, 1739–1743. [CrossRef]
38. Vondracek, M.; Xi, Z.; Larsson, P.; Baker, V.; Mace, K.; Pfeifer, A.; Tjalve, H.; Donato, M.T.; Gomez-Lechon, M.J.; Grafstrom, R.C. Cytochrome P450 expression and related metabolism in human buccal mucosa. *Carcinogenesis* **2001**, *22*, 481–488. [CrossRef]
39. Haiyarit, P.; Ma, N.; Hiraku, Y.; Pinlaor, S.; Yongvanit, P.; Jintakanon, D.; Murata, M.; Oikawa, S.; Kawanishi, S. Nitrative and oxidative DNA damage in oral lichen planus in relation to human oral carcinogenesis. *Cancer Sci.* **2005**, *96*, 553–559. [CrossRef]
40. Ma, N.; Tagawa, T.; Hiraku, Y.; Murata, M.; Ding, X.; Kawanishi, S. 8-Nitroguanine formation in oral leukoplakia, a premalignant lesion. *Nitric Oxide* **2006**, *14*, 137–143. [CrossRef]
41. Kawanishi, S.; Hiraku, Y.; Pinlaor, S.; Ma, N. Oxidative and nitrative DNA damage in animals and patients with inflammatory diseases in relation to inflammation-related carcinogenesis. *Boil. Chem.* **2006**, *387*, 365–372. [CrossRef] [PubMed]
42. Rasheed, M.H.; Beevi, S.S.; Geetha, A. Enhanced lipid peroxidation and nitric oxide products with deranged antioxidant status in patients with head and neck squamous cell carcinoma. *Oral Oncol.* **2007**, *43*, 333–338. [CrossRef] [PubMed]
43. Korde, S.D.; Basak, A.; Chaudhary, M.; Goyal, M.; Vagga, A. Enhanced Nitrosative and Oxidative Stress with Decreased Total Antioxidant Capacity in Patients with Oral Precancer and Oral Squamous Cell Carcinoma. *Oncology* **2011**, *80*, 382–389. [CrossRef] [PubMed]
44. Beevi, S.S.S.; Rasheed, A.M.H.; Geetha, A. Evaluation of Oxidative Stress and Nitric Oxide Levels in Patients with Oral Cavity Cancer. *Jpn. J. Clin. Oncol.* **2004**, *34*, 379–385. [CrossRef]
45. Warnakulasuriya, S.; Parkkila, S.; Nagao, T.; Preedy, V.R.; Pasanen, M.; Koivisto, H.; Niemelä, O. Demonstration of ethanol-induced protein adducts in oral leukoplakia (pre-cancer) and cancer. *J. Oral Pathol. Med.* **2007**, *37*, 157–165. [CrossRef]
46. Ogden, G.R.; Wight, A. Aetiology of oral cancer: Alcohol. *Br. J. Oral Maxillofac. Surg.* **1998**, *36*, 247–251. [CrossRef]
47. Wight, A.; Ogden, G.R. Possible mechanisms by which alcohol may influence the development of oral cancer—a review. *Oral Oncol.* **1998**, *34*, 441–447. [CrossRef]

48. Imanowski, U.A.; Stickel, F.; Maier, H.; Gärtner, U.; Seitz, H.K. Effect of alcohol on gastrointestinal cell regeneration as a possible mechanism in alcohol-associated carcinogenesis. *Alcohol* **1995**, *12*, 111–115. [CrossRef]
49. Theruvathu, J.A.; Jaruga, P.; Nath, R.G.; Dizdaroglu, M.; Brooks, P.J. Polyamines stimulate the formation of mutagenic 1,N2-propanodeoxyguanosine adducts from acetaldehyde. *Nucleic Acids Res.* **2005**, *33*, 3513–3520. [CrossRef]
50. Yamaguchi, H.; Hosoya, M.; Shimoyama, T.; Takahashi, S.; Zhang, J.F.; Tsutsumi, E.; Suzuki, Y.; Suwa, Y.; Nakayama, T. Catalytic removal of acetaldehyde in saliva by a Gluconobacter strain. *J. Biosci. Bioeng.* **2012**, *114*, 268–274. [CrossRef]
51. Setshedi, M.; Wands, J.R.; De Monte, S.M. Acetaldehyde Adducts in Alcoholic Liver Disease. *Oxidative Med. Cell. Longev.* **2010**, *3*, 406524. [CrossRef] [PubMed]
52. Wang, M.; Mcintee, E.J.; Cheng, G.; Shi, Y.; Villalta, P.W.; Hecht, S.S. Identification of DNA adducts of acetaldehyde. *Chem. Res. Toxicol.* **2000**, *13*, 1149–1157. [CrossRef] [PubMed]
53. Yu, H.-S.; Oyama, T.; Matsuda, T.; Isse, T.; Yamaguchi, T.; Tanaka, M.; Tsuji, M.; Kawamoto, T. The effect of ethanol on the formation of N 2-ethylidene-dG adducts in mice: Implications for alcohol-related carcinogenicity of the oral cavity and esophagus. *Biomarkers* **2012**, *17*, 269–274. [CrossRef] [PubMed]
54. Balbo, S.; Meng, L.; Bliss, R.L.; Jensen, J.A.; Hatsukami, R.K.; Hecht, S.S. Kinetics of DNA adduct formation in the oral cavity after drinking alcohol. *Cancer Epidemiol. Biomark. Prev.* **2012**, *21*, 601–608. [CrossRef] [PubMed]
55. Balbo, S.; Meng, L.; Bliss, R.L.; Jensen, J.A.; Hatsukami, D.K.; Hecht, S.S. Time course of DNA adduct formation in peripheral blood granulocytes and lymphocytes after drinking alcohol. *Mutagenesis* **2012**, *27*, 485–490. [CrossRef] [PubMed]
56. Boy, S.C. Leukoplakia and erythroplakia of the oral mucosa-a brief overview. *Clin. Rev.* **2012**, *67*, 558–560.
57. Feller, L.; Lemmer, J. Oral Squamous Cell Carcinoma: Epidemiology, Clinical Presentation and Treatment. *J. Cancer Ther.* **2012**, *3*, 263–268. [CrossRef]
58. Mahomed, F. Oral submucous fibrosis - a potentially malignant condition of growing concern. *Clin. Rev.* **2012**, *67*, 562–565.
59. Scully, C.; Bagan, J. Oral squamous cell carcinoma overview. *Oral Oncol.* **2009**, *45*, 301–308. [CrossRef]
60. Van Der Waal, I. Potentially malignant disorders of the oral and oropharyngeal mucosa; terminology, classification and present concepts of management. *Oral Oncol.* **2009**, *45*, 317–323. [CrossRef]
61. Fukuda, M.; Kusama, K.; Sakashita, H. Molecular insights into the proliferation and progression mechanisms of the oral cancer: Strategies for the effective and personalized therapy. *Jpn. Dent. Sci. Rev.* **2012**, *48*, 23–41. [CrossRef]
62. Roepman, P.; A Wessels, L.F.; Kettelarij, N.; Kemmeren, P.; Miles, A.J.; Lijnzaad, P.; Tilanus, M.G.J.; Koole, R.; Hordijk, G.-J.; Van Der Vliet, P.C.; et al. An expression profile for diagnosis of lymph node metastases from primary head and neck squamous cell carcinomas. *Nat. Genet.* **2005**, *37*, 182–186. [CrossRef] [PubMed]
63. Macigo, F.G.; Mwaniki, D.L.; Guthua, S.W. The association between oral leukoplakia and use of tobacco, alcohol and that based on relative risks assessment in Kenya. *Eur. J. Oral Sci.* **1995**, *103*, 268–273. [CrossRef] [PubMed]
64. Lee, C.-H.; Ko, Y.-C.; Huang, H.-L.; Chao, Y.-Y.; Tsai, C.-C.; Shieh, T.-Y.; Lin, L.-M. The precancer risk of betel quid chewing, tobacco use and alcohol consumption in oral leukoplakia and oral submucous fibrosis in southern Taiwan. *Br. J. Cancer* **2003**, *88*, 366–372. [CrossRef] [PubMed]
65. Petti, S.; Scully, C. Association between different alcoholic beverages and leukoplakia among non- to moderate-drinking adults: A matched case–control study. *Eur. J. Cancer* **2006**, *42*, 521–527. [CrossRef] [PubMed]
66. Morse, D.E.; Psoter, W.J.; Cleveland, D.; Cohen, N.; Mohit-Tabatabai, M.; Kosis, D.L.; Eisenberg, E. Smoking and drinking in relation to oral cancer and oral epithelial dysplasia. *Cancer Causes Control.* **2007**, *18*, 919–929. [CrossRef] [PubMed]
67. Jaber, M.A.; Porter, S.; Gilthorpe, M.; Bedi, R.; Scully, C. Risk factors for oral epithelial dysplasia—the role of smoking and alcohol. *Oral Oncol.* **1999**, *35*, 151–156. [CrossRef]
68. Kulasegaram, R.; Downer, M.; Jullien, J.; Zakrzewska, J.M.; Speight, P. Case-control study of oral dysplasia and risk habits among patients of a dental hospital. *Oral Oncol.* **1995**, *31*, 227–231. [CrossRef]

69. E Morse, D.; Katz, R.V.; Pendrys, D.G.; Holford, T.R.; Krutchkoff, D.J.; Eisenberg, E.; Kosis, D.; Mayne, S.T. Smoking and drinking in relation to oral epithelial dysplasia. *Cancer Epidemiol. Biomark. Prev.* **1996**, *5*, 769–777.
70. Li, L.; Psoter, W.J.; Buxó, C.J.; Elias, A.; Cuadrado, L.; Morse, D.E. Smoking and drinking in relation to oral potentially malignant disorders in Puerto Rico: A case-control study. *BMC Cancer* **2011**, *11*, 324. [CrossRef]
71. Purdue, M.P.; Hashibe, M.; Berthiller, J.; La Vecchia, C.; Maso, L.D.; Herrero, R.; Franceschi, S.; Castellsagué, X.; Wei, Q.; Sturgis, E.M.; et al. Type of Alcoholic Beverage and Risk of Head and Neck Cancer—A Pooled Analysis Within the INHANCE Consortium. *Am. J. Epidemiol.* **2008**, *169*, 132–142. [CrossRef] [PubMed]
72. Waterhouse, A.L.; Sacks, G.L.; Jeffery, D.W. Introduction to Phenolics. In *Understanding Wine Chemistry*; Wiley: Hoboken, NJ, USA, 2016; pp. 99–104.
73. Soleas, G.J.; Diamandis, E.P.; Goldberg, D.M. Wine as a biological fluid: History, production, and role in disease prevention. *J. Clin. Lab. Anal.* **1997**, *11*, 287–313. [CrossRef]
74. Golan, R.; Gepner, Y.; Shai, I. Wine and Health–New Evidence. *Eur. J. Clin. Nutr.* **2018**, *72*, 55–59. [CrossRef] [PubMed]
75. Yang, C.S.; Wang, H. Cancer Preventive Activities of Tea Catechins. *Molecules* **2016**, *21*, 1679. [CrossRef] [PubMed]
76. Gutiérrez-Venegas, G.; Sánchez-Carballido, M.A.; Suárez, C.D.; Gómez-Mora, J.A.; Bonneau, N. Effects of flavonoids on tongue squamous cell carcinoma. *Cell Boil. Int.* **2020**, *44*, 686–720. [CrossRef] [PubMed]
77. Belobrov, S.; Seers, C.; Reynolds, E.; Cirillo, N.; McCullough, M. Functional and molecular effects of a green tea constituent on oral cancer cells. *J. Oral Pathol. Med.* **2019**, *48*, 604–610. [CrossRef] [PubMed]
78. Masuda, M.; Suzui, M.; Weinstein, I.B. Effects of epigallocatechin-3-gallate on growth, epidermal growth factor receptor signaling pathways, gene expression, and chemosensitivity in human head and neck squamous cell carcinoma cell lines. *Clin. Cancer Res.* **2001**, *7*, 4220–4229. [PubMed]
79. Elattar, T.M.; Virji, A.S. Effect of tea polyphenols on growth of oral squamous carcinoma cells in vitro. *Anticancer. Res.* **2000**, *20*, 3459–3465. [PubMed]
80. López, E.P.-F.; Wang, Q.-T.; Wei, W.; Jornet, P.L. Potential chemotherapeutic effects of diosgenin, zoledronic acid and epigallocatechin-3-gallate on PE/CA-PJ15 oral squamous cancer cell line. *Arch. Oral Boil.* **2017**, *82*, 141–146. [CrossRef]
81. Yoshimura, H.; Yoshida, H.; Matsuda, S.; Ryoke, T.; Ohta, K.; Ohmori, M.; Yamamoto, S.; Kiyoshima, T.; Kobayashi, M.; Sano, K. The therapeutic potential of epigallocatechin-3-gallate against human oral squamous cell carcinoma through inhibition of cell proliferation and induction of apoptosis: In vitro and in vivo murine xenograft study. *Mol. Med. Rep.* **2019**, *20*, 1139–1148. [CrossRef]
82. Li, A.; Gu, K.; Wang, Q.; Chen, X.; Fu, X.; Wang, Y.; Wen, Y. Epigallocatechin-3-gallate affects the proliferation, apoptosis, migration and invasion of tongue squamous cell carcinoma through the hippo-TAZ signaling pathway. *Int. J. Mol. Med.* **2018**, *42*, 2615–2627. [CrossRef] [PubMed]
83. Mohan, K.C.; Gunasekaran, P.; Varalakshmi, E.; Hara, Y.; Nagini, S. In vitro evaluation of the anticancer effect of lactoferrin and tea polyphenol combination on oral carcinoma cells. *Cell Boil. Int.* **2007**, *31*, 599–608. [CrossRef] [PubMed]
84. Ramshankar, V.; Krishnamurthy, A. Chemoprevention of oral cancer: Green tea experience. *J. Nat. Sci. Boil. Med.* **2014**, *5*, 3–7. [CrossRef] [PubMed]
85. Yuan, C.-H.; Horng, C.-T.; Lee, C.-F.; Chiang, N.-N.; Tsai, F.-J.; Lu, C.-C.; Chiang, J.-H.; Hsu, Y.-M.; Yang, J.-S.; Chen, F.-A. Epigallocatechin gallate sensitizes cisplatin-resistant oral cancer CAR cell apoptosis and autophagy through stimulating AKT/STAT3 pathway and suppressing multidrug resistance 1 signaling. *Environ. Toxicol.* **2016**, *32*, 845–855. [CrossRef] [PubMed]
86. Kim, J.W.; Amin, A.R.; Shin, D.M. Chemoprevention of head and neck cancer with green tea polyphenols. *Cancer Prev. Res.* **2010**, *3*, 900–909. [CrossRef] [PubMed]
87. Lee, U.-L.; Choi, S.-W. The Chemopreventive Properties and Therapeutic Modulation of Green Tea Polyphenols in Oral Squamous Cell Carcinoma. *Isrn Oncol.* **2011**, *2011*, 1–7. [CrossRef] [PubMed]
88. Chan, C.-Y.; Lien, C.-H.; Lee, M.-F.; Huang, C.-Y. Quercetin suppresses cellular migration and invasion in human head and neck squamous cell carcinoma (HNSCC). *Biomedicine* **2016**, *6*, 15. [CrossRef] [PubMed]
89. Haghiac, M.; Walle, T. Quercetin Induces Necrosis and Apoptosis in SCC-9 Oral Cancer Cells. *Nutr. Cancer* **2005**, *53*, 220–231. [CrossRef]

90. Yuan, Z.; Wang, H.; Hu, Z.; Huang, Y.; Yao, F.; Sun, S.; Wu, B. Quercetin Inhibits Proliferation and Drug Resistance in KB/VCR Oral Cancer Cells and Enhances Its Sensitivity to Vincristine. *Nutr. Cancer* **2014**, *67*, 126–136. [CrossRef]
91. Chen, S.F.; Nieh, S.; Jao, S.W.; Liu, C.L.; Wu, C.H.; Chang, Y.C.; Yang, C.Y.; Lin, Y.S. Quercetin suppresses drug-resistant spheres via the p38 MAPK-Hsp27 apoptotic pathway in oral cancer cells. *PLoS ONE* **2012**, *7*, e49275. [CrossRef]
92. Kang, J.W.; Kim, J.H.; Song, K.; Kim, S.H.; Yoon, J.-H.; Kim, K.-S. Kaempferol and quercetin, components of Ginkgo biloba extract (EGb 761), induce caspase-3-dependent apoptosis in oral cavity cancer cells. *Phytother. Res.* **2009**, *24*, S77–S82. [CrossRef] [PubMed]
93. Lai, W.W.; Hsu, S.C.; Chueh, F.S.; Chen, Y.Y.; Yang, J.S.; Lin, J.P.; Lien, J.C.; Tsai, C.H.; Chung, J.G. Quercetin inhibits migration and invasion of SAS human oral cancer cells through inhibition of NF-kappaB and matrix metalloproteinase-2/-9 signaling pathways. *Anticancer Res.* **2013**, *33*, 1941–1950. [PubMed]
94. Ma, Y.; Yao, C.; Liu, H.; Yu, F.; Lin, J.; Lu, K.; Liao, C.; Chueh, F.; Chung, J. Quercetin induced apoptosis of human oral cancer SAS cells through mitochondria and endoplasmic reticulum mediated signaling pathways. *Oncol. Lett.* **2018**, *15*, 9663–9672. [CrossRef] [PubMed]
95. Zhao, J.; Fang, Z.; Zha, Z.; Sun, Q.; Wang, H.; Sun, M.; Qiao, B. Quercetin inhibits cell viability, migration and invasion by regulating miR-16/HOXA10 axis in oral cancer. *Eur. J. Pharm.* **2019**, *847*, 11–18. [CrossRef] [PubMed]
96. Huang, C.-Y.; Chan, C.-Y.; Chou, I.-T.; Lien, C.-H.; Hung, H.-C.; Lee, M.-F. Quercetin induces growth arrest through activation of FOXO1 transcription factor in EGFR-overexpressing oral cancer cells. *J. Nutr. Biochem.* **2013**, *24*, 1596–1603. [CrossRef] [PubMed]
97. Prasad, R.; Katiyar, S.K. Bioactive phytochemical proanthocyanidins inhibit growth of head and neck squamous cell carcinoma cells by targeting multiple signaling molecules. *PLoS ONE* **2012**, *7*, e46404. [CrossRef] [PubMed]
98. Yang, N.; Gao, J.; Cheng, X.; Hou, C.; Yang, Y.; Qiu, Y.; Xu, M.; Zhang, Y.; Huang, S. Grape seed proanthocyanidins inhibit the proliferation, migration and invasion of tongue squamous cell carcinoma cells through suppressing the protein kinase B/nuclear factor-kappaB signaling pathway. *Int. J. Mol. Med.* **2017**, *40*, 1881–1888. [CrossRef]
99. Baba, A.B.; Nivetha, R.; Chattopadhyay, I.; Nagini, S. Blueberry and malvidin inhibit cell cycle progression and induce mitochondrial-mediated apoptosis by abrogating the JAK/STAT-3 signalling pathway. *Food Chem. Toxicol.* **2017**, *109*, 534–543. [CrossRef]
100. Qi, C.; Li, S.; Jia, Y.; Wang, L. Blueberry anthocyanins induce G2/M cell cycle arrest and apoptosis of oral cancer KB cells through down-regulation methylation of p53. *Yi Chuan Hered.* **2014**, *36*, 566–573.
101. Seeram, N.P.; Adams, L.S.; Zhang, Y.; Lee, R.; Sand, D.; Scheuller, H.S.; Heber, D. Blackberry, Black Raspberry, Blueberry, Cranberry, Red Raspberry, and Strawberry Extracts Inhibit Growth and Stimulate Apoptosis of Human Cancer Cells In Vitro. *J. Agric. Food Chem.* **2006**, *54*, 9329–9339. [CrossRef]
102. Seeram, N.P.; Adams, L.S.; Hardy, M.L.; Heber, D. Total Cranberry Extract versus Its Phytochemical Constituents: Antiproliferative and Synergistic Effects against Human Tumor Cell Lines. *J. Agric. Food Chem.* **2004**, *52*, 2512–2517. [CrossRef] [PubMed]
103. Han, C.; Ding, H.; Casto, B.; Stoner, G.D.; D'Ambrosio, S.M. Inhibition of the Growth of Premalignant and Malignant Human Oral Cell Lines by Extracts and Components of Black Raspberries. *Nutr. Cancer* **2005**, *51*, 207–217. [CrossRef] [PubMed]
104. Rodrigo, K.A.; Rawal, Y.; Renner, R.J.; Schwartz, S.J.; Tian, Q.; Larsen, P.E.; Mallery, S.R. Suppression of the tumorigenic phenotype in human oral squamous cell carcinoma cells by an ethanol extract derived from freeze-dried black raspberries. *Nutr. Cancer* **2006**, *54*, 58–68. [CrossRef] [PubMed]
105. Zhang, Y.; Seeram, N.P.; Lee, R.; Feng, L.; Heber, D. Isolation and Identification of Strawberry Phenolics with Antioxidant and Human Cancer Cell Antiproliferative Properties. *J. Agric. Food Chem.* **2008**, *56*, 670–675. [CrossRef] [PubMed]
106. Fan, M.-J.; Wang, I.-C.; Hsiao, Y.-T.; Lin, H.-Y.; Tang, N.-Y.; Hung, T.-C.; Quan, C.; Lien, J.-C.; Chung, J. Anthocyanins from Black Rice (*Oryza sativa* L.) Demonstrate Antimetastatic Properties by Reducing MMPs and NF-?B Expressions in Human Oral Cancer CAL 27 Cells. *Nutr. Cancer* **2015**, *67*, 327–338. [CrossRef] [PubMed]

107. Yue, E.; Tuguzbaeva, G.; Chen, X.; Qin, Y.; Li, A.; Sun, X.; Dong, C.; Liu, Y.; Yu, Y.; Zahra, S.M.; et al. Anthocyanin is involved in the activation of pyroptosis in oral squamous cell carcinoma. *Phytomedicine* **2019**, *56*, 286–294. [CrossRef] [PubMed]
108. Mallery, S.R.; Stoner, G.D.; Larsen, P.E.; Fields, H.W.; Rodrigo, K.A.; Schwartz, S.J.; Tian, Q.; Dai, J.; Mumper, R.J. Formulation and In-Vitro and In-Vivo Evaluation of a Mucoadhesive Gel Containing Freeze Dried Black Raspberries: Implications for Oral Cancer Chemoprevention. *Pharm. Res.* **2007**, *24*, 728–737. [CrossRef]
109. Vervandier-Fasseur, D.; Latruffe, N. The Potential Use of Resveratrol for Cancer Prevention. *Molecules* **2019**, *24*, 4506. [CrossRef]
110. Tian, Y.; Song, W.; Li, D.; Cai, L.; Zhao, Y. Resveratrol As A Natural Regulator Of Autophagy For Prevention And Treatment Of Cancer. *Onco Targets Ther.* **2019**, *12*, 8601–8609. [CrossRef]
111. Perrone, D.; Fuggetta, M.P.; Ardito, F.; Cottarelli, A.; De Filippis, A.; Ravagnan, G.; De Maria, S.; Muzio, L.L. Resveratrol (3,5,4′-trihydroxystilbene) and its properties in oral diseases. *Exp. Ther. Med.* **2017**, *14*, 3–9. [CrossRef]
112. Kim, S.-H.; Kim, H.-J.; Lee, M.-H.; Yu, S.-K.; Kim, C.S.; Kook, J.-K.; Chun, H.S.; Park, E.; Lee, S.-Y.; Kim, S.-G.; et al. Resveratrol induces apoptosis of KB human oral cancer cells. *J. Korean Soc. Appl. Boil. Chem.* **2011**, *54*, 966–971. [CrossRef]
113. Yu, X.D.; Yang, J.L.; Zhang, W.L.; Liu, D.X. Resveratrol inhibits oral squamous cell carcinoma through induction of apoptosis and G2/M phase cell cycle arrest. *Tumour Biol.* **2016**, *37*, 2871–2877. [CrossRef] [PubMed]
114. Yagi, A.; Gu, M.; Takahata, T.; Frederick, B.; Agarwal, C.; Siriwardana, S.; Agarwal, R.; Sclafani, R. Resveratrol selectively induces DNA Damage, independent of Smad4 expression, in its efficacy against human head and neck squamous cell carcinoma. *Clin. Cancer Res.* **2011**, *17*, 5402–5411. [CrossRef]
115. Lin, F.-Y.; Hsieh, Y.-H.; Yang, S.-F.; Chen, C.-T.; Tang, C.-H.; Chou, M.-Y.; Chuang, Y.-T.; Lin, C.-W.; Chen, M.-K. Resveratrol suppresses TPA-induced matrix metalloproteinase-9 expression through the inhibition of MAPK pathways in oral cancer cells. *J. Oral Pathol. Med.* **2014**, *44*, 699–706. [CrossRef]
116. Shan, Z.; Yang, G.; Xiang, W.; Pei-Jun, W.; Bin, Z. Effects of resveratrol on oral squamous cell carcinoma (OSCC) cells in vitro. *J. Cancer Res. Aclin. Oncol.* **2014**, *140*, 371–374. [CrossRef] [PubMed]
117. Ko, S.Y.; Ko, H.-A.; Shieh, T.-M.; Chi, T.-C.; Chen, H.-I.; Chen, Y.-T.; Yu, Y.-H.; Yang, S.-H.; Chang, S.-S. Advanced glycation end products influence oral cancer cell survival via Bcl-xl and Nrf-2 regulation in vitro. *Oncol. Lett.* **2017**, *13*, 3328–3334. [CrossRef] [PubMed]
118. Mohan, A.; Narayanan, S.; Balasubramanian, G.; Sethuraman, S.; Krishnan, U.M. Dual drug loaded nanoliposomal chemotherapy: A promising strategy for treatment of head and neck squamous cell carcinoma. *Eur. J. Pharm. Biopharm.* **2016**, *99*, 73–83. [CrossRef] [PubMed]
119. Ho, Y.; Wu, C.-Y.; Chin, Y.-T.; Li, Z.-L.; Pan, Y.-S.; Huang, T.-Y.; Su, P.-Y.; Lee, S.-Y.; Crawford, D.R.; Su, K.-W.; et al. NDAT suppresses pro-inflammatory gene expression to enhance resveratrol-induced anti-proliferation in oral cancer cells. *Food Chem. Toxicol.* **2019**, *136*, 111092. [CrossRef]
120. Lin, C.-C.; Chin, Y.-T.; Shih, Y.-J.; Chen, Y.-R.; Chung, Y.-Y.; Lin, C.-Y.; Hsiung, C.-N.; Whang-Peng, J.; Lee, S.-Y.; Lin, H.-Y.; et al. Resveratrol antagonizes thyroid hormone-induced expression of checkpoint and proliferative genes in oral cancer cells. *J. Dent. Sci.* **2019**, *14*, 255–262. [CrossRef]
121. Chen, Y.-R.; Chen, Y.-S.; Chin, Y.-T.; Li, Z.-L.; Shih, Y.-J.; Yang, Y.-C.S.; Changou, C.A.; Su, P.-Y.; Wang, S.-H.; Wu, Y.-H.; et al. Thyroid hormone-induced expression of inflammatory cytokines interfere with resveratrol-induced anti-proliferation of oral cancer cells. *Food Chem. Toxicol.* **2019**, *132*, 110693. [CrossRef]
122. Hayashi, F.; Kasamatsu, A.; Endo-Sakamoto, Y.; Eizuka, K.; Hiroshima, K.; Kita, A.; Saito, T.; Koike, K.; Tanzawa, H.; Uzawa, K. Increased expression of tripartite motif (TRIM) like 2 promotes tumoral growth in human oral cancer. *Biochem. Biophys. Res. Commun.* **2019**, *508*, 1133–1138. [CrossRef] [PubMed]
123. Elattar, T.M.; Virji, A.S. Modulating effect of resveratrol and quercetin on oral cancer cell growth and proliferation. *Anti-Cancer Drugs* **1999**, *10*, 187–194. [CrossRef] [PubMed]
124. Wang, Y.; Horng, C.; Hsieh, M.; Chen, H.; Huang, Y.; Yang, J.; Wang, G.; Chiang, J.; Chen, H.; Lu, C.; et al. Autophagy and apoptotic machinery caused by Polygonum cuspidatum extract in cisplatin-resistant human oral cancer CAR cells. *Oncol. Rep.* **2019**, *41*, 2549–2557. [CrossRef] [PubMed]

125. Hsieh, M.-J.; Chin, M.-C.; Lin, C.-C.; His, Y.-T.; Lo, Y.-S.; Chuang, Y.-C.; Chen, M.-K. Pinostilbene Hydrate Suppresses Human Oral Cancer Cell Metastasis by Downregulation of Matrix Metalloproteinase-2 Through the Mitogen-Activated Protein Kinase Signaling Pathway. *Cell. Physiol. Biochem.* **2018**, *50*, 911–923. [CrossRef] [PubMed]
126. De Moura, C.F.G.; Soares, G.R.; Ribeiro, F.A.P.; Silva, M.J.D.; Vilegas, W.; Santamarina, A.B.; Pisani, L.P.; Estadella, D.; Ribeiro, D.A. Evaluation of the Chemopreventive Activity of Grape Skin Extract Using Medium-term Oral Carcinogenesis Assay Induced by 4-Nitroquinoline 1-Oxide. *Anticancer. Res.* **2018**, *39*, 177–182. [CrossRef] [PubMed]
127. Srinivasan, P.; Sabitha, K.E.; Shyamaladevi, C.S. Therapeutic efficacy of green tea polyphenols on cellular thiols in 4-Nitroquinoline 1-oxide-induced oral carcinogenesis. *Chem. Interact.* **2004**, *149*, 81–87. [CrossRef]
128. Zhang, W.; Yin, G.; Dai, J.; Sun, Y.U.; Hoffman, R.M.; Yang, Z.; Fan, Y. Chemoprevention by Quercetin of Oral Squamous Cell Carcinoma by Suppression of the NF-kappaB Signaling Pathway in DMBA-treated Hamsters. *Anticancer Res.* **2017**, *37*, 4041–4049.
129. Casto, B.C.; Kresty, L.A.; Kraly, C.L.; Pearl, D.K.; Knobloch, T.J.; A Schut, H.; Stoner, G.D.; Mallery, S.R.; Weghorst, C. Chemoprevention of oral cancer by black raspberries. *Anticancer. Res.* **2003**, *22*, 4005–4015.
130. Chen, K.-M.; Sun, Y.-W.; Kawasawa, Y.I.; Salzberg, A.C.; Zhu, J.; Gowda, K.; Aliaga, C.; Amin, S.; Atkins, H.; El-Bayoumy, K. Black Raspberry Inhibits Oral Tumors in Mice Treated with the Tobacco Smoke Constituent Dibenzo(def,p)chrysene Via Genetic and Epigenetic Alterations. *Cancer Prev. Res.* **2020**, *13*, 357–366. [CrossRef]
131. Berta, G.N.; Salamone, P.; Sprio, A.E.; Di Scipio, F.; Marinos, L.M.; Sapino, S.; Carlotti, M.E.; Cavalli, R.; Di Carlo, F. Chemoprevention of 7,12-dimethylbenz[a]anthracene (DMBA)-induced oral carcinogenesis in hamster cheek pouch by topical application of resveratrol complexed with 2-hydroxypropyl-β-cyclodextrin. *Oral Oncol.* **2010**, *46*, 42–48. [CrossRef]
132. Zheng, T.; Feng, H.; Liu, L.; Peng, J.; Xiao, H.; Yu, T.; Zhou, Z.; Li, Y.; Zhang, Y.; Bai, X.; et al. Enhanced antiproliferative effect of resveratrol in head and neck squamous cell carcinoma using GE11 peptide conjugated liposome. *Int. J. Mol. Med.* **2019**, *43*, 1635–1642. [CrossRef] [PubMed]
133. Tsao, A.S.; Liu, D.; Martin, J.; Tang, X.-M.; Lee, J.J.; El-Naggar, A.K.; Wistuba, I.; Culotta, K.S.; Mao, L.; Gillenwater, A.; et al. Phase II randomized, placebo-controlled trial of green tea extract in patients with high-risk oral premalignant lesions. *Cancer Prev. Res.* **2009**, *2*, 931–941. [CrossRef] [PubMed]
134. Li, N.; Sun, Z.; Han, C.; Chen, J. The chemopreventive effects of tea on human oral precancerous mucosa lesions. *Proc. Soc. Exp. Boil. Med.* **1999**, *220*, 218–224.
135. Yoon, A.J.; Shen, J.; Santella, R.M.; Philipone, E.M.; Wu, H.-C.; Eisig, S.B.; Blitzer, A.; Close, L.G.; Zegarelli, D.J. Topical Application of Green Tea Polyphenol (−)-Epigallocatechin-3-gallate (EGCG) for Prevention of Recurrent Oral Neoplastic Lesions. *J. Orofac. Sci.* **2012**, *4*, 43–50. [CrossRef] [PubMed]
136. Shumway, B.S.; Kresty, L.A.; Larsen, P.E.; Zwick, J.C.; Lu, B.; Fields, H.W.; Mumper, R.J.; Stoner, G.D.; Mallery, S.R. Effects of a topically applied bioadhesive berry gel on loss of heterozygosity indices in premalignant oral lesions. *Clin. Cancer Res.* **2008**, *14*, 2421–2430. [CrossRef] [PubMed]
137. Mallery, S.R.; Zwick, J.C.; Pei, P.; Tong, M.; Larsen, P.E.; Shumway, B.S.; Lu, B.; Fields, H.W.; Mumper, R.J.; Stoner, G.D. Topical application of a bioadhesive black raspberry gel modulates gene expression and reduces cyclooxygenase 2 protein in human premalignant oral lesions. *Cancer Res.* **2008**, *68*, 4945–4957. [CrossRef] [PubMed]
138. Knobloch, T.J.; Uhrig, L.K.; Pearl, D.K.; Casto, B.C.; Warner, B.M.; Clinton, S.K.; Sardo-Molmenti, C.L.; Ferguson, J.M.; Daly, B.T.; Riedl, K.M.; et al. Suppression of pro-inflammatory and pro-survival biomarkers in oral cancer patients consuming a black raspberry phytochemical-rich troche. *Cancer Prev. Res.* **2015**, *9*, 159–171. [CrossRef] [PubMed]
139. Benito, A.S.; Zanuy, M.; Ángeles, V.; Cano, M.A.; Alonso, A.R.; Bravo, I.A.; Blanco, E.R.; Jiménez, M.M.; Sanz, M.L. Adherence to Mediterranean diet: A comparison of patients with head and neck cancer and healthy population. *Endocrinol. Diabetes Y Nutr.* **2019**, *66*, 417–424.

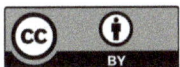

© 2020 by the authors. Licensee MDPI, Basel, Switzerland. This article is an open access article distributed under the terms and conditions of the Creative Commons Attribution (CC BY) license (http://creativecommons.org/licenses/by/4.0/).

MDPI
St. Alban-Anlage 66
4052 Basel
Switzerland
Tel. +41 61 683 77 34
Fax +41 61 302 89 18
www.mdpi.com

Molecules Editorial Office
E-mail: molecules@mdpi.com
www.mdpi.com/journal/molecules